THE EVALUATION OF NEW ANTIARRHYTHMIC DRUGS

W0106415

DEVELOPMENTS IN CARDIOVASCULAR MEDICINE

VOLUME 11

Other volumes in this series:

1. Lancée CT, ed: Echocardiology. 1979. ISBN 90-247-2209-8
2. Baan J, Arntzenius AC, Yellin EL, eds: Cardiac dynamics. 1980. ISBN 90-247-2212-8.
3. Thalen HJ Th, Meere CC, eds: Fundamentals of cardiac pacing. 1979. ISBN 90-247-2245-4.
4. Kulbertus HE, Wellens HJJ, eds: Sudden death. 1980. ISBN 90-247-2290-X.
5. Dreifus LS, Brest AN, eds: Clinical applications of cardiovascular drugs. 1980. ISBN 90-247-2295-0.
6. Spencer MP, Reid JM, eds: Cerebrovascular evaluation with Doppler Ultrasound. 1980. ISBN 90-247-2384-1.
7. Zipes DP, Bailey JC, Elharrar V, eds: The slow inward current and cardiac arrhythmias. 1980. ISBN 90-247-2380-9.
8. Kesteloot H, Joossens JV, eds: Epidemiology of arterial blood pressure, 1980. ISBN 90-247-2386-8.
9. Wackers FJ Th, ed: Thallium-201 and technetium-99-m-pyrophosphate myocardial imaging in the coronary care unit. 1980. ISBN 90-247-2396-5.
10. Maseri A, Marchesi C, Chierchia S, Trivella MG, eds: Coronary care units. ISBN 90-247-2456-2.

Series ISBN: 90-247-2336-1

THE EVALUATION OF NEW ANTIARRHYTHMIC DRUGS

Proceedings of the Symposium on How to Evaluate a New Antiarrhythmic Drug: The Evaluation of New Antiarrhythmic Agents for the Treatment of Ventricular Arrhythmias, held at Philadelphia, Pennsylvania, October 8-9, 1980

edited by

JOEL MORGANROTH, M.D.
The Lankenau Hospital,
Philadelphia, Pennsylvania

E. NEIL MOORE, D.V.M., Ph. D.
School of Veterinary Medicine,
University of Pennsylvania,
Philadelphia, Pennsylvania

LEONARD S. DREIFUS, M.D.
The Lankenau Hospital,
Philadelphia, Pennsylvania

ERIC L. MICHELSON, M.D.
The Lankenau Hospital,
Philadelphia, Pennsylvania

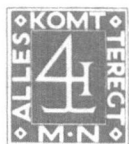

1981

MARTINUS NIJHOFF PUBLISHERS
THE HAGUE / BOSTON / LONDON

Distributors:

for the United States and Canada

Kluwer Boston, Inc.
190 Old Derby Street
Hingham, MA 02043
USA

for all other countries

Kluwer Academic Publishers Group
Distribution Center
P.O. Box 322
3300 AH Dordrecht
The Netherlands

This volume is listed in the Library of Congress Cataloging in Publication Data

ISBN-13: 978-94-009-8272-7   e-ISBN-13: 978-94-009-8270-3
DOI: 10.1007/ 978-94-009-8270-3

PREFACE

In March of 1980, it was evident that a host of new
antiarrhythmic agents were being evaluated in the United
States and that most were proceeding down very different
pathways in their process of evaluation. In part, this was
due to a lack of preciseness of the Food and Drug Administration's guidelines for the evaluation of new antiarrhythmic
agents and in larger part, to the different approaches of
investigators who were usually infatuated with a particular
model of study. Thus, the setting was ripe for similar
antiarrhythmic agents to be studied using markedly different
methods causing confusion and possible delay in their approval
by the Federal Government for marketing. Pre-clinical animal
models of a variety of types were utilized in different ways
by different scientists as was the primary thrust of clinical
evaluation with some centers being limited to invasive electrophysiologic studies while others used primarily noninvasive
ambulatory monitoring and exercise testing models.

Since the United States' physicians have a rather limited
drug armamentarium to treat patients with cardiac arrhythmias,
we feel, as do others, that a concerted effort should be made
to speed the process of obtaining approval of new antiarrhythmic
agents. Such agents are needed not only for the treatment of
patients with life-threatening ventricular arrhythmias but also,
potentially most important, for the prophylaxis of sudden cardiac
death in a high-risk population with electrical instability.

The following manuscripts represent the collective effort of physicians and scientists from the United States and abroad as well as members of the Food and Drug Administration and the pharmaceutical industry to address this problem. The state-of-the-art has been addressed by those active in a particular field in the individual manuscripts which are followed by topical discussions in which all participants were able to express their viewpoints about the important issues raised. While we did not anticipate that this Symposium would evolve a simplified methodology with unanimous consensus to evaluate a new antiarrhythmic agent, the Symposium did identify important research questions yet to be answered and has clarified particularly the inter-relationships between the different models of study in both the pre-clinical and clinical arenas. We hope that this book can be used as a reference for those individuals who design study protocols and define guidelines to determine the suitability of new antiarrhythmic agents for marketing.

Joel Morganroth, M.D.

E. Neil Moore, D.V.M., Ph.D.

Leonard S. Dreifus, M.D.

Eric L. Michelson, M.D.

Philadelphia, Pennsylvania

U.S.A.

CONTENTS

Study Designs: Chronic Patients

*Acute Studies in Patients with Hemodynamically Significant
Significant Ventricular Arrhythmias*

Special Considerations

LIST OF CONTRIBUTORS

R.S. Aronson, M.D.
Assistant Professor of Medicine
Albert Einstein College of Medicine
1300 Morris Park Avenue
New York, NY 10461

R.W.F. Campbell, M.D.
Hon. Consultant Cardiologist
Department of Cardiology
Freeman Hospital, High Heaton
Newcastle-upon-Tyne
England NE 7 7DN

J.R. Crout, M.D.
Director Bureau of Drugs FDA
5600 Fishers Lane
Rockville, MD 20857

L.S. Dreifus, M.D.
Chief, Cardiovascular Division
Lankenau Hospital
Lancaster Avenue & City Line Avenue
Philadelphia, PA 19151

S.J. Ehrreich, Ph.D.
Deputy Director
Division of Cardio-Renal Drugs
FDA HFD-110
5600 Fishers Lane
Rockville, MD 20857

C.L. Feldman, M.D.
Research Professor of Cardiovascular Medicine
University of Massachusetts Medical School
Worcester, Massachusetts 01605

(mail: 56 Union Avenue
Sudbury, MA 10776)

B.F. Hoffman, M.D.
David Hosack Professor of Pharmacology
Chairman, Pharmacology Department Columbia University
630 W. 168th Street
New York, NY 10032

E. Kaplinsky, M.D.
Associate Professor of Cardiology
Meir General Hospital
Kfar-Saba, Israel

J.S. Karliner, M.D.
Director, Clinical Cardiology
University Hospital
225 W. Dickinson Street
San Diego, CA 92103

R.E. Kates, Ph.D.
Assistant Professor of Medicine
Stanford University Medical Center
Division of Cardiology C-2E
Stanford, CA 94305

Helena C. Kraemer, Ph.D.
Associate Professor of Biostatistics in Psychiatry
Stanford University
Department of Psychiatry and Behavioral Sciences
Stanford University
Stanford, CA 94305

D. Krikler, M.D.
Consultant Cardiologist
Royal Postgraduate Medical School
Hammersmith Hospital
London W. 12 OHS England

E.L. Michelson, M.D.
Director, Clinical Research Unit
Department of Research
Lankenau Hospital
Lancaster Avenue & City Line Avenue
Philadelphia, PA 19151

E. Neil Moore, D.V.M., Ph.D.
Professor of Physiology in Medicine
School of Veterinary Medicine
University of Pennsylvania
3800 Spruce Street H1
Philadelphia, PA 19174

J. Morganroth, M.D.
Chief, Cardiac Research and Education
Cardiovascular Division
Lankenau Hospital
Lancaster Avenue & City Line Avenue
Philadelphia, PA 19151

L. Naggan, M.D.
Meir General Hospital
Kfar-Saba
Israel

M. Naito, M.D.
Cardiology Research
Lankenau Hospital
Lancaster & City Line Avenue
Philadelphia, PA 19151

Ph.J. Podrid, M.D.
Research Associate Harvard School of Public Health
Associate in Medicine, Peter Bent Brigham Hospital
665 Huntington Avenue
Boston, MA 02114

K.M. Rosen, M.D.
Chief of Cardiology, Professor of Medicine
Abraham Lincoln School of Medicine
University of Illinois
Box 6998
Chicago, IL 60680

E.H. Sonnenblick, M.D.
Professor of Medicine
Chief, Division of Cardiology
Albert Einstein College of Medicine
1300 Morris Park Avenue
Bronx, New York 10461

J.F. Spear, Ph.D.
Professor of Physiology
University of Pennsylvania School of Medicine
Philadelphia, PA 19104

S. Susskind, M.D.
Albert Einstein College of Medicine
1300,Morris Park Avenue
Bronx, NY 10461

R. Temple, M.D.
Director, Cardio-Renal Division
Food and Drug Administration
5600 Fishers Lane
Rockville, MD 20857

A. Watanabe, M.D.
Professor of Medicine and Pharmacology
Indiana University School of Medicine
1100 W. Michigan Street
Indianapolis, IN 46223

R.A. Winkle, M.D.
Associate Professor of Medicine
Stanford Hospital
Division of Cardiology
Stanford, California 94305

D.P. Zipes, M.D.
Professor of Medicine
Director of Cardiovascular Research
Division of Cardiology
Indiana University School of Medicine
Senior Research Associate
Krannert Institute of Cardiology
1100 W. Michigan Street
Indianapolis, IN 46223

HOW TO EVALUATE A NEW ANTIARRHYTHMIC DRUG: THE CHALLENGE OF
SUDDEN CARDIAC DEATH

JOEL MORGANROTH, M.D.

    The solution to the problem of sudden cardiac death is the
leading challenge to cardiology today. This problem is
epidemic in the United States where approximately one sudden
cardiac death is reported every minute. Thus, over 350,000
individuals succumb per year from this sudden unpredictable
event which usually occurs without warning or clear precipi-
tating factors. Even more disheartening is the fact that
most sudden deaths occur prematurely in life and this malady
is the leading cause of death in the 20 to 64-year old age
group.
    To prevent sudden cardiac death, one can try to
resuscitate the victim immediately after it has occurred,
usually in the home or at work. About one-fifth of these
individuals have acute myocardial infarction though most have
underlying coronary artery disease. Sudden cardiac death is
not a manifestation of advanced irreversible cardiac disease
since long-term survival may occur in many of these individuals.
Potentially more important is the prevention of sudden
cardiac death by identifying high-risk individuals who are
candidates for a prophylactic intervention, such as an antiarrhythmic agent.
    Sudden cardiac death is usually due to a ventricular
tachyarrhythmia, such as ventricular fibrillation. The
ventricular premature complex has been known for a long
time to be an important marker for ventricular tachyarrhythmias. The Coronary Care Unit experience of the 1960's
suggested such a marker and epidemiologic studies during the
1970's have clearly identified ventricular premature complexes

as important predictors of sudden cardiac death. The mere
presence of ventricular premature complexes does not necessarily provide high predictability for sudden cardiac death
but more often the pattern of ventricular premature complex
(e.g., complex forms) and the underlying milieu (e.g., the
extent of structural heart disease) are powerful factors.

Ventricular premature complexes occur in the clinical
area in two important settings. The first is that of
non-hemodynamically significant premature ventricular contractions in which the patient is bothered by occasional
vague, mildly bothersome symptoms such as dizziness and
palpitations or most often no symptoms at all. The concern
of clinical investigation today is that the occurrence of
such ventricular premature contractions, particularly in the
presence of underlying structural heart disease, may place
an individual at high risk of sudden cardiac death, thus
warranting antiarrhythmic suppressive therapy. To test
the efficacy of new antiarrhythmic agents in such individuals,
placebo periods are possible, prolonged outpatient studies
feasible, and non-invasive testing methodology is logical.

The second setting is the presence of hemodynamically
significant ventricular arrhythmias (usually paroxysmal
ventricular tachycardia or fibrillation) which cause immediate
serious symptoms requiring mandatory suppressive therapy.
This relegates such patients to the study of new antiarrhythmic drugs in which placebo periods are not often
possible, inpatient studies are usually required, and
invasive testing methodology reasonable.

The title of this Symposium is "How to Evaluate a New
Antiarrhythmic Drug". Its purpose is to arrive at more
precise and helpful guidelines to determine how to evaluate
such new antiarrhythmic drugs for both efficacy and safety
in the most expeditious manner. This Symposium will not
address the important issues of whether or not ventricular
premature complex suppression is definitely necessary to
prevent sudden death, nor will it debate the precise indications for the treatment of patients with ventricular

arrhythmias since these areas are not resolved and are themselves areas of active investigation.

This Symposium was organized by investigators and has no political affiliation. It, therefore, has no official advisory status. The funding for this Symposium was achieved by educational grant requests from over two dozen members of the pharmaceutical and related healthcare industries.

The organization of this Symposium was in four parts: Part one emphasized the pre-clinical evaluation of anti-arrhythmic agents: what electrophysiologic parameters can be used to screen for new antiarrhythmic drugs that are likely to be efficacious and in which experimental models should such agents be tested? How to define antiarrhythmic efficacy in such models and how to define pre-clinical toxicity and how to evaluate pharmacokinetics and pharmaco-dynamic data were also included in this section.

Part two of the Symposium addressed the study of patients with non-hemodynamically significant ventricular premature complexes and particularly looked at the issues of long-term electrocardiographic monitoring techniques, definitions of antiarrhythmic drug efficacy, and classification of ventricular premature complexes in terms of efficacy measures. A discussion of whether parallel vs. crossover design studies are most applicable to this field of pharmacologic research will also be found in this part of the Symposium.

Part three was devoted to a discussion of how to study patients with hemodynamically significant ventricular arrhythmias. The use of invasive methodology to determine drug efficacy and safety parameters was discussed. The design of studies in critically-ill patients with acute myocardial infarction or digitalis toxicity was also covered.

The fourth part of the Symposium discussed special topics such as: How to monitor and detect electrophysiologic and hemodynamic drug effects, how to detect long-term drug toxicity, how to study atrial arrhythmias, and the appropriate use of emergency data and drug study data obtained outside the U.S.A. in developing the New Drug Application.

The discussions following each of the Symposium sections are attempts to answer each of the questions posed and were derived by active discussion between academic investigators in the United States and abroad, scientists and advisors from the Food and Drug Administration and National Institutes of Health, and representatives of the pharmaceutical and healthcare industry. It is our hope that this information can be used to establish new guidelines which will be used as the basis for an efficient and safe means of providing to the American Public effective and safe antiarrhythmic agents which can eventually be used to prevent or decrease the epidemic of sudden cardiac death.

RELATIONSHIPS BETWEEN EFFECTS ON CARDIAC ELECTROPHYSIOLOGY AND ANTIARRYTHMIC EFFICACY

BRIAN F. HOFFMAN, M.D.

In order to determine what actions of an antiarrhythmic
drug might be required to convert an arrhythmia to normal
rhythm one would have to know what functional and structural
abnormalities were responsible for the arrhythmia, whether or
not these abnormalities could be changed so that essential
parameters approached normal and, if this were not possible,
what other induced changes might adequately compensate for the
abnormality. Unfortunately, in developing a new antiarrythmic
agent it is not possible to fulfill these criteria because
many different mechanisms can cause cardiac arrhythmias; it
is necessary, therefore, to look for effects of a new drug
that cause predictable alterations in certain aspects of
cellular electrophysiology with the expectation that the
variables influenced by the drug are causally related to one
or another mechanism for disturbances of rhythm. The problem
is complicated further by the fact that the abnormalities of
cellular electrophysiology which cause an arrhythmia in a
diseased heart may be uniquely related to the disease process
and thus may not have a reasonable counterpart in the hearts
of experimental animals. Finally, the same considerations
apply to so-called side effects or toxic effects which may
not be particularly troublesome when the drug acts on a
normal heart but which may present a significant problem
when the drug acts on a diseased heart.

In spite of these difficulties it probably is possible
to develop a reasonably logical approach to screening for
antiarrythmic action - an approach that provides a good
chance of evaluating potential antiarrythmic efficacy and

also of identifying a major likelihood of serious undesirable effects on the heart. To do this it first is necessary to have some understanding of the several mechanism that almost certainly can and very likely do cause many common disturbances of rhythm in the human heart and also of the manner in which drug effects depend on the electrophysiological state of the cardiac fibers.

In recent years there has been a marked advance in our understanding of the cellular electrophysiological mechanisms that cause disturbances of cardiac rhythm (1, 2, 3). Nevertheless, the general classification of mechanisms has not changed significantly. Most arrhythmias can be said to arise because of abnormalities either of impulse generation or impulse conduction or because of simulataneous disturbances of both impulse generation and conduction. Abnormal impulse generation can be the result of abnormal automaticity or triggering. The latter term (1) indicates that the abnormal impulse depends on a prior impulse and thus is not truly automatic. Arrhythmias due to automaticity can be attributed either to enhancement of the normal automatic mechanism in specialized cardiac fibers or to the development of an abnormal automatic mechanism. The first, enhancement of normal automaticity, is the result of an increase in the slope of phase 4 depolarization in fibers which show normal automaticity because of the presence of a membrane conductance for potassium, $g_{K,2}$, which decreases with time after the fibers have attained a sufficiently negative transmembrane potential. The decrease in K+ conductance causes a progressive decrease in transmembrane potential; if transmembrane potential attains the threshold value with sufficient rapidity a new impulse is generated. Abnormal automaticity is seen not only in specialized cardiac fibers but also in atrial and ventricular muscle fibers if they fail to attain a normal maximum diastolic potential or resting potential. Abnormal automaticity also results from phase 4 depolarization; it differs from normal automaticity because the mechanism for the phase 4 depolarization is different. In partially depolarized fibers the gradual depolarization during phase 4

does not depend on the $g_{K,2}$ channel but rather results from a
gradual decay in the outward K+ current $I_{x,1}$ that causes
repolarization and a simultaneous increase in inward current
that in many instances flows predominantly in the slow inward
channel, g_{si}.

There are two major causes of triggered rhythms, early
afterdepolarization (EAD) and delayed afterdepolarization (DAD).
The former appear as a new depolarization which interrupts
phase 3 of repolarization; the latter appears as a transient
depolarization during phase 4 and usually is coupled in a rate-
and rhythm-dependent manner to the preceeding action potential.
The mechanism for the EAD has not been studied in detail but
it is likely that two different changes in membrane electrophysiology can result in EAD. It has been shown that agents
like aconitine which attenuate the voltage- and time-dependent
inactivation of the fast inward current, I_{Na}, cause EAD. In
this case it would be reasonable to attribute the new depolarization that consitutes the EAD to an abnormal inward current
in the fast channels. Also, drugs or interventions that
markedly delay the onset of repolarization, such as N-acetylprocainamide, can cause EAD. In this case the primary cause
of the EAD would be either a decrease in outward current in
$I_{x,1}$ or perhaps an augmented and persistent slow inward current
(I_{si}). Finally, since the EAD interrupts repolarization, the
fiber is in a condition which favors abnormal automaticity
as described above. The mechanism for DAD is described subsequently.

The other major cause of arrhythmias is reentrant
excitation. The electrophysiological basis for reentrant
excitation has been known for many years. In reentry the
impulse blocks in some part of the cardiac syncytium, propagates past the area of block in other normally excitable
fibers, then returns to and propagates through the area of
block to cause reexcitation. The anatomical paths and
functional abnormalities that can cause reentrant excitation
are quite varied. The best known example is the heart in
which an anomalous atrioventricular pathway results in the

arrhythmias typical of the Wolff-Parkinson-White syndrome.

Other examples are provided by hearts in which there has
been infarction (4). Here the impulse spreads slowly in
fibers damaged by ischemia, blocks in some and propagates
slowly in others and ultimately reexcites the heart. For
these and most other cases the basic requirements are for an
area of unidirectional block, a circumscribed path over which
there is slow conduction and a transit time for the impulse
that exceed the effective refractory period of tissues proximal
to the area of block. A special case of reentrant excitation
has been termed reflection (5,6). In this case the impulse
propagates up to an area in which excitability is reduced
and spreads with considerable delay to distal fibers. Transmission may be due to electrotonic interaction across an
inexcitable segment. Reentrant excitation occurs because
when fibers distal to the area of reduced excitability develop
an active response, the electrotonic effect of this causes
reexcitation of fibers proximal to the area of diminished
excitability. This mechanism differs from classical reentry
only in that a loop of tissue is not required. Classical
reentry can be described as circus movement but reentry due
to reflection can not. For reentrant excitation to occur
some fibers must demonstrate a change in excitability and
responsiveness such that impulse propagation is impaired.
In some cases it is likely that the slow conduction and
unidirectional block result from partial depolarization
which cases inactivation of I_{Na}. In other cases it is likely
that the loss of transmembrane potential is sufficient to
largely eliminate fast inward current; in this case spread
of the impulse very likely depends on generation of slow
responses due to current in g_{si} (7).

The variety of arrhythmias due to reentrant excitation
is rather large and some additional comments are needed to
identify several main types. There is little doubt that in
many cases atrial flutter is caused by reentry. In most
cases the impulse circulates around an inexcitable obstacle.
This obstacle may be an anatomical entity such as a scar or

the junction of the venae cavae with the right atrium; in
other instances it may be a region in which depolarization is
maintained by elctrotonic effects of the circulating wave
front (8). A number of atrial tachyarrhythmias probably are
due to reentry with the reentrant path including either the
sinoatrial or atrioventricular nodes. In this case the area
of unidirectional block and slow conduction depends on the
special properties of the nodal fibers and in particular on
the fact that their action potentials are generated primarily
by current in slow channels. Fibrillation of either the
atria or ventricles results from random reentry of the impulse
over multiple paths which probably change with time. In all
cases, nevertheless, the requirements for local block and
slow conduction are maintained.

In relation to this brief description of some of the main
mechanisms that cause disturbances of rhythm it is possible
to outline how a drug might exert antiarrhythmic action.
Since many of the commonly used antiarrhythmic drugs are local
anesthetics it is appropriate to begin with a consideration
of this class.

The effect shared by all the local anesthetic antiarrhythmic drugs is an ability to block the fast inward channel
in a dose-dependent manner and thus modify the excitability
of all cardiac fibers that develop a regenerative response as
a result of an inward Na^+ current. Partial block of the fast
inward channel will have a number of predictable effects on
electrical activity. The threshold potential will be shifted
to more positive values and as a result excitability will be
reduced. In addition, for normally polarized fibers which
generate impulses due to normal phase 4 depolarization, the
partial block of fast inward channels will decrease the rate
or abolish spontaneous activity. Block of fast inward channels
also will modify the action potential generated by the fibers
and its propagation. Action potential amplitude and $\dot{V}_{max}$
will decrease and after sufficient change the impulse will
propagate less rapidly and become a less effective stimulus
for adjacent fibers. These effects can result in suppression

of some types of arrhythmias. The change in threshold potential might slow or stop an automatic focus. The decrease in
excitability, coupled with the decrease in effectiveness of
the action potential as a stimulus, might convert an area of
unidirectional block into an area of bidirectional block and
thus interrupt a reentrant rhythm. The shift in threshold
potential to more positive values might prevent DAD from
attaining threshold. Also, all of these actions have the
potential for causing impaired conduction and perhaps initiating an arrhythmia.

The effects of the local anesthetics may be more complex
than this. For some if not all drugs in this class the extent
to which they block fast inward channels is a function of
membrane potential so that block is intensifed by partial
depolarization. Because of this drug effects are more intense
in cells which do not have a normal resting potential or
maximum diastolic potential. For example, it can be shown
that in partially depolarized ischemic areas of the ventricle
a reasonable concentration of lidocaine has much more intense
effects than on normally polarized areas. This property seems
useful in that abnormalities of rhythm probably arise in
abnormal cells and these very likely are partially depolarized.
One might assume that in the case of classical reentry the
segment exhibiting unidirectional block before drug administration would show complete block afterwards with abolition
of reentrant excitation. Similarly, one might assume that if
a parasystolic focus were protected by entry block fibers in
the area in which this condition obtained would be partially depolarized. They thus might show an increased susceptibility
to the effect of a local anesthetic antiarrythmic drug and
develop bidirectional block.

Another aspect of the modulation of the effect of local
anesthetic drugs by membrane potential is shown by their
effects on recovery of responsiveness after an action potential. For a number of agents recovery of the fast channel
from inactivation is delayed considerably and because of this
the duration of the effective refractory period is increased.

This effect is independent of the change- increase or decrease-
in action potential duration. Finally, the intensity of block
by local anesthetics may show what is called use dependence.
The intensity of block is a function of the number of action
potentials per unit time, increasing with more rapid activation.
This effect would tend to make the effects of the drug more
intense when the rhythm is rapid.

In addition to effects on the rapid inward current, and
thus on the action potential upstroke and excitability, antiarrhythmic drugs may influence other of the transmembrane
ionic conductances that underlie electrical activity. A
number of antiarrhythmic drugs decrease the slope of normal
phase 4 depolarization either by increasing outward K+ current,
decreasing inward background current or both. If a focus
were generating impulses at a rapid rate, this effect would
tend to slow or stop impulse generation. Fortunately, in
most cases the properties associated with the effect are not
those that significantly slow impulse generation by the sinus
node. At the same time this action has the potential for
causing undesirable effects. If because of disease or drug
action atrioventricular transmission is blocked, drugs that
slow impulse generation by the normal automatic mechanism
will tend to slow or arrest pacemakers in the His-Purkinje
system. Finally, this drug action would not be expected to
significantly influence rhythms caused by the major abnormal
automatic mechanism except by attenuating inward background
current.

For many years emphasis was placed on the effects of
antiarrythmic drugs on action potential duration and related
changes in the duration of refractoriness. The importance of
these changes is not clear. Most rhythms due to abnormal
impulse generation are not so rapid that a modest increase
in action potential duration would be expected to have a
significant effect. Indeed, a number of quite effective
antiarrhythmic drugs may decrease action potential duration.
An increase in action potential duration and duration of
refractoriness might prevent reentrant excitation if the

transit time in the reentrant circuit was almost equal to the duration of refractoriness at the exit from the reentrant path. Some evidence that this may be the case for ventricular premature depolarizations and procainamide has been provided (9).

Through a careful study of the effects of an antiarrhythmic drug on the transmembrane potentials and membrane ionic currents it often is possible to predict reasonably effectively what actions the drug is likely to exert on selected arrhythmias and on cardiac electrical activity. The actions of the local anesthetic antiarrhythmics, summarized above, provide some examples. In addition, other types of drugs can be expected to modify certain arrhythmias. The so-called calcium channel blockers, drugs that act to block the slow inward channels, have a number of actions which permit a correlation between effect on the cardiac cell membrane and antiarrhythmic efficacy. Verapamil is the best known representative of this group. Verapamil has relatively weak effects on the fast inward channel but decreases current in slow inward channels in a predictable dose-dependent manner. This action should modify those aspects of electrical activity that depend on the slow inward current. Several examples can be presented. There is reasonable evidence that when abnormal automaticity is present in fibers which have a maximum diastolic potential more positive than -55 mV, the action potential upstroke is caused primarily by slow inward current. A drug that was able to block the slow inward channel would be expected to terminate automatic inpulse generation in a focus of this sort. It has been shown both for verapamil and other blockers of the slow inward channel such as nifedipine that this is the case. If perpetuation of a reentrant rhythm depends on slow propagation in tissues in which the action potential is due largely to I_{si}, action of a slow channel blocker would be expected to interrupt the reentrant path. When reentry depends on the impulse traversing some part of either the sinus node or atrioventricular node, the needed slow conduction probably comes about in this manner and for both types of reentry verapamil seems effective. Finally, there is considerable

evidence that delayed afterdepolarizations occur because of
an excessive increase in calcium activity within cardiac
fibers. This, in turn, causes what appears to be an oscil-
latory uptake and release of Ca^{++} by the sarcotubular system
(10). Because of the transient changes in calcium activity
inside the fiber there is a transient increase in membrane
ionic conductance, a transient inward current and a DAD.
Exposure of the fiber to verapamil would be expected to reduce
the Ca^{++} influx through slow channels during each action
potential and in this manner reduce intracellular calcium
activity. This should interrupt the chain of events leading
to DAD. In fact, this very often is the case.

Finally, it often is possible to make some predictions
about toxic or undesirable effects of antiarrhythmic drugs
from a study of their actions on transmembrane potentials of
isolated preparations of cardiac tissue. Clearly, drugs that
block the fast inward channel will reduce excitability, slow
conduction and have the potential for causing serious disturbances of electrical activity either when the drug acts in
too high a conentration or when some fibers in the heart are
partially depolarized. For drugs of this class one should
expect an interaction with serum potassium concentration
since membrane resting potential is strongly dependent on
small changes in this parameter in the normal range of serum
$[K^+]$. If a drug exerts a strong effect on the slope of phase
4 depolarization in vitro it should be expected to have the
potential for limiting the ability of subsidiary pacemakers
to provide an adequate cardiac rate in vivo; if the slope of
phase 4 is unchanged, pacemaker activity in the His-Purkinje
system would be expected to be less depressed. That this is
the case can be shown by comparison of the effects of lidocaine
and ethmozine (11) on transmembrane potentials of Purkinje
fibers and on ventricular rate in dogs with chronic heart
block (12).

In summary, even though the actual mechanisms for specific
arrhythmias in patients may not be known with certainty, our
understanding of cardiac electrophysiology and the general

14

mechanisms for arrhythmia production is sufficient to make quite reasonable and accurate predictions about the therapeutic and toxic effects of new antiarrhythmic drugs from data obtained through studies in membrane electrical activity of cardiac cells.

REFERENCES

1. Cranefield PF. 1977. Action potentials, afterpotentials and arrhythmias. Circ Res 41:415-423.

2. Cranefield PF. 1975. The Slow Response and Cardiac Arrhythmias. Mt. Kisco, Futura Press.

3. Wit AL, Rosen MR, Hoffman BF. 1974. Electrophysiology and pharmacology of cardiac arrhythmias. II. Relationship of normal and abnormal electrical activity of cardiac fibers to the genesis of arrhythmias. B. Re-entry, Section 1. Am Heart J 88:664-670.

4. Janse MJ, van Capelle FJL, Morsink J, Keleber AG, Wilms-Schopman F, Cardinal R, Naumann d'Alnoncourt C, Durrer D. 1980. Flow of "injury" current and patterns of excitation during early ventricular arrhythmias in acute regional myocardial ischemia in isolated porcine and canine hearts. Evidence for 2 different arrhythmogenic mechanisms. Circ Res 47:151-165.

5. Cranefield PF, Klein HO, Hoffman BF. 1971. Conduction of the cardiac impulse. I. Delay, block and one-way block in the depressed Purkinje fiber. Circ Res 28:199-219.

6. Antzelevitch C, Jalife J, Moe GK. 1980. Characteristics of reflection as a mechanism of reentrant arrhythmias and its relationship to parasystole. Circulation 61:182-191.

7. Wit AL, Cranefield PF. 1977. Triggered and automatic activity in the canine coronary sinus. Circ Res 41:435-445.

8. Allessie MA, Bonke FIM, Schopman FJG. 1977. Circus movement in rabbit atrial muscle as a mechanism of tachycardia. III. The "leading circle" concept: a new model of circus movement in cardiac tissue without the involvement of an anatomical obstacle. Circ Res 41:9-18.

9. Giardina EGV, Bigger JT, Jr. 1973. Procaine amide against re-entrant ventricular arrhythmias. Circulation 48:959-966.

10 Kass R, Tsien R, Weingart R. 1978. Ionic basis of transient inward current induced by strophanthidin in cardiac Purkinje fibers. J Physiol 281:209-226.

11 Danilo P, Jr., Langan WB, Rosen MR, Hoffman BF. 1977. Effects of the phenothiazine analog, EN-313, on ventricular arrhythmias in the dog. Eur J Pharm 45:127-139.

12 Ilvento J, Provet J, Rosen M. 1979. Accelerated idoventri-
   cular rhythm: A study of its mechanism in conscious dogs.
   Circulation Vols. 56-60 (Suppl.II):II-86.

WHAT ANIMAL MODELS SHOULD BE USED TO DEFINE ANTIARRHYTHMIC
EFFICACY?   ACUTE DOG MODELS

Leonard S. Dreifus, M.D., Masahito Naito, M.D., Eric L.
Michelson, M.D.

The number and diversity of animal models used to study
the effectiveness of antiarrhythmic agents attests to the
inadequacy of any one model to closely simulate the most
frequent and important cause of sudden death in man.[1]
Obviously each model is able to imitate certain aspects of
the arrhythmias seen in the presence of ischemic heart disease,
but significant problems have been identified in relating
the arrhythmias induced in these models to those resulting
from acute or chronic ischemia in man. In general, these
models do not take into account such factors as prior coronary
and cardiac disease, neurohumoral influences, collateral
circulation, or the anatomical locations of the diseased
vessels and infarcted zones, each of which may influence the
susceptibility for ventricular arrhythmias to culminate in
ventricular fibrillation. While the Harris[2-4] 1 stage and
2 stage coronary artery ligation models introduced more than
30 years ago remain most popular for the study of ventricular
arrhythmias associated with myocardial ischemia and infarction,
they have not been completely satisfactory as models for antiarrhythmic drug testing.

Since an ideal model of sudden death has not been clearly

established, merits and limitations of the present techniques should be examined. Overall however, it appears that previous extensive research on the effectiveness of antiarrhythmic drugs in reducing the number of incidences of ventricular arrhythmias associated with ouabain, epinephrine, isopreterenol, halothane anesthetics and hydrocarbons as well as the arrhythmias which appear in the subacute stages of coronary occlusion may have only limited relevance in the pharmacologic quest to identify effective antiarrhythmic agents in the prevention of sudden cardiac death. Specifically, canine models used for the study of antiarrhythmic agents must address the arrhythmias, 1) associated with sudden death (ventricular tachycardia or ventricular fibrillation), and 2) ventricular premature complexes that are harbingers of sudden death. In contrast, models that evaluate antiarrhythmic agents that reduce the number of so-called innocent complexes are interesting as far as ventricular premature beat screening purposes are concerned, but will add little to the development of truly effective antiarrhythmic drug therapy.

ANTIARRHYTHMIC DRUG TESTING MODELS

Harris Two Stage Ligation

Most early investigations of antiarrhythmic drugs utilized the simple 2 stage ligation of the left anterior descending coronary artery [4-8] (Table 1). In the first stage the left anterior descending coronary artery was ligated incompletely by placing a 20 gauge needle within the ligature along side the coronary artery and then removing the needle after securing the ligature. Some 10 to 30 minutes later the artery was then totally ligated.[3] Although a very high incidence of cardiac arrhythmias was noted beginning 4-6 hours following the ligation and lasting 24-48 hours the nature of this arrhythmia did not represent the fatal mechanisms usually associated with sudden cardiac death. Furthermore, all antiarrhythmic agents, particularly those of the fast sodium channel variety were effective in reducing the number of premature ventricular systoles and intermittent runs of accelerated automatic ventricular tachycardia.[4-8] Hence, while this model was useful in identifying those drugs with any potential ability to suppress abnormal automaticity it did not have validity in relation to the experimental question of sudden cardiac death due to ventricular fibrillation. Ventricular fibrillation was rarely observed in these animals and the ventricular arrhythmias were not due to either an acute ischemic issue or relief of that ischemia (i.e., reperfusion). Most investigators have attributed these arrhythmias to automatic mechanisms localized to Purkinje fibers in proximity to areas of recent myocardial infarction,[1,9-11] rather than reentry.

Sequential Coronary Artery Ligation/Reperfusion

A number of investigators[12-14] have performed studies using multiple 1 stage ligations of the left anterior descending coronary artery in which antiarrhythmic drugs were given either prophylactically or just subsequent to each of the multiple ligations in the same animal. Ligations however, were sustained for only 5-6 minutes and then the vessel was released allowing reperfusion. After a 20-30 minute

stabilization period, a second or third ligation was then
performed often using a second or third antiarrhythmic
drug so that the animal could serve as its own control.

In view of what is now recognized as the 2 distinct phases
of immediate ventricular arrhythmias that occur at 2-12
minutes ("immediate" or IVA) and 13-30 minutes ("delayed" or
DVA) following sudden acute ligation it is obvious that the
time for the development of the first phase is insufficient
and certainly the second phase would be totally missed by
such a maneuver.[15]   It is also well known that reperfusion
after such a short period of ligation was invariably never
followed by any serious arrhythmias so that this model had
no utility as a reperfusion arrhythmia model. Furthermore,
analysis of the electrophysiologic consequences of sequential
ligations revealed a conspicuous inconsistency in the electrophysiologic parameters of the ischemic and border zone tissues
from one ligation to the next, even in the absence of drug
therapy.[16,17]   Hence, the nonuniformity of the electrophysiologic events and the unfortunate selection of the
short period of ligation followed by the reperfusion phase
invalidate comparison of both the arrhythmic events and drug
effects.[12,16,17]

Harris 1 Stage Ligation With or Without Reperfusion

Acute proximal ligation of the left anterior descending
or circumflex coronary artery in the open chested dog appears
to be the simplest infarction-arrhythmia model.[3,17,28]
Unfortunately, this procedure results in a variably high
incidence (10-90%) of ventricular fibrillation or ventricular

tachycardia depending on how proximal the vessel is ligated,

how much the vessel is manipulated prior to ligation, the

neurohumoral and autonomic state of the animal, its heart

as well as other technical factors. Using their own versions

of 1 stage LAD occlusion models Stephenson et al,[19]

reported the effectiveness of quinidine and procainamide;

and Verdouw et al[27] noted the effectiveness of aprindine,

although Elharrar and workers[12] noted worsening of the

ventricular arrhythmias with the use of aprindine.

Kniffen et al[25] found bretylium to be effective against

single stage ligation arrhythmias. Gamble and Cohn[19]

reported that procainamide, lidocaine and propranolol were

all effective in preventing fatal reentrant arrhythmias as

well as automatic arrhythmias in a comparable feline model.

However, the relative advantages of each of these drugs

was relatively small and none was optimally protective.

Rosenbaum et al[26] noted the marked effectiveness of

amiodarone following acute ligation of the left anterior

descending coronary artery.

Acute Coronary Artery Reperfusion Model

The most malignant arrhythmia model is that of 1 stage

proximal LAD occlusion followed by acute release and reper-

fusion after 20-30 minutes of ligation. This results in

the highest (50-100%) incidence of ventricular fibrillation

and tachyarrhythmias. Stephenson[19] reported the effective-

ness of procainamide, and more particularly quinidine, during

both the ligation phase and reperfusion stage using this

model. However, Naito et al[28] failed to confirm the

efficacy of a variety of agents in this model, and noted that
when appropriate statistical methods were used, lidocaine
and procainamide administered either prophylactically and/or
prior to release were each ineffective in preventing fatal
ventricular fibrillation. Furthermore, verapamil also had
no effect in preventing reperfusion or ventricular fibrillation,
nor did 2 weeks of pretreatment with amiodarone.

Several comments appear necessary to qualify the results
of acute one stage ligation and reperfusion. Williams
et al [29] first commented that the occurrence of ventricular
tachycardia and fibrillation following reperfusion could be
related to the ventricular arrhythmias produced by the antecedent ligation. This has subsequently been confirmed by
Naito et al. [28] Thus the electrophysiologic events of
ligation and subsequent reperfusion are closely associated
and the effects of reperfusion antiarrhythmic interventions
must be interpreted in this light. It must also be pointed
out that nearly every laboratory has varied at least some
aspect of either the occlusion or reperfusion procedure so
it is difficult to compare the results of different investigators with respect to relative drug efficacies.

It remains to be determined if the one stage ligation,
followed by release and reperfusion after 30 minutes, is
an ideal test to adequately identify antiarrhythmic drugs
that could be used prophylactically to prevent sudden death
due to ventricular fibrillation. This model may offer too
severe a test of a potential antiarrhythmic agent, but this
also needs further evaluation. Furthermore, human hearts

have been usually damaged by prior coronary obstruction and
infarction with and without various degrees of ischemia, and
variable degrees of collateral circulation. Moreover, the
predictability of ventricular fibrillation following coronary
reperfusion appears linked to electrophysiologic derenagements
and ventricular arrhythmias which occur during the antecedent
ligation period.[28] Hence, any analysis of reperfusion
arrhythmias must take into consideration the precise electrophysiologic events both of the ligation period as well as
the reperfusion period. These models have other limitations.
For example they do not take into consideration the status
of left ventricular function, other hemodynamic parameters
such as the state of the peripheral vascular resistance,
the effects of heart rate during the course of ischemia and
infarction as well as various neurohumoral and autonomic
influences that may be relevant clinically in the sudden
cardiac death syndrome.

The subacute 2 stage Harris model has been useful in
drug testing because dogs survive the acute procedure and
because of the high incidence of premature ventricular complexes which occur during the one to two days following
infarction. All potential antiarrhythmic agents if administered in the appropriate manner appear effective in decreasing the incidence of these ventricular arrhythmias.
Unfortunately these delayed automatic arrhythmias apparently
bear little relevance to the electrophysiologic events
occurring at the time of coronary occlusion and possible
reperfusion in the human situation. Hence, these subacute

models do not represent the human problem of either sudden death nor necessarily the problem of chronic PVCs. Therefore, subacute models should probably be used only for initial drug screening purposes.

Finally, for the evaluation of an antiarrhythmic drug using any given arrhythmia model it is important first that sufficieint numbers of control animals be studied so that the mean frequency of arrhythmias as well as the variability around the mean can be defined.[30] Studies must be designed prospectively and the appropriate rigorous statistical methods applied to confirm possible drug efficacy. This will lead ultimately to the earlier recognition of both potentially effective and ineffective agents and will result in the more effective utilization of those limited resources available to new antiarrhythmic drug development and testing.

In conclusion: 1) Acute ligation animal models with or without reperfusion techniques are available for anti-arrhythmic drug testing; 2) These are sudden death models although they are of unproven value in the study of acute spontaneously occurring sudden death. They do not simulate chronic ischemic heart disease with prior infarction/ischemia, and do not consider various modifiers such as innate collateral circulation status, left ventricular function, heart rate effects, and neurohumoral influences; 3) Any ideal drug should protect against sustained ventricular tachycardia and fibrillation resulting from ligation and reperfusion; 4) To date, no available antiarrhythmic agent has proven unequivocal and substantial efficacy in these models. Thus, they may be too severe a test of most drugs; 5) Subacute ligation models are also available but they are of unproven value in the determination of a new antiarrhythmic drug's effectiveness in reducing acute spontaneously occurring sudden death but are useful in initial drug screening.

REFERENCES

1. Fozzard HA: Validity of myocardial infarction models. Circulation Supplement III 51,52:III-131-137, 1975
2. Harris AS, Rojas AG: The initiation of ventricular fibrillation due to coronary occlusion. Exp Med Surg 1:105, 1943
3. Harris AS: Delayed development of ventricular ectopic rhythms following experimental coronary occlusion. Circulation 1:1318, 1950
4. Harris AS, Estandia A, Ford TJ Jr, Smith HT, Olsen RW, Tillotson RR: Effect of intravenous procainamide (Pronestyl) upon ectopic ventricular tachycardia accompanying acute myocardial infarction. Circulation 5:551-558, 1952
5. Mokler CM, Van Arman CG: Pharmacology of a new anti-arrhythmic agent, -Diisopropyl-amino- -phenyl- (2 pyridyl)-butyramede (SC-7031). J Pharm and Experimental Therap 131:114-124, 1962
6. Lucchesi BR, Whitsitt LS: Antiarrhythmic effects of beta adrenergic blocking agents. Ann NY Acad Sci 139:940-951, 1967
7. Allen JD, Shanks RG, Zaidi SA: Effects of lignocaine and propranolol on experimental cardiac arrhythmias. Br J Pharm 42:1-12, 1971
8. Danilo P Jr, Langan WB, Rosen MR, Hoffman BF: Effects of the phenothiazine analog, EN-313, on ventricular arrhythmias in the dog. Europ J of Pharm 45:127-139, 1977
9. Friedman PL, Stewart JR, Fenoglio JJ Jr, Wit AL: Survival of subendocardial Purkinje fibers after extensive myocardial infarction in dogs: In vitro and in vivo correlations. Circ Res 33:597-611, 1973
10. Friedman PL, Stewart JR, Wit AL: Spontaneous and induced cardiac arrhythmias in subendocardial Purkinje fibers surviving extensive myocardial infarction in dogs. Circ Res 33:612-626, 1973
11. Horowitz LN, Spear JF, Moore EN: Subendocardial origin of ventricular arrhythmias in 24 hour old experimental myocardial infarction. Circulation 53:56-63, 1976
12. Elharrar V, Gaum WE, Zipes DP: Effect of drugs on conduction delay and the incidence of ventricular arrhythmias induced by acute coronary occlusion in dogs. Am J Cardiol 39:544-549, 1977
13. Battle WE, Naimi S, Avitall B, Brilla AH, Banas JS Jr, Bate JM, Levine HG: Distinctive time course of ventricular vulnerability to fibrillation during and after release of coronary ligation. Am J Cardiol 34:42-47, 1974
14. Williams DO, Scherlag BJ, Hope RR, El Sherif N, Lazzara R: The pathophysiology of malignant ventricular arrhythmias during acute myocardial ischemia. Circulation 50:1163-1172, 1974

15. Kaplinsky E, Ogawa S, Balke CW, Dreifus LS: Two periods of early ventricular arrhythmias in the canine acute myocardial infarction model. Circulation 60:397-403, 1979

16. Corbalan R, Verrier RL, Lown B: Differing mechanisms for ventricular vulnerability during coronary artery occlusion and release. Am Heart J 92:223-229, 1976

17. Balke CW, Kaplinsky E, Michelson EL, Dreifus LS: Limitations of sequential coronary reperfusion as a model for antiarrhythmic drug evaluation. Circulation Suppl II:II-87, 1979

18. Laadt JR, Allen JB: The effect of quinidine on ventricular fibrillation induced by coronary ligation. Am Heart J 39:279-282, 1950

19. Stephenson SE, Cole RK, Parrish TF, et al: Ventricular fibrillation during and after coronary occlusion: Incidence and protection afforded by various drugs. Am J Cardiol Jan:77-87, 1960

20. Weisse AB, Moschos CB, Passannante AJ, Khan MI, Regan TJ: Relative effectiveness of three antiarrhythmic agents in the treatment of ventricular arrhythmias in experimental acute myocardial ischemia. Am Heart J 81:503-510, 1971

21. Gamble OW, Cohn K: Effect of propranolol, procainamide and lidocaine on ventricular automaticity and reentry in experimental myocardial infarction. Circulation 46:498-506, 1972

22. Khan MI, Hamilton JT, Manning GW: Early arrhythmias following experimental coronary occlusion in conscious dogs and their modification of beta adrenoceptor blocking drugs. Am Heart J 86:347-358, 1973

23. Myers RW, Pearlman AS, Hymen RM, et al: Beneficial effects of vagal stimulation and bradycardia during experimental acute myocardial ischemia. Circulation 49:943-947, 1974

24. Borer JS, Kent KM, Goldstein RE, Epstein SE: Nitro-glycerine induced reduction in the incidence of spontaneous ventricular fibrillation during coronary occlusion in dogs. Am J Cardiol 33:517, 1974

25. Kniffen FJ, Lomas TE, Counsell RE, Lucchesi BR: The antiarrhythmic and antifibrillatory actions of bretylium and its 0-iodobenzyl trimethylammonium analog, UM-360. J Pharm and Exper Therap 92:120-128, 1975

26. Rosenbaum MB, Chiale PA, Halpern MS, Nau G, et al: Antiarrhythmic efficacy of amiodarone. Am J Cardiol 38:934-944, 1976

27. Verdouw PD, Remme WJ, Hugenholtz PG: Cardiovascular and antiarrhythmic effects of aprindine (AC 1802) during partial occlusion of a coronary artery in the pig. Cardiovasc Res 11:317-323, 1977

28. Naito M, Michelson EL, Kmetzo JJ, Kaplinsky E, Dreifus LS: Failure of antiarrhythmic drugs to prevent experimental reperfusion ventricular fibrillation. Circulation 63:Jan, 1981 (In Press)

29. Williams DO, Scherlag BJ, Hope RR, El Sherif, N, Lazzara R: The pathophysiology of malignant ventricular arrhythmias during acute myocardial ischemia. Circulation 50:1163-1172, 1964
30. Balke CW, Kaplinsky E, Michelson EL, Naito M, Dreifus LS: Reperfusion ventricular arrhythmias: Correlation with antecedent coronary artery ligation arrhythmias and duration of acute ligation. Am Heart J (submitted)

ADREN	Adrenalin
AMI	Amiodarone
AP	Aprindine
Auto	Automaticity
Brady	Bradycardia
BRET	Bretylium
CC	Closed chest
COAG	Coagulation
DISO	Disopyramide
DPH	Phenytoin
E	Effective
ETH	Ethmozin
HAL	Halothane
Immed	Immediate
ISO	Isoproterenol
L	Lidocaine
LAD	Left anterior descending coronary artery
LCx	Left circumflex coronary artery
MEX	Mexiletine
NE	Not effective
NTG	Nitroglycerin
OC	Open chest
Occl	Occlusion
OUAB	Ouabaine
P	Procaine
PA	Procainamide
PRO	Propranolol
PRACT	Practolol
Prox	Proximal
Prox Seg	Proximal segment
Q	Quinidine
Reent	Reentry
Rep	Reperfusion
SCO	Sequential coronary occlusion
SCOR	Sequential occlusion and reperfusion
SOT	Sotalol
TOC	Tocainide
V	Verapamil
VAG-STIM	Vagal stimulation
VF	ventricular fibrillation
VT	Ventricular tachycardia
VPC	Ventricular premature complex

AUTHOR	ANIMAL	MODEL	TYPE OF LIGATION	STUDY PERIOD	END POINT	DRUG	RESULTS
Harris[4] Estandia Ford, et al 1952	Dog	CC	LAD 2 Stage Prox Occl	16-20 hrs	VT	P PA	P-NE PA-E
Mokler[5] VanArman 1960	Dog	CC	A) LAD 2 Stage Prox Occl B) OUAB	24 hrs	VT	DISO PA Q	DISO-E PA-E Q-E
Lucchesi[6] Whitsitt Stickney 1967	Dog	CC	A) LAD 2 Stage Prox Occl B) OUAB	48-72 hrs	VPC VT	dl PRO l PRO	dl PRO-E d PRO-NE
Allen[7] Shanks Zaidi 1971	Dog	CC	LAD 2 Stage Prox Occl HAL-ADREN OUAB	20-44 hrs	VT	L PRO	L-E PRO-E PRO>L
Danilo[8] Rosen Hoffman 1977	Dog	CC	LAD 2 Stage Occl	22-26 hrs	VPC,VT	ETH Q	ETH-E Q-E ETH>Q
Elharrar[12] Gaum Zipes 1977	Dog	OC	LAD 1 Stage Prox Seg Occl Rep	Immed; 6min Occl 30min Rep	VT VF	AP V V+ISO Q	AP-worsens V-NE V+ISO-NE Q-NE

AUTHOR	ANIMAL	MODEL	TYPE OF LIGATION	STUDY PERIOD	END POINT	DRUG	RESULTS
Laadt[18] Allen 1950	Dog	CC	LAD 1 Stage Prox Occl	20-30 hrs	VF	Q	Q-NE
Stephenson[19] et al 1960	Dog	OC	LAD 1 Stage Prox Occl + Rep	Immed Occl + 30 min Rep	VF	Q P PA L	Q>others
Weisse[20] Maschos Passannante 1971	Dog	CC	LAD LCx Prox COAG	4 hrs	VT	PA L DPH	PA-E L-E DPH-E
Gamble[21] Cohn 1972	Cat	OC	LAD 1 Stage Prox Occl	45 min- 3 hrs	VT VF	PA L PRO	Auto PA-E PRO-E L-E Reent PA-NE PRO-NE L-worse
Khan[22] Hamilton Manning 1973	Dog	CC	LAD 1 Stage Prox Occl	Immed to 2 hrs	VF VT	d PRO SOT d PRO PRACT	d PRO-E SOT-E d PRO-NE PRACT-E
Meyers[23] Pearlman Hyman, et al 1974	Dog	OC	LAD Septal 1 Stage Occl	30 min	VF	VAG	VAG STIM-E Brady-E

AUTHOR	ANIMAL	MODEL	TYPE OF LIGATION	STUDY PERIOD	END POINT	DRUG	RESULTS
Borer[24] Kent Goldstein et al 1974	Dog	OC	LAD + Septal 1 Stage Occl	30 min	VF	NTG	NTG-E
Kniffen[25] Lomas Counsell Lucchesi 1975	Dog	OC	LAD 1 Stage Prox Occl	20 min Occl + Rep ISO+CaCl2 Stellate ganglion stimulation	VF	BRET	BRET-E
Rosenbaum[26] Chiale Halpern et al 1977	Dog	CC	LAD 1 Stage Prox Occl	Immed	VF	AMI	AMI-E
Verdouw[27] Remme Hugenholtz 1977	Pig	OC	LAD 1 Stage Prox Occl (75%)	Immed	VF	AP	AP-E
Naito[28] Michelson Kmetzo 1981	Dog	OC	LAD 1 Stage Prox Occl + Rep	Immed Rep at 30 min	VT VF	L PA V AMI	L-NE PA-NE V-NE AMI-NE

DESCRIPTION OF CHRONIC CANINE MYOCARDIAL INFARCTION MODELS SUITABLE
FOR THE ELECTROPHARMACOLOGIC EVALUATION OF NEW ANTIARRHYTHMIC DRUGS

E.L. Michelson, M.D., J.F. Spear, Ph.D., E.N. Moore, D.V.M., Ph.D.

INTRODUCTION

Numerous acute and subacute animal models of myocardial infarction
have been developed for the purpose of studying the malignant ventricular
arrhythmias that contribute to sudden death in patients with ischemic
heart disease. Much has been learned about arrhythmia mechanisms from
these studies.[1-13] In addition, as detailed elsewhere in this symposium
by Drs. Dreifus and Moore, some of these models have also proven useful
in the evaluation of new antiarrhythmic agents. For example, during the
period from 12 to 72 hours following canine coronary artery occlusion,
animals remain otherwise stable but manifest frequent premature ventricular complexes (PVCs). These arrhythmias apparently result from the increased automaticity of surviving Purkinje fibers in proximity to areas
of recent infarction.[5,8,9] Virtually every potential antiarrhythmic agent,
when administered in an appropriate dosage, has been successful in suppressing these arrhythmias. Although failure to suppress these arrhythmias
would render a potential antiarrhythmic agent suspect, little can be
deduced about a drug's ultimate utility either in the treatment of human
PVCs or in the prevention of sudden death from its effectiveness in
this subacute myocardial infarction model.

At present, there are no established models of chronic myocardial
infarction that have demonstrated utility in the evaluation of potential
antiarrhythmic agents. Although "chronic" coronary artery ameroid constrictor and balloon occlusion models have been described, it appears that
these models are more accurately characterized as ongoing acute and subacute preparations rather than "chronic". However, several laboratories
have recently developed chronic canine models in which sustained ventricular tachyarrhythmias are inducible days to weeks and longer following
experimental myocardial infarction.[14-16] These models have been based on
the observations by previous investigators that release of a canine

coronary artery occlusion, after a period ranging from 40 minutes to 3 hours, was capable of salvaging jeopardized myocardium.[17-19] Subsequent work has demonstrated that the anatomic and electrophysiologic milieu resulting from coronary occlusion followed by reperfusion in these animals remains arrhythmogenic well past the acute and subacute phases of the infarction.[14-16] More recently, Garan and coworkers[20] have developed an alternative chronic canine infarction-ventricular tachyarrhythmia model. By occluding the mid-left anterior descending coronary artery and all other epicardial vessels coursing to the left ventricular apex, dogs develop chronic lesions which simulate human "aneurysms", and are also prone to pacing-induced arrhythmias.

In the canine models presently described, arrhythmias can be initiated and terminated by methods of programmed stimulation comparable to those used in the clinical catheterization laboratory in man.[21-27] In addition, evidence suggests that the arrhythmias initiated in both man and these chronic models have a similar "localized reentrant mechanism".[26] Moreover, the apparent stability and reproducibility of the induced arrhythmias make these chronic myocardial infarction models ideal for evaluating potential diagnostic and therapeutic interventions designed to reduce the incidence of sudden cardiac death in man. The results of recent initial, provocative electropharmacologic studies done using these canine chronic infarction models will be presented.

METHODS

In our laboratory, studies have been performed on more than 50 healthy adult mongrel dogs weighing 8 to 16 kg. Animals were anesthetized with intravenous sodium pentobarbital (30 mg/kg body weight) and then ventilated with room air through a cuffed pharyngeotracheal tube using a volume-cycled positive pressure respirator. Body temperature was maintained with a thermal mattress and the heart was exposed through a limited left thoracotomy using aseptic techniques. The mid or distal left anterior descending coronary artery was occluded by the Harris two-stage procedure. The ligature was then released two hours after complete occlusion and the vessel massaged gently. Re-establishment of pulsatile arterial blood flow distal to the site of occlusion was evident in each case.

The chests were closed and routine post-operative care was administered including prophylactic antibiotic therapy. At 3 to 30 days after initial occlusions, when the animals were in otherwise clinically stable condition, and the accelerated ventricular arrhythmias of the first 24 to 48 hours had subsided, dogs were anesthetized with sodium pentobarbital (10 mg/kg) plus diazepam (1 to 2 mg/kg), each intravenously, or 30 mg/kg intravenous sodium pentobarbital. Ventilation and body temperature were maintained as before, and the heart was exposed through a left lateral thoracotomy. Intra-aortic pressure was monitored via catheters introduced via either the femoral or carotid vessels. With the use of 22 gauge needles, Teflon-coated stainless steel plunge (hook) wire electrodes (0.10 mm in diameter) were placed in multiple subepicardial, intramyocardial and subendocardial sites within the distribution of both occluded and non-occluded vessels. The plunge electrodes were insulated except at the tip. Routine methods of programmed electrical stimulation [21-27] were performed using either unipolar cathodal or bipolar stimulation to determine whether sustained ventricular tachyarrhythmias could be induced. Rectangular current pulses of 2 milliseconds (ms) duration were delivered by an optically-isolated constant current source that was continuously variable from 0 to 10 milli-amps (mA). For unipolar cathodal stimulation, the indifferent anode was a stainless steel rib spreader having an approximately 8 cm^2 surface in contact with the chest wall. Programmed electric stimulation was performed using a custom-designed digital stimulator (Bloom Associates, Narberth, PA).

Protocol of Programmed Electric Stimulation

To evaluate the propensity to sustained ventricular tachyarrhythmias, ventricular extrastimuli were introduced during ventricular pacing at a cycle length of 300 ms. This cycle length was chosen to facilitate con-sistent ventricular capture in each of the animals studied. In animals with less than 1:1 retrograde ventriculo-atrial conduction during ven-tricular drive pacing, simultaneous left atrial pacing was done to pre-vent interference from intermittent supraventricular capture beats. Both basic drive pacing and extrastimuli were applied at the same ventricular site using constant current pulses of twice diastolic threshold intensity. Scanning of diastole was initiated with the introduction of a single ven-tricular extrastimulus after 8 paced beats. If a sustained ventricular tachyarrhythmia was not elicited, double and, if necessary, triple ventricu-lar extrastimuli were then introduced during ventricular pacing. "Sustained" was defined as more than one minute of ventricular tachycardia or

nonself-terminating ventricular flutter or fibrillation requiring countershock. After a sustained ventricular tachyarrhythmia was induced, random
ventricular pacing or programmed single or double ventricular extrastimuli
were introduced in an attempt to terminate the tachycardia. If these
modalities were not successful or hemodynamic deterioration was evident,
rapid burst pacing and/or countershock was used to terminate sustained
tachyarrhythmias. In selected animals, arrhythmia initiation was also
studied using endocardial catheter techniques via electrode catheters with
a 1 cm interelectrode distance introduced via the jugular and/or carotid
vessels. This was done to more closely simulate the techniques used in the
clinical cardiac electrophysiology laboratory in man.

All experiments conformed to the "Guiding Principles in the Care and
Use of Animals" approved by the Council of the American Physiological
Society and with the Animal Care Policies of the University of Pennsylvania
and Lankenau Hospital.

RESULTS

Patterns of Arrhythmias

We have recently reviewed our results in the first 38 animals studied
3 to 30 days following the two-stage coronary occlusion and reperfusion
procedure. Sustained ventricular tachyarrhythmias could be initiated in
35 using programmed stimulation. Fourteen dogs had inducible sustained
ventricular tachycardia, 9 had inducible flutter, and 12 had pacing-induced
fibrillation. Ventricular tachycardia was defined as an accelerated ventricular rhythm with a basic cycle length of greater than or equal to 120 ms.
Ventricular tachycardia was also characterized by an isoelectric baseline
between successive QRS complexes on the scalar electrocardiogram. In
general, episodes of sustained ventricular tachycardia could be initiated
with either single or double extrastimuli, and subsequently could be
terminated with either one or two programmed ventricular extrastimuli, or
with short 3 to 5 beat bursts of rapid pacing. Hemodynamically, ventricular
tachycardia was usually well-tolerated in the open chest, anesthesized dog
with a variable mechanical alternans often maintaining arterial blood
pressure.

At cycle lengths shorter than 120 ms, an organized, regular arrhythmia
was defined as ventricular flutter. During a typical episode of flutter,
there was no isoelectric baseline discernible between successive QRS

complexes on the scalar electrocardiogram. Double or triple extrastimuli were usually required for initiation of flutter, but extrastimuli were less consistently successful than rapid pacing in arrhythmia termination. Ventricular flutter was less stable hemodynamically than tachycardia, and rapid burst pacing was just as likely to facilitate degeneration of flutter into fibrillation as it was to terminate the arrhythmia.

Ventricular fibrillation (VF) was defined as a chaotic, incoordinate and irreversible ventricular rhythm confirmed electrocardiographically as well as visually. Although an occasional animal had VF initiated reproducibly with a single extrastimulus, double or triple extrastimuli were usually necessary to initiate fibrillation, and countershock was required for termination.

While different animals showed different patterns of ventricular tachyarrhythmias, in a given animal there was considerable reproduciblity in the rate and morphology of the arrhythmia which could be induced. This pattern however, could be changed by various pacing and pharmacologic interventions as detailed below. In addition, in a minority of animals, more than one distinct tachyarrhythmia was initiated reproducibly.

Anatomic Findings and Correlates

In each of the 35 experimental animals with inducible ventricular tachyarrhythmias, a "mottled", patchy infarction was present upon gross examination with close interspersing of normal and abnormal myocardium within the area of infarction. Although there was a tendency to subepicardial sparing, there was no gradient of injury from one layer to the next transmurally.

There were three animals with no inducible arrhythmias: Two dogs had small mottled infarctions with multiple 1 mm x 1 mm punctate areas of necrosis dispersed over 2 cm x 3 cm areas, and one animal had an isolated dense 5 mm x 5 mm area of infarction.

It was our impression that in dogs with larger infarcts (e.g. $\geq$ 3 cm x 3 cm), the initiation of ventricular tachycardia was more likely than VF, and in dogs with smaller infarcts (e.g. < 1 cm x 2 cm) the initiation of VF was more likely. Furthermore, for any given infarct size, the greater the degree of mottling within that area (i.e., the extent of interspersing of normal and abnormal myocardium), the more likely it was to initiate ventricular tachycardia or flutter rather than fibrillation. However, even the largest infarcts produced by our occlusion-reperfusion methods involved less than 25% of the left ventricle, were patchy within involved areas, and did not result in hemodynamic embarrassment.

Arrhythmia Inducibility

In our experiments, the ability to induce ventricular tachyarrhythmias in individual animals depended on the site of stimulation.[28] In a given animal, we were not able to induce ventricular tachyarrhythmias from all sites tested. In addition, while some sites required only a single ventricular extrastimulus to be successful, other sites which were successful required two or three ventricular extrastimuli for arrhythmia initiation. This variability in inducibility was dependent on both the local properties of excitability and refractoriness at the site of stimulation, as well as the anatomic relationship of a site with respect to the area of infarction.[15,28]

Overall, in the 24 animals in which this was studied in detail, the most successful sites tended to be those intramyocardial sites exhibiting normal excitability and refractoriness within 2 cm of the border of the area of infarction. Out of 44 such sites tested, 27 (61%) were successful in initiating ventricular arrhythmias. In comparison, normal left ventricular sites > 2 cm from an area of infarction, normal right ventricular sites, endocardial catheter sites, and left ventricular infarct sites were each successful at $\leq$ 25% of the sites attempted in initiating arrhythmias. Thus, in doing serial electropharmacologic studies, it is important to attempt arrhythmia initiation from a sufficiently large number of sites; and if feasible, the same sites that initiated arrhythmias before drug administration should be evaluated again after drug administration.

Effect of Antiarrhythmic Agents

In 19 animals 20-25 mg/kg procainamide (mean plasma level at time of study 12.5 μg/ml) was administered intravenously after the basic pattern of ventricular tachyarrhythmia was determined. In each case, the severity of arrhythmia was reduced. In 4 of 9 animals in which ventricular fibrillation could be induced before procainamide, no arrhythmias were inducible following procainamide. In the other five animals with ventricular fibrillation, only sustained tachycardia (3 animals) or non-sustained ventricular tachycardia (2 animals) could be initiated after procainamide. This ability of procainamide to prevent the re-initiation (6 dogs) or to reduce the severity (4 dogs) of the arrhythmia was also true for animals which had ventricular flutter or ventricular tachycardia.

In 10 other animals, a 2-3 mg/kg bolus of lidocaine was given intravenously after the completion of baseline studies and a 0.07 mg/kg/minute infusion initiated. After lidocaine administration, it was still possible to re-initiate the same ventricular tachyarrhythmia in each case. In individual animals the cycle length of the pacing-induced tachyarrhythmia was variably either prolonged, shortened or unchanged after lidocaine was administered. In addition, in 6 animals, a 2-3 mg/kg lidocaine bolus was also given intravenously during an episode of sustained ventricular tachycardia. Lidocaine was only successful in one of these 6 cases in terminating an arrhythmia that was already established and in 2 cases apparently facilitated acceleration rather than slowing of the tachycardias. Notably, these effects of both procainamide and lidocaine in this model mimicked closely those effects reported in patients with recurrent sustained ventricular tachyarrhythmias studied in the clinical electrophysiology laboratory.[21-27,29]

In addition, we have also studied the antiarrhythmic activity of the non-neuronal blocking, bethanidine derivative, meobentine sulfate in our chronic model. Antiarrhythmic efficacy was demonstrated in all 10 dogs studied after intravenous administration of 20 mg/kg meobentine over 30 minutes. In the 9 dogs with VF initially, re-initiation was prevented for as long as 6 to > 12 hours.

Other Chronic Myocardial Infarction-Ventricular Tachyarrhythmia Models

Other chronic canine myocardial infarction-ventricular tachyarrhythmia models have been developed independently by several investigators. Their methods are compared to ours in Table I. In brief, their methods and results have been as follows: Karagueuzian, et al[14] studied conscious closed chest 12-17 kg dogs using programmed pacing via sewn-on epicardial plaque electrodes. They reported the ability to initiate "protracted tachycardias" (> 10 sec) consistently with a single extrastimulus in dogs 3 to 5 days after a two-stage--two hour occlusion then reperfusion of the proximal left anterior descending coronary artery. Presumably with more aggressive pacing techniques (e.g. use of more sites, use of double or triple extrastimuli) arrhythmia susceptibility could also have been demonstrated after day 5 in their animals. In contrast, other dogs subjected to permanent occlusion without reperfusion by these authors, had protracted arrhythmias only infrequently. Using this model, Glassman, et al[30]

reported that the intravenous administration of (a) 5-10 mg/kg lidocaine
was ineffective in preventing arrhythmia initiation; (b) 25-30 mg/kg procainamide markedly prolonged the cycle length of inducible arrhythmias
(190 → 261 ms) but did not prevent their re initiation; and (c) 0.4 mg/kg
verapamil was not only ineffective but actually increased the incidence
of inducible VF. Of note, their results with procainamide were somewhat
less favorable than we have observed.

Lucchesi and coworkers[16,31,32] have used a similar model, but they
retain a partial coronary occlusion after a 1½-2 hour period of two-stage
proximal left anterior descending coronary artery occlusion. They have
done serial electropharmacologic studies in awake 14-18 kg dogs 3-10 days
after infarction via chronically-implanted intramyocardial electrodes.
Dogs have either pacing-induced sustained tachycardia, VF or non-sustained
tachycardia (approximately one-third each) using their methods. They
have found the following: (a) Disopyramide at plasma levels of 1.0 µg/ml
actually increased the rate and prolonged the duration of inducible tachyarrhythmias; whereas at 2.0-4.0 µg/ml, the tachycardia rate and duration
were decreased. However, only at plasma levels $\geq$ 7.0 µg/ml was arrhythmia
initiation prevented.[31] (b) Chronic bretylium studied $\geq$ 3 hours after
administration of 5 mg/kg intravenously was effective in preventing re-
initiation of ventricular tachycardia and VF;[32] and (c) intravenous administration of 5 mg/kg pranolium (N-dimethylpropranolol, UM-272), a non-beta-
blocking, non-membrane active derivative of propranolol, either prevented
arrhythmia re-initiation or prolonged the cycle length of those tachyarrhythmias still inducible.[16]

Anecdotally, (personal communication) and of considerable importance,
Lucchesi has also observed that both the superimposition of an otherwise
non-lethal ischemic lesion,as well as the stress of maximal physical exertion, may each be sufficient to precipitate PVCs and subsequently VF in
their chronic model. This is of particular interest since *none of the
chronic models described in this presentation is characterized by chronic,
spontaneously-occurring PVCs.*

Garan, et al[20] have developed an alternative arrhythmia model which
simulates chronic anterior myocardial infarction with aneursym formation.
They ligate the mid-left anterior descending coronary artery and all other
epicardial vessels coursing to the left ventricular apex. The majority
of their dogs have survived this procedure (20/25, 80%) and the majority

of these dogs had inducible tachycardia (16/20, 80%). Dogs were studied open-chested 5-28 days after infarction, and many of these dogs (11/20, 55%) had inducible sustained ventricular tachyarrhythmias with programmed or burst ventricular pacing. The rates of the tachyarrhythmias in their model, using 15-25 kg dogs, were often in the range of 200-300 beats/minute. They found verapamil (1.5-10.0 mg/kg intravenously) to be an ineffective antiarrhythmic agent.[20]

Historically, it should be noted that much of our insight into what is now considered strong evidence that a reentrant mechanism underlies these arrhythmias has been based on important studies by El-Sherif, Scherlag, Lazzara and coworkers.[6,7] Their work was done in dogs 3-7 days after occlusion of the proximal left anterior descending coronary artery. In a series of reports they correlated the antiarrhythmic activity of various drugs with the effects of these drugs on delayed epicardial electrical activity, a presumptive marker for reentry. In their model, intravenous lidocaine (2 mg/kg)[33] diphenylhydantoin (5-10 mg/kg)[34] and procainamide (5-10 mg/kg)[35] all slowed conduction in the ischemic zone and all prevented reentrant beats; whereas verapamil (0.5 mg/kg)[36] and propranolol (0.2 mg/kg)[36] were each without effect. However, their model was not one of reproducibly inducible sustained ventricular tachyarrhythmias, and it is not clear how the findings in their model relate to the chronic human situation.

TABLE I

Chronic Canine Myocardial Infarction-Arrhythmia Models

Investigators (ref)	Methods			Drugs Tested
El-Sherif, Lazzara and coworkers [33,36]	LIG	3-7d	O/C	DPH, L, PA, Pr, V
Karagueuzian, Wit and coworkers [14,30]	LIG/R	3-5d	Awake	L, PA, V
Patterson, Gibson, Lucchesi, et al [16,31,32]	LIG/R⁻	3-10d	Awake	Br, Diso, Pra
Michelson, Spear, Moore [15,28]	LIG/R	3-30d⁺	O/C	L, M, PA
Garan, Fallon, Ruskin [20]	LIG/L	5-28d	O/C	V

Abbreviations

Methods: d = days; LIG = ligation; LIG/L = multiple ligations; O/C = open chest, anesthetized; R = reperfusion, R⁻ = partial reperfusion. *Drugs Tested:* Br = bretylium; DPH = diphenylhydantoin; Diso = disopry-amide; M = meobentine; PA = procainamide; Pr = propranolol; Pra = pranolium; (ref): references, indicated by superscripts.

SUMMARY

Thus, there are now several chronic canine myocardial infarction-ventricular tachyarrhythmia models which are available for the evaluation of new antiarrhythmic drugs (Table I). The available models fulfill many, but not all of the requirements for an ideal chronic arrhythmia model (Table II). The sustained arrhythmias initiated in these models using programmed pacing presumably have the same localized reentrant mechanism that characterizes chronic human myocardial infarction and chronic coronary artery disease.[26] However, these models are not suitable for determining whether a new drug will abolish spontaneously-occurring PVCs. In addition, these models are of unproven value in the study of acute spontaneously-occurring sudden death; although recently initiated, provocative work may shed further light on this subject. Most importantly, the available models do seem well-suited to the evaluation of new drugs intended for use in chronic coronary artery disease patients at risk for sustained reentrant ventricular tachycardia or VF. Notably, the results of preliminary electropharmacologic studies in these canine models parallel closely those findings reported in human patients with sustained life-threatening ventricular tachyarrhythmias (Table III). Therefore, increased use of these chronic models for new antiarrhythmic drug testing is strongly recommended.

TABLE II

Ideal vs Available Chronic Canine - Arrhythmia Models

Ideal	Available
1. (a) Arrhythmia mechanism comparable to patients with chronic CAD: Reentry	Yes
(b) Pathophysiology similar (e.g., atherogenic CAD)	No
2. Susceptible to:	
(a) spontaneous PVCs	No
(b) spontaneous VT/VF	No[1]
(c) inducible VT/VF	Yes
3. Technically feasible	Yes
4. (a) Stable - short term: hours, days	Yes
(b) Stable - long term: weeks, months	Yes[2]
(c) Open-chest and closed chest	Yes
5. Effects and dosages of antiarrhythmic drugs parallel man	Yes[2]

Abbreviations

CAD = coronary artery disease; PVCs = premature ventricular complexes; VT/VF = ventricular tachycardia/fibrillation; No[1]: may be susceptible with exertion or superimposed mild ischemia; Yes[2] = needs further evaluation.

TABLE III

Comparison of Anti-VT/VF Drug Efficacy Evaluated by
Programmed Pacing in Chronic Dog Models vs Man

Chronic Dog Models	Efficacy	Man	Efficacy
Lidocaine	+/-		+/-
Procainamide	YES, ↓ VT rate		YES, ↓ VT rate
DPH	yes		yes
Disopyramide	YES ↓ VT rate		YES, ↓ VT rate
Propranolol	NO		NO
Bretylium (chronic)	YES, ↓ VT rate		yes ↓ VT rate
Verapamil	NO		NO
Pranolium	YES		?
Meobentine	YES, ↓ VT rate		?

Abbreviations

DPH = diphenylhydantoin; Efficacy: YES = often; yes = occasional;
+/- = infrequent; VT = ventricular tachycardia; VF = ventricular
fibrillation; ↓ = decrease; ? = unknown.

Acknowledgments

    We thank Ralph Iannuzzi, C. William Balke, Rita Falcone,
Mark Schaffenburg and Thomas Blenko for skilled technical assistance,
Susan Sabol for help with data analysis, and Ann Hagan for assistance in
manuscript preparation.

From the Division of Cardiology, Departments of Research and Medicine,
Lankenau Hospital, and the School of Veterinary Medicine, University of
Pennsylvania, Philadelphia, Pennsylvania

Supported in part by a Grant-in-Aid Award from the Lancaster Chapter,
Pennsylvania Affiliate, American Heart Association; and by Grants HL23071,
HL16076, HL19045 from the National Heart Lung and Blood Institute,
National Institutes of Health, Bethesda, Maryland

Dr. Michelson is recipient of Clinical Investigatorship Award IK08 HL 00709
from the National Heart, Lung and Blood Institute, National Institutes of
Health, Bethesda, Maryland.

REFERENCES

1. Harris AS, Rojas AG. Initiation of ventricular fibrillation due to
    coronary occlusion. Exp Med Surg 1943;1:1-105-22
2. Waldo AL, Kaiser GA. A study of ventricular arrhythmias associated
    with acute myocardial infarction in the canine heart. Circulation
    1973;47:1222-8
3. Boineau JP, Cox JL. Slow ventricular activation in acute myocardial
    infarction: a source of reentrant premature ventricular contractions.
    Circulation 1973;48:702-13

4. Scherlag BJ, El-Sherif N, Hope R, Lazzara R. Characterization and localization of ventricular arrhythmias resulting from myocardial ischemia and infarction. Circ Res 1974;35:372-83
5. Wit AL, Bigger JT Jr. Possible electrophysiological mechanisms for lethal arrhythmias accompanying myocardial ischemia and infarction. Circulation 1975;51,52:Suppl III:III:96-115
6. El-Sherif N, Scherlag BF, Lazzara R, Hope RR. Reentrant arrhythmias in the late myocardial infarction period. I. Conduction characteristics in the infarct zone. Circulation 1977;55:686-702
7. El-Sherif N, Hope RR, Scherlag BF, Lazzara R. Reentrant arrhythmias in the late myocardial infarction period. II. Patterns of initiation and termination of reentry. Circulation 1977;55:702-19
8. Horowitz LN, Spear JF, Moore EN. Subendocardial origin of ventricular arrhythmias in 24-hour old experimental myocardial infarction. Circulation 1975;53:56-62
9. Spear JF, Michelson EL, Spielman SR, Moore EN. The origin of ventricular arrhythmias 24 hours following experimental anterior septal coronary artery occlusion. Circulation 1977;55:844-52
10. Kaplinsky E, Ogawa S, Balke CW, Dreifus LS. Two periods of early ventricular arrhythmia in the canine acute myocardial infarction model. Circulation 1979;60:397-403
11. Levites R, Banka VS, Helfant RH. Electrophysiologic effects of coronary occlusion and reperfusion: observations on dispersion of refractoriness and ventricular automaticity. Circulation 1975;52:760-5
12. Ramanathan KB, Bodenheimer MM, Banka VS, Helfant RH. Electrophysiologic effects of partial coronary occlusion and reperfusion. Am J Cardiol 1977;40:50-4
13. Janse MJ, van Capelle JL, Morsink H, et al. Flow of "injury" current and patterns of excitation during early ventricular arrhythmias in acute regional myocardial ischemia in isolated procine and canine hearts. Evidence for two different arrhythmogenic mechanisms. Circ Res 1980;47:151-165
14. Karagueuzian HS, Fenoglio JJ, Weiss MB, Wit AL. Protracted ventricular tachycardia induced by premature stimulation of the canine heart after coronary artery occlusion and reperfusion. Circ Res 1979;44:833-46
15. Michelson EL, Spear JF, Moore EN. Electrophysiologic and anatomic correlates of sustained ventricular tachyarrhythmias in a model of chronic myocardial infarction. Am J Cardiol 1980;45:583-90
16. Gibson JK, Lucchesi BR. Electrophysiologic actions of UM-272 (pranolium) on reentrant ventricular arrhythmias in postinfarction canine myocardium. J Pharmacol Exp Ther 1980;214:347-53
17. Maroko PR, Libby P, Ginks WR, et al. Coronary artery reperfusion I. Early effects on local myocardial function and the extent of myocardial necrosis. J Clin Invest 1972;51:2710-16
18. Ginks WR, Sybers HD, Maroko PR, Covell JW, Sobel BE, Ross J Jr. Coronary artery reperfusion. II. Reduction of myocardial infarct size at 1 week after the coronary occlusion. J Clin Invest 1972;51:2717-23
19. Reimer KA, Lowe VE, Rasmussen MM, Jennings RB. The wavefront phenomenon of ischemic cell death: I. Myocardial infarct size vs duration of coronary occlusion in dogs. Circulation 1977;56:786-94
20. Garan H, Fallon JT, Ruskin JN. Sustained ventricular tachycardia in recent myocardial infarction. Circulation 1980, in press

21. Denes P, Wu D, Dhingra RC, et al. Electrophysiologic studies in patients with chronic recurrent ventricular tachycardia. Circulation 1976;54:229-36
22. Wellens HJJ, Düren DR, Lie KI. Observations on mechanisms of ventricular tachycardia in man. Circulation 1976;54:237-44
23. Fisher JD, Cohen HL, Mehra R, Altschuler H, Escher DJW, Furman S. Cardiac pacing and pacemakers. II. Serial electrophysiologic-pharmacologic testing for control of recurrent tachyarrhythmias. Am Heart J 1977;93:658-68
24. Josephson ME, Horowitz LN, Farshidi A, Kastor JA. Recurrent sustained ventricular tachycardia. 1. Mechanisms. Circulation 1978;57:431-40
25. Wellens HJJ. Value and limitations of programmed electrical stimulation of the heart in the study and treatment of tachycardias. Circulation 1978;57:845-53
26. Josephson ME, Horowitz LN, Farshidi A, Spielman SR, Michelson EL, Greenspan AM. Sustained ventricular tachycardia: evidence for protected localized reentry. Am J Cardiol 1978;42:416-23
27. Mason JW, Winkle RA. Electrode-catheter arrhythmia induction in the selection and assessment of antiarrhythmic drug therapy for recurrent ventricular tachycardia. Circulation 1978;58:971-85
28. Michelson EL, Spear JF, Moore EN. Initiation of sustained ventricular tachyarrhythmias in a model of chronic infarction: importance of the site of stimulation. Am J Cardiol 1980;45:II:II-494 (abstr)
29. Greenspan AM, Horowitz LN, Spielman SR, Josephson ME. Large dose procainamide therapy for ventricular tachyarrhythmia. Am J Cardiol 1980;46:453-62
30. Glassman RD, Davis JC, Wit AL. Effects of antiarrhythmic drugs on sustained ventricular tachycardia induced by a premature stimulus in dogs after coronary artery occlusion and reperfusion. Fed Proc 1978;37:730 (abstr)
31. Patterson E, Gibson JK, Lucchesi BR. The electrophysiologic effects of disopyramide phosphate upon reentrant ventricular arrhythmias in conscious dogs after myocardial infarction. Am J Cardiol 1980, in press
32. Patterson E, Gibson JK, Lucchesi BR. Chronic canine ventricular tachyarrhythmias - prevention by bretylium tosylate administration. In press
33. El-Sherif N, Scherlag BJ, Lazzara R, Hope RR. Reentrant ventricular arrhythmias in the late myocardial infarction period. 4. Mechanism of action of lidocaine. Circulation 1977;56:395-402
34. El-Sherif N, Lazzara R. Reentrant ventricular arrhythmias in the myocardial infarction period. 5. Mechanism of action of diphenylhydantoin. Circulation 1978;57:465-72
35. El-Sherif N. Electrophysiologic basis of procainamide therapeutic and toxic effects on ischemia-related reentrant ventricular arrhythmias. Am J Cardiol 1979;43:429 (abstr)
36. El-Sherif N, Lazzara R. Reentrant ventricular arrhythmias in the late myocardial infarction period. 7. Effect of verapamil and D-600 and the role of the "slow channel". Circulation 1979;60:605-15
37. Wellens HJJ, Bär FWHM, Lie KI, Düren DR, Dohmen HJ. Effect of procainamide, propranolol and verapamil on mechanism of tachycardia in patients with chronic recurrent ventricular tachycardia. Am J Cardiol 1977;40:579-85

38. Horowitz LN, Josephson ME, Farshidi A, Spielman SR, Michelson EL, Greenspan AM. Recurrent sustained ventricular tachycardia. 3. Role of the electrophysiologic study in selection of antiarrhythmic regimens. Circulation 1978;58:986-97
39. Anderson JL, Patterson E, Wagner JG, Johnson TA, Lucchesi BR, Pitt B. Clinical pharmacokinetics of intravenous and oral bretylium tosylate in survivors of ventricular tachycardia or fibrillation. In press

NON-CANINE ANIMAL MODELS FOR EVALUATING ANTIARRHYTHMIC EFFICACY

E. Neil Moore, D.V.M., Ph.D., Joseph F. Spear, Ph.D. and Eric L.
Michelson, M.D., University of Pennsylvania, School of Veterinary
Medicine, Philadelphia, Pa.

The most important question in deciding which animal model to employ
for a study on the efficacy of an antiarrhythmic agent concerns whether
one is screening for a potential antiarrhythmic compound or is testing and
evaluating an already proven antiarrhythmic agent. In "screening," one
may have hundreds of agents to analyze and therefore an inexpensive,
simple and quick animal model is needed. However, if one is "testing"
an already known antiarrhythmic agent then one must use more sophisticated
animal models. An important criterion for any non-canine model employed
in antiarrhythmic testing is that the model have some direct relationship
to the human clinical situation. For example, the antivivisectionists have
suggested that tissue cultures of cardiac cells should be utilized for
evaluation of antiarrhythmic agents and indeed one can record cardiac
pacemaker activity, and even simulated reentry by growing a circuit loop
of tissue cultured cardiac cells. Although it is possible to do tissue
culture studies on the effects of antiarrhythmic agents, I still believe
there are questions as to the relevance of such studies to the clinical
situation in man.

Another question that one must ask when using a non-canine model is
whether or not potential drug side effects can be tested. Everyone is
well aware that undesireable side effects are the major problem with the
antiarrhythmic agents that we currently have. If a non-canine model does
not permit the evaluation of potential side effects of an agent on blood
pressure, contractility, the central nervous system, gastrointestinal
system and other undesirable effects, then such a non-canine model may be
inappropriate for testing and evaluating the potentially useful mechanisms
in many antiarrhythmic agents.

One non-canine animal model that has been used for screening antiarrhythmic agents is the mouse chloroform arrhythmia model. The mouse

chloroform arrhythmia model is one that concerns sensitizing the myocardium to catecholamines by the presence of chloroform. The model has
been suggested to test for both antiarrhythmic and/or beta blocking
activity. However, the mouse chloroform arrhythmia model seems to be a
much better test for beta blockers than for testing antiarrhythmic drugs.
Although it has been suggested that ventricular fibrillation occurs in the
mouse chloroform arrhythmia model, the possibility that skeletal muscle
tremors results in apparent ventricular fibrillation in the recorded ECG
also seems a possibility.

Another frequently used non-canine animal model is the rat. The rat
is employed for most toxicology studies and has been used for coronary
occlusion-reperfusion studies (1). In rat coronary occlusion-reperfusion
studies there have been reports where blood pressures and contractility
were recorded as well as blood plasma samples taken for drug concentration
evaluations. In addition to the limitations of the canine acute occlusion-
reperfusion arrhythmia model that Dr. Dreifus has already alluded to,
there are even more fundamental problems in using the rat. For example,
the rat electrocardiogram is different from most other mammals in that no
ST segment is present. Also, the transmembrane potential of ventricular
muscle fibers in most mammals exhibit a prominent plateau phase which
results in an isoelectric ST segment. In contrast, the transmembrane
potentials from the ventricular muscle of rat are triangulated with no
plateau phase. Consequently, the T wave in the rat electrocardiogram
arises immediately following the QRS complex and there is no isoelectric
ST phase (2). Dr. Hoffman has already mentioned that antiarrhythmic
agents work via influencing membrane conductances to the various ions
that are concentrated in different gradients across cardiac membranes.
Since rat myocardial transmembrane potentials are different from most
other mammalian cardiac fibers the associated membrane ionic conductances
must also be different. Therefore, evaluation of an antiarrhythmic
agent in the rat may not predict its effect in other mammals due to
differences in membrane ionic permeability characteristics. We know
that the rat is insensitive to a number of cardioactive agents. For
example, very large doses of digitalis in the rat do not cause the
arrhythmias and conduction problems observed in man and other mammals.

Guinea pigs have been used for evaluating the effects of antiarrhythmic agents in suppressing cardiac dysrhythmia associated with digitalis

toxicity. The effects of antiarrhythmic agents in suppressing these predominantly automatic rhythms of digitalis cardiotoxicity have also been
evaluated in the dog (3). However the dog differs from man in that the dog
arrhythmias caused by cardiac glycoside toxicity are not easily suppressed
by beta blockers; in the guinea pig and man, beta blockers do suppress
the digitalis cardiotoxicity arrhythmias. The digitalis cardiotoxicity
technique for evaluating antiarrhythmic activity requires giving small
sequential doses of ouabain (or other glycoside) until over 50% of the
beats are ventricular extrasystoles. Once the rhythm reaches this
percentage of extrasystoles then a test antiarrhythmic compound is administered to determine the drug's efficacy in the suppression of PVC's.
The guinea pig appears to be an economical digitalis cardiotoxicity
animal model.

The rabbit is another economical animal model for antiarrhythmic
drug testing and has been employed particularly for evaluating effects on
AV conduction. Small catheters have been employed to record electrograms
from atrium, bundle of His and ventricles as commonly done in man in
investigations designed to evaluate the effects of antiarrhythmic compounds. Langendorf perfused rabbit hearts also have been used. The
superficial location of both the SA and AV nodes into the rabbit heart
permit recording transmembrane potentials simultaneously from the pacemaker regions as well as from the other cardiac tissues. Thus, most
microelectrode studies concerning effects of antiarrhythmic compound on
sinus node and AV node have been completed in rabbit hearts. The rabbit
heart also has been used to analyze and precisely map ST segment alterations resulting from coronary occlusion (4).

The cat is becoming a more commonly used antiarrhythmia test animal
being used both for evaluating suppression of arrhythmias due to digitalis
cardiotoxicity and myocardial infarction. Myerburg and colleagues at the
University of Miami were the first to develop a chronic myocardial infarction model using multiple occlusions or multiple terminal branches of the
left anterior descending coronary artery (LAD) (5). One month to six
months after ligation, spontaneous PVC's develop in this chronic cat
infarction model. These findings in the cat suggested the possibility
of developing a canine model as well that would have chronic spontaneous
tachyarrhythmias. However, as Dr. Michelson stated, the dog chronic
infarct model differs from the cat in that the dog models do not have

spontaneous PVC's.

One technique that has been extensively used for evaluating antiarrhythmic agents is the ventricular fibrillation threshold (VFT) technique.
Although the VFT technique is most commonly used in the dog, the cat, pig
and monkey and even man have been the subject of VFT investigations (6).
This technique consists of stepwise increasing the amount of current
delivered during the ventricular vulnerable period (latter part of the T
wave). The ventricular fibrillation threshold is measured as the minimal
amount of current required to cause ventricular fibrillation (3). Two
methods of determining VFT are used. The first consists of scanning the
vulnerable period with a single 10 msec pulse which is progressively
increased in intensity until fibrillation occurs. Since the single
pulse method is tedious and time-consuming, a second VFT method was
developed which employs a 120 msec long 100 Hz train of 4 msec pulses.
The train VFT method does not require time scanning the vulnerable period
and only the intensity of the pulses within the train need to be increased
until fibrillation results. The ventricular fibrillation technique is a
technique that we believe provides an idea if an antiarrhythmic agent is
increasing the electrical stability of the ventricles. For example, if
in the presence of an antiarrhythmic agent twice as much current is
required to initiate fibrillation, then that agent must have enhanced the
electrical stability of the heart. Thus, the ventricular fibrillation
technique is another technique for evaluating antiarrhythmic efficacy
and although usually carried out in the dog, can equally well be carried
out in other animals.

A number of investigators are now using the pig for electrophysiological and electropharmacological studies since the pig is reported to
have very few coronary collaterals. Thus the pig coronary circulation
seems more similar to man than the dog where extensive coronary collaterals
are present. However, the pig heart does have a number of other differences
from man. The pig is an ungulate and as most ungulates, its ventricular
specialized conduction system (Purkinje fibers) are very different than
man. The porcine EKG is also different from man and the dog in that there
is a more rapid activation sequence of the ventricles than in man and the
dog. However, with the increasing price of dogs, pigs are becoming a more
economical experimental animal. Jaok Han and colleagues in Albany developed
a chronic porcine infarct model (7). They irradiated a discrete region of

a coronary artery and then fed the pigs on a severe high cholesterol diet. On the high cholesterol diet in the presence of the damaged coronaries, the pigs eventually developed spontaneous ventricular tachycardia and/or ventricular fibrillation (VT/VF). The Albany group actually set up a "porcine coronary care unit" and monitored the pigs for development of VT/VF and evaluated the effects of antiarrhythmic agents. Janse and colleagues in Amsterdam also have done many elegant electrophysiological studies in the pig during myocardial infarction (8). They have completed activation mapping and analyzed the mechanism of genesis of tachyarrhythmia in the pig during acute occlusion and reperfusion. Janse's studies have included in vivo microelectrode recordings during ischemia, the collection of ischemic coronary perfusate and the effects of this coronary perfusate on cardiac transmembrane potentials, etc. Thus, the pig is becoming a more commonly used experimental animal model and although not having the extensive data banks of electrophysiological information available for the dog, does have advantages for evaluations of antiarrhythmic agents and agents designed to salvage ischemic myocardial tissue in danger of cell death.

In summary, there really is not any single animal model that can predict the potential antiarrhythmic activity and potential effectiveness of that agent for use in man. Thus, there is no simple answer to the question, "What is the most ideal model in which one can test antiarrhythmic agents?" There are many animal models that tell you different things; the only way to test a new antiarrhythmic agent is to obtain an electrophysiological-electropharmacological profile by evaluating the agent in different test models and in different animals. Almost all animal studies have limitations since they are done using non-atherogenic coronary ischemia, usually are performed in anesthetized animals and usually are carried out using a non-primate animal. When one asks the only really important question of whether a given agent is an antiarrhythmic compound that prevents sudden death, I always recall the famous statement attributed to Galen who said, "All who drink of this remedy recover in a short time, except those it does not help, who all die. Therefore, it is obvious that it fails only in incurable diseases."

REFERENCES

1. W.F. Lubbe, P.S. Daries and L.H. Opie. Ventricular arrhythmias associated with coronary artery occlusion and reperfusion in the isolated perfused rat heart: a model for assessment of antifibrillatory action of antiarrhythmic agents. Cardiovasc. Res. 12:212-220, 1978.

2. Spear, J.F. Relationship between the scaler electrocardiogram and cellular electrophysiology of the rat heart. In: International Workshop on the Rat Electrocardiogram in acute and chronic pharmacology and toxicology. R. Budden, D.K. Detweiler and G. Zbinden (Eds.), in press, 1981.

3. Moore, E.N., Spear, J.F., Feldman, H.S., Moller, R. Electrophysiological properties of a new antiarrhythmic drug - Tocainide. Am. J. Physiol. 41:703, 1978.

4. Simson, M.B., Harden, W.R., Barlow, C.H., Harken, A.H. Epicardial ischemia as delineated with epicardial ST segment mapping and nicotainamide adenine dinucleotide (NADH) fluorescence photography. Am. J. Cardiol. 44:263, 1979.

5. Myerburg, R.J., Gelband, H., Nilsson, A., Sung, R.J., Thurer, R.J., Morales, A.R., Bassett, A.L. Long-term electrophysiological abnormalities resulting from experimental myocardial infarction in the cat. Circ. Res. 41:738, 1977.

6. Horowitz, L.N., Spear, J.F., Josephson, M.E., Kastor, J.A., MacVaugh, H., Moore, E.N. Ventricular fibrillation threshold in man. Am. J. Physiol. 39:274, 1977.

7. Lee, K.T., Lee, W.M., Han, J., Jarmolych, J., Bishop, M.B., and Goel, B.G. Experimental model for study of "sudden death" from ventricular fibrillation of asystole. Am. J. Cardiol. 32:62, 1973.

8. Janse, M.J., van Capelle, F.J.L., Morsink, H., Kleber, A.G., Wills-Schopman, F., Cardinale, R., Naumann, e, Alnoncourt, C. and Durrer, D. Flow of injury current in pattern of excitation during early ventricular arrhythmias and acute regional myocardial ischemia in isolated porcine and canine hearts: evidence for two different arrhythmogenic mechanisms. Circ. Res. 47:151, 1980.

GENERAL GROUP DISCUSSION: ANIMAL MODELS

Dr. Brian Hoffman: The presentations dealing with animal models have focused
ery strongly on identification of drugs which might be effective in preventing
sudden death in patients with coronary artery disease. That is an extremely
important role. However, one must realize that there are other important
arrhythmias in humans, particularly supraventricular arrhythmias. We not only
need better animal models for screening agents designed to prevent sudden
death but also better animal models to screen for drugs which would be effective
in dealing with the supraventricular arrhythmias. As our population gets
older these supraventricular arrhythmias are becoming very bothersome and
important.

In relation to the Harris one-stage coronary artery ligation technique
or any other canine model which is uniformly lethal, one really is limited
to determining if the drug prevents ventricular fibrillation. On the other
hand, Dr. Dreifus, isn't it possible in using some of the non-lethal acute
canine models to not only look for antiarrhythmic efficacy, but also to
determine whether a drug either increases the severity of the arrhythmias
or the incidence of sudden death. I think in screening that it is important
to know whether or not a drug makes degeneration of ventricular tachycardia
into ventricular fibrillation more probable.

Dr. Dreifus: Yes, this is a very important point. I glossed over the
differences for instance between procainamide, lidocaine, and amiodarone.
There are very classical differences among the drugs, some of which could
be potentially dangerous in particular patients, and indeed could result in
ventricular tachycardias becomine more rapid or even fibrillation developing.
There are many new directions that we need to go in evaluating the electrophysiological properties of antiarrhythmic drugs. For example, how does
the fractionated activity which is continuous during diastole get into the normal myocardium? No one has the foggiest idea what happens there. We need
to know to prevent this rapid activity from causing the arrhythmia to become

more dangerous.

Dr. Wellens: Dr. Dreifus talked about arrhythmias in the setting of acute
occlusion and release of a coronary artery. My question is, do you believe
that arrhythmias occurring on release of the coronary artery are relevant
for the human heart. We have observed spasms of coronary arteries where
arrhythmias develop at the time of the spasm but not at the release of the
spasm. Perhaps the time interval between the spasm and the release is too
short to have these release arrhythmias. However, studies with streptokinase
infusion in patients with acute myocaridal infarction have resulted in
perfusion being restored after 1 to 3 hours after the acute occlusion and
arrhythmias were not observed. Perhaps in this case you get a gradual opening
up of the coronary vessel of increased collateral circulation and consequently
reperfusion arrhythmias are not observed. I would like to hear your comments
about the use of release arrhythmias as useful for understanding clinical
arrhythmias.

Dr. Dreifus: A very important question. Let me first restate what I said. I
mentioned that occlusion and release within a finite period of time such as 5
or 6 minutes missed the early arrhythmias. It certainly missed the late
arrhythmias. The period of ligation was too short. Thus, we picked 20 to
30 minutes. Why? Becuase that gave us the highest incidence of the
ventricular fibrillation. If you look between 60 minutes and 2 hours, there are
really no arrhythmias. And finally, you have answered your own question,
that in the human model, there may be slow release and consequently spasm
doesn't suddenly result in reperfusion. However, we really do not know what
happens within the coronary circulation at the moment of sudden death in man.
That is a very important question to answer and the results may not be too
different from our animal models when we finally have the answer.

Dr. Wellens: Dr. Moore, you discussed the fact that in studies of digitalis
toxicity that you see marked differences between the dog heart versus other
animal hearts. in the ability of beta blockers to suppress or treat arrhythmias
caused by digitalis toxicity. We have just finished a study where different
breeds of dogs exhibited tremendous differences as far as the sensitivity
to digitalis was concerned. I am of course interested in the relevancy
of this information in treating our patients. It is obvious that different
techniques are being used at different institutions. This causes great
difficulty in interchaning information and in applying information to the human
situation. Is it possible in this point of time to come up with recommendations

as to the models that should be used to bring some uniformity and clarity to this situation.

Dr. Moore: Of course, we also see differences in different dogs. However, this probably is no different than man where equally variable results are found with digitalis. I have heard it stated that before we were able to monitor digitalis serum levels, that digitalis may have killed as many people as it saved due to the inability to correlate dose levels with therapeutic effects.

Dr. Wellens: Is it possible at this point to bring some order in the chaos? I realize that we do not have the ideal arrhythmia model at this time, but at leaset I think we should give some guidelines to give some order.

Dr. Moore: I agree, one has to realize too that the cardiac digitalis toxicity arrhythmias as well as the arrhythmias with the Harris 2-stage coronary ligation are due to altered automaticity rather than reentry. I think that most lethal arrhythmias in man are not due to altered automaticity. What we really need are good models that have reentry as their basis. It would be very nice if the chronic dog model with "reentrant" tachyarrhythmias which Eric Michelson just discussed had spontaneous arrhythmias and even sudden death. However, even after 9-10 months following two-stage occlusion-reperfusion we have not seen sudden death nor are we seeing PVC's at all. One point that is interesting is that patients rescusitated from primary ventricular fibrillation often have no electrocardiographic changes nor demonstrable lesions and yet they are very prone to sudden cardiac death within the first year. Perhaps such patients may have very small lesions, because we have been impressed that with very small mottled infarction ($\overset{<}{-}$ 1.5 cm^2) that our chronic infarct dogs are very prone to VF following programmed electrical stimulation. I don't think Hein that we have an ideal model, but the chronic dog model I believe is going to be very helpful.

Dr. Hoffman: I think that Dr. Wellens did make two very important points. I would certainly support what Neil said. We ought to standardize as much as possible among dogs, among laboratories and that means not only watching the breed but also size. We know that arrhythmias in the ventricle are strongly dependent upon ventricular mass. We also have to standardize in terms of age, young dogs respond very differently to drugs from older dogs, as do people. I think that one has to watch for other factors even dietary com-position. For lidocaine and similar drugs, intensity of effect is quite steeply dependent on serum K concentration between 2.5 and 5 meq/L. If you use fasted dogs, you get very different dose response curves from fed dogs.

So we have a lot of tidying up to do and we'll try to do it.

Dr. Hai: My question is addressed to Dr. Dreifus. You mention the acute occlusion-release model and the fact that many of the conventional anti-arrhythmic drugs that are available are not effective in preventing the ventricular arrhythmias following occlusion or release. Are beta blockers an exception to that rule?

Dr. Dreifus: In our studies thus far, we did not study beta blockers so this is still an area to be examined.

Dr. Michelson: Another important consideration with ligation arrhythmias is heart rate. Dr. Lazzara, Hope and others showed 7-8 years ago that the major mediating effect of beta blockers is presumably becuase of its heart rate effects not because of an antiarrhythmic effect. For example, if a dog has a heart rate of 90 or 100 open-chest, when you ligate, that dog survives, whereas if the dog's heart rate is 160 or 150 under anesthetic, it does not. There are a number of other mediating effects. The problem with acute occlusion/release models has been that everyone has used a different time, ligated at a different place, and no one has sacrificed the 30-50 dogs required to figure out the mean frequency, the mean indicence of VF and what the variability is around that mean. Thus, a study of 10 control versus 10 test dogs doesn't mean anything. You have to know what the range of spontaneous variability is and that's difficult.

Dr. Hoffman: If I could make one more comment. We have suffered with the same problem in chronic studies on 2-stage Harris dog where the efficacy of any particular drug clearly is dependent upon the severity of the ventricular arrhythmia. If you have 2-stage Harris dogs in which 40 to 50% of impulses are ventricular premature beats, you can find that at a particular dose and serum concentration of adrug may be 80% effective. You test the same drug in other dogs with a more rapid VT and you may find that your drug is totally ineffective. Evaluation of a drug in comparison among drugs somehow has to be quantified in terms of the severity of the arrhythmia even in a constant model.

Dr. Zipes: What is the relevance of a ventricular fibrillation threshold (VFT)? What does it mean when the VFT doubles in a normal dog with an intervention and a normal dog doesn't fibrillate anyway. I don't understand what a twice normal VFT means. In regards to Dr. Wellens comments on reperfusion arrhythmias, actually Dr. Hildred Muller and Dr. W. Ganz both have demonstrated the development of ventricular arrhythmias in man on reperfusion following streptokinase infusion. One possible mechanism for reperfusion arrhythmias is a heterogenous restoration of flow upon reperfusion. It is quite clear that the majority of patients who have sudden death have ischemia related disease. Yet 15 to 20% of Cobb's patients rescusitated from out of hopsital primary VF do not have significant coronary disease. In addition, patients who have coronary disease and have sudden death have the coronary disease 24 hours a day, yet only at 12:30 do they develop ventricular fibrillation. There must be another ingredient on top of the chronic coronary disease that causes this sudden development of a ventricular tachyarrhythmia. What I am suggesting is that the role of the autonomic nervous system and central nervous system need to be addressed as well. Perhaps the panel could comment.

Dr. Michelson: I would like to address the next to last point Dr. Zipes made. Patients with WPW syndrome for example or dual AV nodal pathways, always have a fixed structural mileau throughout their lifetime which presumably predisposes them to sustained reentrant arrhythmias. You know that the structure is present and is abnormal, het such patients are not in continuous incessant tachyarrhythmias. What is required is some generator as well as some perpetuator. For example, the chronic canine model is merely a model of a perpetuator and it is limited to that. It is limited to a structural mileau which is useful for studying perpetuators. Patients with chronic coronary artery disease presumably have a certain fixed mileau which functionally becomes altered during periods of even what would otherwise be non-lethal ischemic events. Much of what we have learned about electrophysiology up until about 2 or 3 years ago when it has become fashionable to study ventricular tachycardia in patients was learned from the human model of WPW and such.

Dr. Hoffman: I would like to extend on that a little bit. I don't think it is a crucial defect in the chronic models that with the exception of Ralph Lazzara's cat, that they do not have recurrent ventricular premature beats. Clearly, patients in whom there are scars due to ischemia are at risk of reentrant excitation and ventricular fibrillation. It would be nice in the dog model if there were spontaneous premature beats to initiate the reentry. This is the initiating factor. But even though you don't as long as you perturb your dog model's heart with rapid pacing and premature beats, you still can see whether or not a drug will decrease the likelihood of reentry given the appropriate initiating event and whether it decreases the likelihood that the arrhythmias will degenerate into fibrillation. I think the chronic models although they are incomplete analogs of the human, still let us ask important questions. It would be nice also to be able to deal with the initiating event but that is so complex, I don't think any single model could do it.

Dr. Dreifus: Dr. Zipes, I think your points are well taken. As far as the neuro-humoral mechanisms, the problem is that we don't have good models. I can just cite one example. There are models in which if you crush the brain, ventricular arrhythmias are very prone. If you inject lidocaine into the 3rd ventricle of the brain, not into the left ventricle, but into the brain, you completely abolish these arrhythmias. The diversity of these models is just enormous. It isn't that we are ignoring the role of the nervous system. It is that is difficult to get a handle on it but hopefully in the near future some investigator will develop a suitable model. As far as Cobb's patients who do not have demonstrable coronary disease, we don't have the foggiest idea what happens. How can we develop a model if we don't know what happens at that event. I am sure as more studies develop and we see the mechanism, we'll develop the model to match that of what Cobb and all of us have observed. There are a tremendous number of models that need to be developed to match the human situation. We now are focalizing in on very severe testing models. Why? Because they are reproducible and easier. I would not like to defend why we only stuck to these for there is no reason to.

Dr. Hoffman: I am going to interject briefly. We also should mention that there are spontaneous animal models of other heart disease with induced arrhythmias. Cats very frequently get a non-specific cardiomyopathy which involves both atrium and ventricle and in which atrial flutter and fibrillation occur as well as ventricular arrhythmias. Dogs very frequently get mitral valve disease that gives them mitral insufficiency and again both ventricular arrhythmias and supraventricular arrhythmias occur. So if one is looking for models that might represent different mechanisms for arrhythmias different from coronary artery disease, then such animal models are available and some of them are very good.

Dr. Moore: I wanted to comment on the ventricular fibrillation threshold (VFT) technique. I am not "married" to this technique as it has an awful lot of problems and requires extensive control of parameters such as block, body temperature, electrode configuration and sets of VFT current, etc. I can make two comments. One is that we did do VFT studies in man and were pleased to find that VFT results in man were similar to our canine VFT

studies. For example, in man we found that the left ventricular VFT's
were higher than the right ventricle and that areas of ischemia had very
low VFT's versus normal myocardium. A second point is that Dave Euler
recently has shown in our lab that the VFT causes fibrillation by initiating
microreentry. The VFT technique is a simple technique that can be used to
obtain an electropharmacological profile of a drug. In regards to the
autonomic nervous system, the fact that our dogs with chronic mottled
infarcts do not have spontaneous PVC's and sudden death may relate to the fact
that they are living out in the peaceful countryside and unlike patients
are not subjected to the stresses that stimulate the autonomic nervous
system. One other point regarding the autonomic nervous system concers
studying a patient in the cath lab under Valium or in the O.R. neither the
cath lab or O.R. present a normal physiological situation and the determination of an effective antiarrhythmic agent in this setting may not assure one
that you have protected that individual during every day life situations.
The autonomic nervous system is very important. Last point. In the reperfusion
arrhythmias, heart rate is very important. If you stimulate the vagus and
slow heart rate just before you allow reperfusion, then you don't see
fibrillation very often.

Dr. Hoffman: Two other things that relate to Doug Zipes' question about
ventricular fibrillation thresholds. I think when one makes these measurements,
it is extremely useful to make the converse measurement and that is the ease
of defibrillation. It is possible that some antiarrhythmic drugs or potential antiarrhythmic drugs might make it more difficult to defibrillate with
countershock. This would be extremely important to know from animal studies
before one goes into human testing. Secondly, I think that if one studies
ventricular fibrillation induced by electric stimuli, one ought to look
not only at the current required but also at the likelihood that a fibrillatory
arrhythmia persists because we really have two chances with respect to
ventricular fibrillation. One can prevent it happening or one could change
conditions in the heart so that even if fibrillation starts, it would terminate
within 10 or 15 seconds. We know that this can happen. It happens in the
small mammalian hearts. It probably happens sometimes in dogs and humans.
A drug that increased the likelihood that fibrillation would be a self-
terminating arrhythmia would be a useful drug. I think studies on
ventricular fibrillation thresholds can be helpful.

Dr. Lucchesi: Isn't it particularly important to consider age and if you

consider age, then you have a technical problem of the size of the animal.
If you have a domestic swine then you're talking 150-200 kg. Miniature
swine are not so miniature. And it would seem that possibility of having
animals with spontaneous atherosclerosis in the older animals would be
quite great and so therefore it could have a great bearing on your models.
Has there been any age-related study?

Dr. Moore: A number of years ago in New Jersey they used to allow garbage
feeding of pigs and in this instance they kept the sows until old age.
Today female pig that is not a prolific breeder is not kept. Hans Luginbuhl
in our lab found that these aged pigs fed on garbage (that's a human diet)
did develop atherosclerosis and had extensive coronary artery disease.

Dr. Wyndham: A number of different factors which might influence the result
of direct studies have been mentioned and I wondered if I could ask a question
to the panel about ventricular function? It's clear that in human spontaneous
paroxysmal sustained ventricular tachycardia, the anatomic basis is frequently ventricular aneurysm, and poor ventricular function relates to
outcome. What can the panel tell us about the present state of knowledge
regarding ventricular function in acute and chronic dog models. and are
there any recommendations to standardize and control the role of ventricular
dysfunction in future models, particularly the chronic canine infarct model.

Dr. Hoffman: We've done some studies in the 2-stage Harris model measuring
left ventricular pressure and systemic arterial pressure and I would say that
the usual dog with the 2-stage Harris infarct has a minimal functional
defect in terms of ventricular function. If one does circumflex occlusions
in the dog, proximal circumflex, of course you have quite marked impairment
of ventricular function, an inability to keep forward flow up at high rates,
and it looks more like humans that have had large ventricular infarcts.
I don't know of any studies done on dogs with large ventricular aneurysms.
These I think are infrequent in dog models. I agree ventricular function is
important: Investigators who try to provoke arrhythmias in surgical patients
so that the aneurysm and the arrhythmogenic area can be excised know that
even though they could provoke the arrhythmia very readily in the cath lab
that as soon as the patient is on the pump and the left ventricle is somewhat
decompressed, it becomes difficult to initiate the arrhythmia, and often
impossible to have it sustained. Early physiologists showed that in the
dog heart ventricular fibrillation would persist with a normal left ventricular and diastolic pressure and often would not persist if the left

ventricle were completely vented. So stretch on the heart fibers is crucial and in our models this factor usually is uncontrolled.

Dr. Michelson: We have a number of observations in our chronic model and I would like to ask that when I'm finished that Dr. Ruskin present some of the observations that he has in his chronic canine model because they have purposely gone after producing infarcts that are more apical aneurysmal that you would otherwise get in a routine dog model where the collaterals are extensive. In our model we started off with proximal LAD occlusion, went to the mid-LAD and finally ended up with an infarct that was essentially 1 cm^2. In this animal there was no hemodynamic compromise and these small infarcts were electrocardiographically silent. Such a model might represent in a sense normal coronary arteries with sudden death in man. These small chronic infarcts were still susceptible to inducible arrhythmias. I will say this: Very, very small infarcts the animals are very highly susceptible to inducible ventricular fibrillation. When the infarcts get a little larger, a little more patchy and mottled, the animals seem to be more susceptible to sustained VT. However, you can put these dogs into VF. These animals with ±15% of the left ventricular mass infarcted are not hemodynamically compromised, and in fact they develop a mechanical alternans with fast ventricular tachycardias and you can leave them in this V-tach for up to one hour. These animals are open-chest and in a recumbent position so they can maintain their hemodynamics.

Dr. Ruskin: Dr. Michelson, I don't think our model in terms of size is that different from what you've seen. The infarcts that we've created are probably an average of 18% of the left ventricular mass, maybe even a little bit larger. So, while our model is a transmural infarct with a clearcut area that is tissue-paper with bulging it still doesn't result in a great deal of hemodynamic compromise. The dogs in fact do very well chronically and what we've found in trying to create bigger infarcts is that we lose them acutely within a day or two or even less time than that. I think that if you get much over 20% of the LV mass that the dogs don't survive. If they are below about 20% they do extremely well. I don't think it's comparable in a functional sense to a patient with a tremendous area of damage and a functionally important left ventricular aneurysm. We also see what you do in the animals with sustained VT, i.e., they will stay in VT for as lon as you leave them there and many of them will maintain fairly reasonable perfusion pressures.

Dr. Hoffman: The dog probably has a better heart than we do. We used a lot of dogs in which we've done a 2-stage LAD ligation high up just below the first diagonal branch and then we have waited 10 days before applying a balloon occluder on the proximal circumflex. You can do a complete circumflex occlusion in that dog 10 days after the first infarct, hold it for 6-10 minutes and in most animals they maintain good systemic arterial pressure and systemic flow. I still am amazed, but they can keep good hemodynamic function with a minimally well perfused left ventricular mass.

Dr. Michelson: Dr. Wyndham's other point, though, is a good point. In managing patients clinically it is obvious always to the patient's advantage to make sure that the patient is functionally maximized. It is a very important clinical consideration that making the patient's ventricular function better may be an effective antiarrhythmic therapy.

Dr. Moore: One must always consider when studying arrhythmias that there are a lot of other causes of arrhythmias other than just myocardial infarction, thyrotoxicosis, CNS lesions, pulmonary disease, etc.

Dr. Hoffman: Yes, these questions bring up the very difficult problem in evaluating long-term efficacy of drugs in man in relation to dose-response because a drug may be found which at a particular dose and blood level is effective in the cath lab while that blood level or that tissue level of drug may not be sufficient when the patient is at home because for some reason, left ventricular and diastolic pressure goes up. So to me, failure of available drugs to exert a prophylactic effect doesn't necessarily prove that they are not potentially efficacious. It may mean that in the usual test situation we don't identify the dose they need for the moment when they are likely to have their lethal arrhythmia.

Dr. Woosley: I'd just like to make a comment about the philosophy of drug screening. I think that as we now study drugs in the various models, drugs that we know have efficacy in certain clinical conditions, we find that they do not have uniform efficacy in all the screening tests. It's also important that as you evaluate a drug in these various screens that you not throw away a drug just because it has adverse effects in one model and also naturally do not accept a drug because it has beneficial effects in only one model. I agree with Dr. Moore that you need a spectrum of actions in these models to help evaluate the drug.

Another point is that the alpha blockers are supposedly very good for reperfusion arrhythmias and Drs. Rosen and Hoffman have looked at alpha receptors in the myocardium. I wonder if there's any other data in these various arrhythmia models or in clinical situations that might tell us more about alpha blockers, alpha receptor and arrhythmias?

Dr. Dreifus: Dr. Woosley, we just don't have enough studies to answer that question. One brief comment to Dr. Wyndham. Many patients with aneurysms don't have arrhythmias, and many who don't have aneurysms have plenty of arrhythmias. So I don't think that we can directly correlate left ventricular function and the problem of ventricular arrhythmias. I think Dr. Hoffman's comments concerning the variability with and without changes in left ventricular function is an important thing to understand.

Dr. Ehrreich, FDA: Dr. Hoffman, I wonder if you have been able to distinguish among the calcium antagonists in your models in terms of predictability for antiarrhythmic purposes in man? And also, whether any of the panelists with their various models have been able to distinguish the so-called vascular type of slow calcium channel blockers from the more cardiac type?

Dr. Hoffman: I think we've made a little progress on the efficacy or lack of efficacy of calcium-blockers as antiarrhythmics. In our studies on transmembrane potentials we find that verapamil has quite prominent effects on electrical activity in sinus node and AV node where action potentials are due to slow inward current. Nifedepine which is a different kind of calcium-blocker, has minimal effects on AV nodal activity and sinus node activity, and I think this difference correlates well with their reported efficacy in superventricular arrhythmias, which probably involve reentry in either AV node or sinus node. We have less information in terms of another arrhythmia that seems to depend on slow inward current, and that's the delayed afterdepolarization induced arrhythmia. I would say that for supraventricular arrhythmias, when we're almost sure they depend upon cells using slow inward channels, we can get a good correlation in terms of whether or not the blocker blocks heart slow channels or primarily vascular slow channels. For ventricular arrhythmias we don't have the correlation yet, but hopefully we will.

Dr. Frommer: I'd like to comment about the importance of statistical analyses and to say that from what we've learned in clinical studies and clinical trials, that we should also in animal studies account for all animals that were started in the protocol in any fashion at all. And secondly, we should give consideration for a random allocation of animals between the therapy under test and the control therapy. Thirdly, to the

extent possible, we should blind the investigator performing the study and
the one analyzing the results from the intervention that was under study.
I think these are things we have learned from the clinical studies, and
are all too often overlooked in the animal laboratory.

Dr. Michelson: Dr. Frommer, you know the principal investigator never
steps into the lab until the results are good.

Dr. Frommer: Point well-taken.

Dr. Hoffman: Dr. Frommer, your point is extremely important. However, it
is very difficult to do, because if you're comparing a new potential antiarrhythmic agent to whatever are the standards for your laboratory, lidocaine and quinidine for example, after the first 2-300 dogs you usually
know whether they've gotten lidocaine, quinidine or something else. So
you really would have to require that the investigator would not be
privied to any events during the investigation, if you want him to be
really blind.

Dr. Dreifus: Louie Katz said never do the second dog.

Dr. Frommer: I think Dr. Katz had a good idea there. I think the comment
is very appropriate that you really cannot do the studies with the investigator totally blind in many, many circumstances. On the other hand, it is
possible to account for all animals that walked or were brought to the
laboratory doors. Second, it is possible to have a formal randomized
allocation between two measurements.

Dr. Hoffman: I support that completely.

Dr. Frommer: I think since dietary regimens may change and the size and
weight of animals may change that a random allocation is important. It is
possible to have blinding in certain kinds of studies, but obviously for
the initial feasibility of studies to look at promise one cannot be too
blinded. But if one takes the next step to say that I have done X number
of animals and thereby propose a definitive animal study, I think it would
be much more pursuasive if those studies were performed as blinded as
"circumstances" permit.

Dr. Lucchesi: With respect to alpha blockade, we have been able to show
as others have shown that phentolamine at least can prevent the reperfusion
arrhythmias after coronary occlusion and reperfusion. One of the interesting
things that we found, however, was that late in the reperfusion stage, that
is 12-18 hours after phentolamine had been discontinued, that almost a
100% mortality occurs in that group of animals due to ventricular fibrilla-

tion. We don't know the reason for this. Secondly, I think it's important in the fibrillation threshold model, not only to study fibrillation thresholds in the non-ischemic heart, but in the regionally ischemic heart. This may help to resolve some of the questions that were raised before.

Dr. Hoffman, do you believe it would be profitable to consider anti-fibrillatory agents as being somewhat different than antiarrhythmic agents, that is, could an agent be strictly anti-fibrillatory without necessarily affecting premature ventricular contractions and maybe even ventricular tachycardia.

Dr. Hoffman: In general, I agree that an antifibrillatory agent need not have any other standard antiarrhythmic effect. I mean, if one makes imaginery computer simulations of hearts which you then can fibrillate, you can change conditions so that fibrillation is highly unlikely or likely to be self-terminating by doing things that you wouldn't think were antiarrhythmic interventions at all. Now that's the imaginery answer. In the real world, even the drugs that seem to be antifibrillatory (take bretyllium for one) also do have other antiarrhythmic action. So we're waiting for better, cleaner, single action molecules. What we need the pharmaceutical industry to do is to give us some molecules that do one thing and only one thing and nothing else. Then we can whittle down and answer some of the many questions that we have.

Dr. Watanabe: I would like to comment on the experimental models that we have been using in the last couple of years. The firstmodel is the isolated, perfused rabbit heart in which we produce ventricular fibrillation by rapid stimulation. I think this model is applicable to study the effects of antiarrhythmic drugs and to study the effects of drugs designed to make defibrillation easier. A second model is the hypoxic canine Purkinje fiber preparation. I think it is important to study the effects of drugs under hypoxic conditions since the results may be quite different than when studied under more normal non-ischemic conditions.

Dr. Morganroth: I don't think there's any question that animal models can be very useful for screening potentially new antiarrhythmic agents, but let me offer this scenario. A few days ago a man from Mars came to visit me. His flying saucer landed in my back yard and he handed me a potion and said, "On Mars this drug is fantastic, it absolutely wipes out all ventricular ectopy. We've stolen some humans and it appears to work in them

also. Please take it to the regulatory agency that exists in your government as I'd like to have this drug sold in all pharmacies in your country."
My point really concerns whether it is necessary to test already proven
antiarrhythmic agents in any of these models prior to testing them in
humans. It has been pointed out that there is no ideal animal model that
can predict what the agent will do in man.

Dr. Hoffman: Yes I think you do have to look at drugs in animal models
before you test them in humans because I believe you owe it to humans,
whether they are volunteers or patients. The probability that a drug
might be effective and also might be safe needs to be tested in animal
models. I think it's impossible to do away with tests in animal models,
and to do tests in tissue culture, or in microbes as Dr. Moore mentioned.
What is the best animal model? I think you cannot answer that, first
without specifying the types of arrhythmias you're concerned with; the
animal model has to be related to the problem that the patient presents.
I think that when clinical cardiologists are better able to tell us the
exact mechanism for the arrhythmias that they must treat, that we can then
probably define the best animal model to test for compounds to prevent
those arrhythmias.

Dr. Morganroth: Once you have demonstrated in animal studies that a drug
is safe the question still remains what one model or two models need to
support antiarrhythmic efficacy before you will allow me to give the drug
to patients?

Dr. Hoffman: Even if we limit the qeustion as to ability to prevent
ventricular ectopy, I still would insist on animal testing. You can investigate many things in animals that you simply cannot study in the clinical
electrophysiology lab. Your animal findings may be very significant. For
example, at normal heart rates N-acetylprocainamide can be given up to
astronomical blood levels and you do not induce arrhythmias. However, if
you give it to dogs with chronic heart block in which heart rate is 40 to
60, then high blood levels of NAPA induce early afterdepolarizations,
runs of premature depolarizations and a high incidence of sudden death
over the next 4-6 hours. One can find out facts about drugs in animal
experiments that you need to know before you are going to study them in
people.

Dr. Michelson: As a clinical cardiologist, the minimal preclinical information that I would accept before clinical trials would include at least a

24-hour PVC infarction model, an abnormal automaticity model (ouabain or catecholamine induced) and at least one chronic reentrant model.

Dr. Moore: As everyone knows, the problem has not been to design agents which will suppress ventricular ectopy due to altered automaticity or reentry. The problem is that the undesirable side effects eliminate most antiarrhythmic agents. I would like to emphasize two points that I think are very important that can be answered in animal models and which are questions that should be answered before one does human studies. First, what happens if one suddenly withdraws a drug or if subtherapeutic levels of the drug are present. Propranolol, anticoagulants and other compounds may actually cause problems upon withdrawal or at subtherapeutic doses. A point that Dr. Hoffman alluded to that I think is very important, is that one can determine if a new compound actually makes the heart more difficult to defibrillate. It has recently been shown that quinidine may actually make the heart more difficult to defibrillate. Also, as observed in the respiratory intensive care unit and in our animal studies, respiratory acidosis may make the heart more difficult to defibrillate. Those are some of the questions that animal studi-s can answer.

Dr. Dreifus: I think there is merit in keeping flexibility in which animal model to use. Obviously, there are many animal models that we haven't even touched upon. One thing is that it is often difficult to stick with one model. You can't imagine in working with these animal models what it costs in both time and money so you can't do everything and use multiple models.

Dr. Hoffman: I was given the impossible charge to summarize. Instead of summarizing I will let you have a few of my somewhat depressed reactions to the morning. Dr. Lucchesi mentioned the effects of alpha blockade on release arrhythmias and this is extremely interesting, but it just opens a host of new problems. The coronary arteries have both alpha constrictor and beta dilator capability and we know that with exercise in normal people as well as animals, reflexly, you activate the sympathetic nervous system and you get alpha constriction and beta dilation and it balances out. If you give an alpha blocker, you certainly are going to modify the perfusion of the normal myocardium and the collateral perfusion of ischemic myocardium. So when you have an antiarrhythmic effect, is it due to an effect on cellular electrical activity, is it due to some change in perfusion, or is it due to both? I think we know far too little about

the set which is most favorable to the development of any type of
arrhythmia. As Dr. Dreifus mentioned, a great deal of money and a lot of
dogs have been used to study reperfusion arrhythmias. We developed a
model in which we could occlude the LAD for 30 minutes and then get
reperfusion arrhythmias, wait an hour, and then occlude again and get
exactly the same effect. Then for a trivial reason, we looked at the
effect of ventilation on the stability of the model and we found that by
varying ventilation and changing arterial pH between about 7.25 and 7.38
we could convert our release arrhythmias to no release arrhythmias as we
went in the acidic direction and back into release fibrillation as we
went in the alkaline direction. Thus, drugs may modify ventilation and
perfusion and therefore modify factors like tissue pH. So it would be
premature to identify as Dr. Morganroth hopes the best animal model to
test for each antiarrhythmic action. Unfortunately I think the physiologists will have to continue to stumble along learning more about mechanisms
for arrhythmias, factors that influence those mechanisms, teach the pharma-
cologists all of that, and then hopefully we may develop some good sure
fire consistent models.

DEFINING THE PHARMACODYNAMICS AND PHARMACOKINETICS OF NEW ANTIARRHYTHMIC DRUGS

Robert E. Kates

The time course of drug transit through the body and the time course of drug effect are closely related phenomena. It is generally assumed that the intensity of the activity of an antiarrhythmic drug is a function of the drug's concentration at an effector site in the myocardium, and that this effector site concentration is in equilibrium with the concentration of the drug in the blood. Therefore, studies to describe the time course of accumulation and disappearance of antiarrhythmic drugs in the blood are helpful in understanding the dynamics of antiarrhythmic drug action. Extensive studies are required to completely understand the pharmacokinetics and pharmacodynamics of drugs and to evaluate the physiologic and pathophysiologic changes which can influence them. However, the evaluation of a new antiarrhythmic drug does not require a complete understanding of all the factors which affect absorption and disposition. This discussion will focus on those aspects of pharmacokinetics and pharmacodynamics which are relevant to the evaluation of the clinical utility and efficacy of new antiarrhythmic drugs.

The pharmacokinetic description of a new drug generally involves the characterization of an elimination half-life, total body clearance, an estimate of bioavailability, and perhaps the description of the blood concentration time course in terms of computer-generated rate constants associated with a two- or three-compartment pharmacokinetic model. These data are useful and interesting, but do not sufficiently answer the underlying questions which need to be addressed. Pharmacokinetic and pharmacodynamic studies need to answer two simple questions: 1) What happens to a drug once administered to a patient? and 2) how does its fate affect clinical efficacy?

Defining the fate of a new antiarrhythmic drug involves both qualitative and quantitative considerations. The fate of a drug in terms of its metabolic byproducts needs to be adequately defined. Most antiarrhythmic drugs are metabolized in the body and are conjugated or converted to nonactive metabolites, which are subsequently eliminated by renal or biliary secretory mechanisms. Several antiarrhythmic drugs, however, are metabolized to compounds which do produce significant cardiac or other effects. Drug metabolites may have activities similar to those of the parent drug with the same or different potency, or they may produce effects (cardiac or other) different from those of the-parent compound. The consequences of drug metabolism may be that a metabolite contributes to the desired effects of the parent drug, is antagonistic, or produces noncardiac side effects which limit the usefulness of the parent agent. Several examples of reported active metabolites of antiarrhythmic drugs are shown in Table I. One of the major difficulties in assessing the clinical relevance of these reported active metabolites, however, is the paucity of studies carried out in human subjects.

Table I: Reported Metabolites of Antiarrhythmic Drugs

Drug	Metabolite
Aprindine	desethylaprindine
Disopyramide	mono-N-dealkylated disopyramide
Encainide	O-demethyl encainide
	3-methyl-O-demethyl encainide
Lidocaine	monoethylglycinexylidide
	glycinexylidide
Procainamide	N-acetyl procainamide
Quinidine	3-hydroxyquinidine
Verapamil	norverapamil

Drug metabolites are generally identified and evaluated in small animal models. Animal studies are of value in helping to identify potential active metabolites in man, but such studies should not be an end in themselves. It must be determined whether these metabolites are formed in humans and to what extent they accumulate. When the accumulation of a suspected metabolite is confirmed, its activity should be evaluated in human subjects, at least in the range of blood concentrations to which it accrues during administration of the parent drug. Not all metabolites of antiarrhythmic drugs which are shown to have pharmacologic activity need to be extensively studied. Only those agents need to be studied which have significant cardiac or other effects, and which accumulate in the plasma to an extent sufficient to produce a clinically relevant effect.

The literature regarding the clinical significance of active drug metabolites is extremely limited. A few examples will suffice to illustrate this point. The N-dealkylated metabolite of lidocaine, monoethylglycine xylidide, is believed to be active in humans and its accumulation may be contributory to the CNS side effects which can occur as a result of lidocaine administration (1). Despite its apparent importance as a modifier of the clinical efficacy of lidocaine, it has not been adequately studied in humans. Another antiarrhythmic drug, lorcainide, is metabolized following oral administration to an N-dealkylated compound, norlorcainide, which has been shown to possess significant antiarrhythmic activity (2). There is evidence to suggest that this important metabolite significantly modifies the clinical efficacy of lorcainide. It clearly needs to be further studied in patients.

N-acetylprocainamide is the only well-studied metabolite of an antiarrhythmic drug (3,4). It appears that this metabolite contributes to the cardiac effects of procainamide. Knowledge of its activity, accumulation, and the role of renal function in the elimination of NAPA is clearly important for the optimal clinical employment of procainamide.

In addition to a qualitative understanding of the metabolic fate of antiarrhythmic drugs, an understanding of the quantitative aspects of absorption, distribution, and elimination is necessary. Bioavailability, the rate and extent to which a drug reaches the systemic circulation, is an important factor which significantly modifies the clinical efficacy of an orally administered drug. Several antiarrhythmic drugs are extensively destroyed in the liver during the first pass through the portal circulation and do not reach the systemic circulation in sufficient amounts to be effective. In some cases, large oral doses can be administered to overcome this problem, but as illustrated by lidocaine, first-pass metabolism of large doses can lead to extensive formation of toxic, undesirable metabolites (5). Administration of large oral doses can also lead to saturation of the hepatic extraction processes. This results in nonlinear bioavailability with disproportionate increases in the amount of drug reaching the systemic circulation as the dose is increased. This has been shown for lorcainide where the fraction of the dose reaching the systemic circulation increases from 27% to 50% when the dose is increased from 150 to 300 mg (6). A doubling of the administered dose results in an increase in the effective dose from 40.5 mg to 150 mg, which is almost a fourfold increase in effective dose. Bioavailability is also very sensitive to formulation variabilities, but this topic will not be considered here.

There are numerous factors which influence drug distribution. Serum

protein binding is one factor which needs to be investigated in the early
stages of new drug evaluation. Serum protein binding, for the most part, is of
academic interest, but can also be of clinical significance.All antiarrhythmic
drugs are bound to some extent to the serum proteins. It is generally accepted
that the drug which is bound to serum proteins is in a storage state and is not
available to cross membranes and subsequently produce effects at effector sites
in the myocardium. If the percentage of the drug in the serum which is bound
to proteins remains constant, independent of total drug concentration, then
this binding is of little consequence. However, if binding to serum proteins
is saturable and influenced by changes in total serum drug concentrations, the
binding can be of significant clinical relevance. This nonlinear binding is
best illustrated by disopyramide. The binding of disopyramide to serum
proteins approaches saturation at low therapeutic levels and the amount of free
drug in the serum increases disproportionately to increases in the total serum
concentration (7). This not only complicates the titration of dosage, but
confuses the interpretation of the meaning of measured serum drug concentration.

An understanding of drug elimination is generally described by drug
clearance and elimination half-life. However, it is important to also know the
route of elimination; whether a drug is metabolized or whether renal
elimination of the parent drug is the predominant route. An investigation of
drug elimination must include studies to determine whether elimination is
linear over the expected clinically useful serum concentration range. If
elimination is nonlinear and clearance decreases with increasing serum
concentration, then this needs to be adequately characterized. Drug
elimination also needs tc be investigated in terms of the patient population
likely to receive the antiarrhythmic drug. This requires that elderly
patients with reduced renal function be studied.

Describing the time course of drug action is more difficult than
describing the absorption and disposition characteristics of a drug. Drug
concentrations can readily be quantitated with a high degree of sensitivity
and specificity. Drug action, on the other hand, is often not directly
measured, but is inferred from measurements of clinical status such as PVC
frequency. Even when more precise measurements of effect can be evaluated,
their relationship to clinical efficacy remains to be defined.

Antiarrhythmic drugs are generally assumed to act reversibly. Their
action is dependent on the formation of a drug-effector site interaction which
obeys the law of mass action. Subsequently, the intensity of response should

correlate with the concentration of free drug in the plasma. For this reason, the pharmacodynamics of antiarrhythmic drugs are generally described in terms of plasma drug concentration. Relationships between intensity of effect and plasma concentration have been described for several antiarrhythmic drugs. In discussing the pharmacodynamics of a drug, however, one must be specific in defining the effect being evaluated; antiarrhythmic drugs produce more than one effect, and drug action can be measured in several ways. Previous studies with lorcainide illustrate this point (2). The pharmacodynamics of lorcainide was studied in patients, and the time course of drug action was described in terms of two measurable parameters, PVC reduction and QRS widening. While both of these observed drug effects are related to drug concentration in the plasma, the time course of these two effects are quite different. In one patient it was shown that QRS widening (expressed as percentage of control) had returned to zero, while PVC's were still totally suppressed. The time for PVC frequency to return to pre-drug levels was several hours following the return of the QRS interval to control. Clearly, when discussing the time course of effect of lorcainide, one must specify the particular effect being considered.

When the time course of antiarrhythmic effect can be correlated with serum drug concentration, the relationship is often summarized in terms of a "therapeutic range." It must be kept in mind that a therapeutic range is simply a statistical attempt to describe the plasma concentrations which correlate with optimal clinical efficacy in most individuals with a particular dysrhythmia. The upper limit of a therapeutic range is defined in terms of an increasing likelihood of occurrence of some unacceptable side effect, and the lower limit implies that plasma drug levels below this limit result in inadequate drug delivery to the myocardium with resulting inadequate arrhythmic suppression. Summarizing drug pharmacodynamics in terms of a therapeutic range is useful, but too often is based on studies in only a small number of patients, and the upper and lower limits are often chosen somewhat arbitrarily.

Drug response, however, does not always correlate with plasma drug concentrations. There are several explanations for this lack of correlation: The measured total plasma drug concentrations may not be representative of the concentration of drug at the effector site due to nonlinear plasma protein binding; the effect of the drug may not be due to a simple reversible interaction at the effector site; or the observed action may be modified by, or entirely due to, a drug metabolite.

In cases where metabolites modify the clinical efficacy, the effect may not be manifest for hours or even days after commencement of a chronic therapy with the parent drug. This is best illustrated by the n-acetyl metabolite of procainamide. Acute pharmacodynamic studies of procainamide are not relevant to the pharmacodynamics of procainamide during chronic administration. Following administration of a single dose of procainamide, very little n-acetylprocainamide is formed and its presence is not sufficient during acute studies to modify the clinical efficacy of the parent drug. During chronic administration of procainamide, n-acetylprocainamide can accumulate substantially due to its slow elimination and it may contribute to clinical efficacy of the parent drug. During chronic oral administration of procainamide, the plasma concentration of n-acetylprocainamide has been shown to be as high as 2.5 times the procainamide concentration (8).

The situation with lorcainide is very similar to procainamide. Norlorcainide is eliminated from the body much more slowly than the parent drug. Subsequently, it accumulates considerably during chronic lorcainide administration, not reaching pseudostate-state levels for days after starting lorcainide therapy. The plasma concentration of norlorcainide is generally 2-4 times the lorcainide concentration once pseudosteady state is achieved (2).

These examples help to point out the need for the evaluation of drug pharmacodynamics during chronic administration. Single-dose studies may be misleading and the contribution of active metabolites may be completely missed.

In summary, several conclusions can be drawn regarding the evaluation of the pharmacodynamics and pharmacokinetics of new antiarrhythmic drugs:

1. The identity, the pharmacologic activity and the extent of accumulation of metabolites of antiarrhythmic drugs need to be determined in humans.

2. Studies to elucidate the quantitative aspects of absorption, distribution and elimination of new antiarrhythmic drugs provide important information and need to be carried out in patients.

3. The possibility of dose, or concentration, dependence in bioavailability, protein binding and elimination needs to be better investigated.

4. The relationship between serum drug concentrations and clinical efficacy needs to be better defined in sufficiently large populations, and the criteria for upper and lower limits of recommended therapeutic levels need to be based on more objective criteria.

5. The time course of effect of new antiarrhythmic drugs needs to be

evaluated during chronic drug studies.

REFERENCES

1. Blumer J, Strong JM, Atkinson AJ: The convulsant potency of lidocaine and its n-dealkylated metabolites. J Pharmacol Exptl Ther 186:31-36, 1973.
2. Meinertz T, Kasper W, Kersting F, Just H, Behtold H, Jahnchem E: Lorcainide II. Plasma concentration-effect relationship. Clin Pharmacol Ther 26: 196-204, 1979.
3. Atkinson AJ, Lee WK, Quinn ML, Kushner W, Nevin MJ, Strong JM: Dose-ranging trial of n-acetylprocainamide in patients with premature ventricular contractions. Clin Pharmacol Ther 21:575-587, 1977.
4. Kates RE, Jaillon P, Rubenson DS, Winkle RA: Intravenous n-acetylprocain-amide disposition kinetics in coronary artery disease. Clin Pharmacol Ther 28:52-57, 1980.
5. Boyes RN, Scott DB,Jebson PJ, Godman MJ, Julian DG: Pharmacokinetics of lidocaine in man. Clin Pharmacol Ther 12:105-116, 1971.
6. Jahnchen E, Bechtold H, Kasper W, Kersting F, Just H, Heykants J, Meinertz T: Lorcainide I. Saturable presystemic elimination. Clin Pharmacol Ther 26: 187-195, 1979.
7. Meffin PF, Robert EW, Winkle RA, Harapat S, Peters FA, Harrison DC: Role of concentration-dependent plasma protein binding in disopyramide disposition. J Pharmacokinet Biopharm 7:29-46, 1979.
8. Reidenberg MM, Dreyer DE, Levy M, Warner H: Polymorphic acetylation of procainamide in man. Clin Pharmacol Ther 17:722-730, 1975.

GENERAL GROUP DISCUSSION: PHARMACOLOGY

Dr. Herling: Can we be sure that serum levels are representative of what
is occurring in an area of compromised blood flow within the peri-ischemic
zone or infarction zone? Are tissue levels more accurate in telling us
where we are going with antiarrhythmic therapy?

Dr. Kates: The answer is probably not. There are investigators working
with animal models looking at myocardial distribution. Dr. Wenger has
published some data on procainamide. Perhaps he would like to comment on
his model using ischemic tissue.

Dr. Wenger: I think it is a good question but I don't have a good
answer. We don't know where to look in myocardium to find the site of
action of many drugs. It is difficult first of all to follow tissue
concentrations and secondly we don't know yet what to look at and what
it means. I think it is an area of great interest and we need to do more
work to find out what it means.

Dr. Herling: Another point is that therapeutic concentrations are given
to us by drug companies and do they mean anything in terms of what we
are shooting for in preventing sudden death or treating arrhythmias.
Should we use those levels or cast them aside and seek an effect before we
see toxic effects?

Dr. Kates: Without pointing fingers, a lot of those levels come out of
academia as well. Several points, first, suggested therapeutic levels are
based on some major pharmacologic effects, not necessarily clinical
efficacy. Second, they are often based on small populations, third, which
is more of a technological question, they are based on various assay
methods. The clinical effect is clearly what we need to determine.

Dr. Lucchesi: I think the discrepancy between plasma concentrations and
myocardial concentrations may account for some of the problems we encounter
in animal models. For example, in the acute ligation model, and the
Harris model, flow to the ischemic area or the peripheral regions of that

ischemic area do not really return until collaterals have opened up to
supply flow to that region. It may account for why an animal at 48 hours
is far more responsive to a given agent than at 24 hours or even earlier.
Also, some drugs gain access to the myocardium very slowly. Dr. Anderson is
in the audience and maybe he would like to comment on some of his human
studies with bretyllium.

Dr. Anderson: I don't really have enough human data, at least quantitative
data to make a comment. We did notice however, in our dog model, that the
kinetics of the antifibrillatory effects of bretyllium seemed to parallel
those of the tissue myocardial levels of the drug rather than serum concentration of the drug. Although I don't want to propose that this is a simple
1:1 relationship. Nevertheless, after a bolus injection there was a rapidly
falling serum level, whereas both the myocardial levels and VF threshold
continued to rise for a period of about 3 hours and then began to decline
thereafter. So at least with that drug which appears to be highly membrane
bound those kinetics seemed to be important, at least in the acute situation.

Dr. Wenger: I would like to ask Dr. Dreifus a question regarding his
amiodarone study. When was the drug actually administered and what evidence
was there that the drug was in the tissue?

Dr. Dreifus: We used chronic oral administration for two weeks and as far
as plasma concentrations was concerned it's not useful because amiodarone
must be in the tissue. Now how did we know it was in the tissue? We found
a markedly different behavior of the arrhythmias in the post release phase
in the amiodarone animals than in all the other animals. What happened
upon reperfusion instead of a sudden burst of ventricular tachycardia and
fibrillation and death in a high percentage of the animals, was that the
amiodarone treated dogs still died but they died much slower, and had many
more ventricular arrhythmias for longer periods of time preceding fibrillation.
They lived for 20-40 minutes and then finally deteriorated. So there was
something different about amiodarone treated animals that needs to be
further explored.

Dr. Zipes: The temporal relationship of drug administration to the time
of coronary occlusion is very critical. For example, a drug given prior
to occlusion can have a much greater increase in tissue concentration
compared to a drug given just after coronary occlusion. The reasons are
self-evident. Indeed, it is probably not an unreasonable extrapolation
to the clinical area. A patient who comes in with crushing chest pain

and is given an I.V. administration of a drug may have a totally different tissue concentration compared to the patient who is on chronic maintenance therapy and develops his myocardial infarction. I think tissue concentrations in certain models are very relevant.

Dr. Kates: One area that I addressed that no one has mumped up to speak about is the area of metabolites. I find it very frustrating that metabolites found in high concentrations during a human drug study cannot be administered to patients without obtaining a new IND. We have to first obtain toxicity data on that metabolite.

Dr. Krikler: As part of our routine electrophysiological study in patients, we re-test the patient an average of 3 days later using a limited electrophysiological study so we do believe that indeed we are looking at the metabolites. Particularly with amiodarone we try and validate the effects at 3 months with a full electrophysiological study. There again we will be looking at metabolites.

Dr. Morganroth: What sort of basic pharmacokinetic data should be required in terms of beginning to use dosage regimens in patients and should plasma levels be determined in patients depending upon the effect of the suppression of arrhythmias?

Dr. Kates: It is difficult from an academic point of view to say what is important initially, what is purely academic and what may be important later. Clearly kinetic studies in patients with renal failure or hepatic dysfunction are important but are they important at the time that we are first evaluating a new drug? I think what you really want me to answer is what is needed to do a phase 2 study. I think we need to know basically what happens to the drug. Is the drug really the agent that we are talking about or is it a metabolite. I think that has to be answered. I think we need to know if the metabolites accumulate. How extensively do they accumulate? How pharmacologically active are they? We would have to know what happened to the drug. In terms of finding a therapeutic range, I don't think that can be done early on. That requires a large population and I don't think that has a place in early studies. People tend to publish therapeutic levels in their initial studies and this information goes into review papers and becomes very hard to revise. I am not sure we need to do pharmacokinetic modeling and come up with a three compartment model and rate constants and alphas and betas.

Dr. Woosley: I would like to jump on the bandstand with you about active metabolites and encourage the drug industry to pursue active metabolites. I think the F.D.A. has encouraged that and has made it possible to do so without the expense incurred with an entirely new entity. N-acetylprocain-amide is the agent I am referring to. However, we learned something with N-acetylprocainamide. It turned out to be an entirely different pharmacologic entity, both electrophysiologically and efficaciously. So we can't take any short cuts when we go to man, but I think there should be some short cuts in toxicology before preceding to man. It should be made possible to reduce the cost to the pharmaceutical industry to allow investigation of metabolites.

Dr. Dingell: It is an accepted fact in circles of drug metabolism, that very often you find not only a change in the rates of metabolism of a compound with prolonged administration, but indeed the pathways and the pathways which are involved in the formation of active metabolites change after a drug is given for a prolonged period of time. The rates of metabolism of the active metabolites themselves and consequently their levels in tissue are also markedly altered. Another point is that I think perhaps we talked a great deal this morning about variability in the animal models. I think probably one of the major causes of this variability can indeed be the species differences in metabolism of compounds both quantitatively and qualitatively as one goes from one species to another. To further complicate the matter there is also the enormous variability between one patient and another and one could develop very elaborate pharmacokinetic models for a relatively small patient population and then find that a considerable number of your patients come in with markedly different responses as far as their metabolism is concerned. So the problem is enormously complicated. I think that whenever we undertake studies on antiarrhythmic drugs we should make sure we have a very strong drug metabolism component in our efforts.

Dr. Temple: I am not quite sure how difficult it has been to study metabolites when anyone wanted to do it. I can't think of any major battles we have had over that issue. The ground rules apply for studying any new agnet and as Dr. Woosley pointed out, a metabolite is a new agent kinetically. The animal studies on the parent compound may very well give you little guidance as to the metabolites in humans. The toxicology ground rules for studying a new agent are pretty straight forward for very short-term studies and not much toxicology is needed. However, for longer term studies, more toxicology is required. I have to see what the people from industry believe. I don't think it is particularly hard to do at least short-term metabolite sutdies of up to say 2 weeks to find out what you need to know. Our position would be that if the previous data serves to define the toxicology of the metabolite, there is no need to do anything else. If it doesn't, then there probably is. Maybe you can be more specific or have some horror stories to enunciate.

Dr. Kates: It is my impression that it is not that simple to do studies on metabolites directly in patients.

Dr. Temple: It's not something that is commonly requested.

Dr. Kates: But if it were requested...

Dr. Temple: If the parent drug is well into clinical studies and someone wanted to do some simple kinetic studies of a metabolite for a duration of a couple of days, then the kind of toxicology that would be necessary as defined in our guidelines involves principally short-term studies, i.e. L.D. 50's, in several species and studies of at most a couple of weeks duration in animals. If someone could show that the metabolite was present in the animal model that had been studied before, even those things might be unnecessary.

Dr. Kates: Thank you.

Dr. Moore: What do you think is the ideal animal model to determine the metabolism and pharmacokinetics of a drug? You have indicated that you don't think the dog is ideal.

Dr. Kates: The best animal model obviously is man. There are questions of ethics perhaps when giving a Cl4 labeled compound to a normal subject or patient and there are difficulties with doing these studies. However, I think that wehn you consider what is involved, that we don't have any choice or alternatives. No animal model is a good predictor of human drug metabolism.

Dr. Temple: We look at a drug in a setting of itself, but as clinicians, we don't use drugs in that manner. We might have someone on an antiarrhythmic and then put them on vasodilators to improve cardiac output. We are not aware of drug interactions nor what happens to metabolism when perfusion to the gut is changed or perfusion to the kidneys is changed. Considering a linear setting is really not appropriate to the patient that you are talking about as the model, when treating a patient with ischemic disease with nitrates, beta blockers and antiarrhythmics and using combinations of all three would likely result in different effects than when any one drug was given individually.

Dr. Kates: I think you have to define the normal before you can define the abnormal. Clearly, we are opening a can of worms when we discuss drug interactions. This is a huge area that would be an incredible burden on the pharmaceutical industry to have to address in early development. There are just so many possibilities. I think this needs to be very carefully addressed and if there are combinations that are always going to occur then they should be evaluated.

Dr. Winkle: Dr Temple, if I have a drug that I have given to a significant number of patients and I know it has a metabolite that has been found at concentration X in all of these patients, what value is an LD50 study in dogs or rats or whatever if I plan to give small doses of the metabolite not to exceed the concentration which has already been achieved in a large number of patients?

Dr. Temple: Well, I think that depends on what study you are planning to do. If it were just that to do a simple kinetic study, there might not be any need to do any further studies. If the metabolite is going to be worked up fully, like a regular drug, you may need to define what its potential toxicities are and the fact that you have achieved low blood levels of it or some blood level of it in the course of giving the parent drug may or may not tell you what would happen when you begin to investigate it as an anti-arrhythmic agent itself. I guess my bottom line is that if a requirement looks stupid, someone in the drug industry or one of their investigators will argue with us about it if they think it is dumb. I don't know whether there have been things like that where someone thought a requirement was foolish but in all probability if no one asks, we will do it in the usual way which is for species LD50's. You could ask what is the value of an LD50 for any drug. You're not going to give 1000 mg of most of these drugs intravenously all at once but the studies are done to define the limits and the potentials. It is a perfectly good question to ask concerning what one learns from those things.

Dr. Winkle: Just for the record then, it might be possible to give metabolites without doing LD50 studies.

Dr. Temple: I think it depends on what you want to do and how much exposure there is. If, for example, the concentrations in human studies of a month are known and the question is what if you give the same amount once, it might not be necessary to go through the usual procedures.

Dr. Winkle: That information on humans is almost always available because it is usually the motivating factor that causes people to want to study metabolites.

Dr. Temple: Most people don't want to study the metabolite in a very short term study. They want to work up the metabolite or at least plan to do that.

Dr. Winkle: I would disagree because I think that the really relevant information we need to find out about metabolites would probably be best identified from fairly short term studies. We need to help understand how the so-called parent drug is acting and most of the time I think that a short-term study would answer those questions.

Dr. Temple: When someone comes with a desire to study a metabolite, it usually has not been anything like that. Maybe it looks so discouraging, no one has tried.

Dr. Winkle: It seems that nobody is trying to do these studies so maybe we should beck up one step and go to the pharmaceutical industry. Obviously they are not coming to you. This is the picture I'm getting.

Dr. Temple: No one has come up and said, look, all we want to do is deliver half the dose that is normally achieved in the course of these chronic studies. We only want to do it once so don't make us repeat the whole chemistry, and the other requirements we just need to find out one thing once. I can tell you I don't recall any instance in my four years' experience where someone has said, this whole thing is crazy, can't we do this? They may be thinking this and not saying it. I don't know.

Dr. Abrams: Since none of my colleagues from industry have stood up I felt that it was appropriate to address some of the questions that were raised. Obviously, pharmaceutical companies differ as much from each other as academic institutions do so no one can speak for all of industry. However, the companies that I am familiar with do intensively investigate metabolites of drugs that are marked for development well before they get into man. The problems for understanding their biology often results from not being able to synthesize enough of the metabolite to do the biology with. There is also very often an assay problem in that you may have an assay for the nature drug but it may not be identical for the metabolite. If there are several metabolites then there are additional problems. Since pharmaceutical companies like any institution have finite resources, a decision has to be

made on what you are going to pursue. Relative to carrying out studies with
metabolites in man, we did have a recent program in which a metabolite was
studied and the F.D.A. interpretation was liberal relative to what needed to
be done to study the metabolite in man. I would like to comment on my
notion of minimal, because with safety assessment studies, nothing is minimal.
The limiting factor isn't how long the animals are treated. The limiting
factor is the fact that you have to study a couple of species, several
doses, do histopathology, and all that takes time, money and people. I
think the best hope for pursuing metabolites in man is a reasonable position
by the F.D.A. and I believe that they are prepared to do that. If you can
show that when the main drug is given to man that this metabolite is indeed
present, that in chronic safety studies in several species, that the metabolite has been shown to be present then previous safety information applies
and studies with the metabolite in question are appropriate. I believe that
is the best hope to quickly get into man and carry out studies relative to
the comments that Dr. Winkle made. However, since you really don't have a
proper safety profile on the metabolite you want to know what it does in
normal volunteers before giving it to people who may be sick. Thus, there
probably isn't any real short cut to a substantial assay of the drug's
behavior in man with very limited safety information available.

Dr. Ehrreich: I just want to comment on what Dr. Abrams said. He took some
of the words right out of my mouth. Having worked at three pharmaceutical
companies myself over a 12-year period, I know that when a drug is discovered
to have an active metabolite that a lot of effort goes into determining the
metabolite's activity and to a certain extent it's relative toxicity to the
parent compound. One of the reasons we at the F.D.A. have had little
problem as Dr. Temple pointed out earlier with these metabolites is that a
lot of information is available on them when we get an application to test
them. So really there is little to do except some short-term toxicity
studies. Certainly in short-term studies carried out for kinetic purposes,
the amount of material that has already been done generally will suffice.
I think there is little chance that an active metabolite will reach our
hands at the F.D.A. with little information and will be asked to be tested
in long-term studies in man.

Dr. Kates: I don't know how long lidocaine has been around but it's before
I got out of school. Lidocaine has two metabolites that are pharmacologically
active in animals. We know from limited data that they seem to be eliminated

very slowly in man. However, no one's given them to a human subject so
we don't know anything about their real contribution. There is a lot of
speculation. It a-cumulates in some patients and not in others and it
appears to be important. I don't think anyone would disagree with that.
What has been the road block that has prevented studies with it.
Dr. Ehrreich: That I can't answer. I don't think we've gotten an application to have those metabolites tested.

HOW SHOULD HOLTER MONITORING ANALYSIS BE PERFORMED?

C.L. FELDMAN

1. INTRODUCTION

As new anti-arrhythmic agents are developed their premarket testing
has become an increasingly scientific and economic challenge. At present,
there are two acceptable techniques for testing new anti-arrhythmic
agents. One of these, acute testing with electrophysiologic measurements, offers substantial advantages because it allows the investigator
to separate "benign" ventricular arrhythmias from those which are self-
perpetuating and potentially result in ventricular fibrillation and
sudden death. This technique will be discussed later in the symposium.
The disadvantages of the electrophysiologic technique are its invasive
nature and possibility that the results may not be representative of
situations that the patient will encounter in normal life.

The ideal measure of an anti-arrhythmic efficacy is its ability
to prevent sudden death. Fortunately, the frequency with which this
measure occurs is very low. Thus, studies of efficacy which depend on
sudden death require large populations and are unreasonably expensive.
The next best measure is the presence of ventricular premature contractions
(VPC), particularly high grade VPCs, which seem to be statistically
predictive of ventricular fibrillation in patients with infarcted,
ischemic, or otherwise inhomogeneous regions of myocardium.

At present, the only reasonably accurate and efficient method of
measuring the effect of an anti-arrhythmic agent is Holter monitoring
with automatic or semi-automatic data reduction. This is especially true
if the tests are to be performed under realistic conditions with
ambulatory patients. As our chairman and others have shown (1, 2, 3) the
statistics of the situation demand that substantial amounts of monitoring
be performed to show efficacy of a particular drug - typically 48 to 72
hours for a control period and a like-time for the test. Usually, this
rules out in-patient monitoring as well as intermittent recording. Be-

cause of the large amount of data, the ideal solution is probably to reduce the data as it is recorded and record only the results. Unfortunately,
the state-of-the-art of such "Smart Recorders" is very primitive and their
accuracy is inadequate for scientific purposes. The only viable technique
is Holter monitoring as we all know it.

2. RECORDERS

Although, for many years, there was only a single manufacturer of
recorders suitable for Holter monitoring, this is no longer the case. The
last ten years have seen the introduction of approximately half a dozen
recorders of satisfactory quality, both reel-to-reel and cassette type.
The cassette types offer the user greater convenience than the reel-to-reel
types but, because they use narrower tape, present some problems in attaining adequate signal-to-noise ratio. Further, the cassettes often seem to
have a tendency to jam - a problem minimized by the use of high quality
cassettes.

As can be seen in Table I, (4) which summarizes the properties of most
available recorders, none of them achieve the specifications recommended
by the American Heart Association for ECG machines or patient monitors.

Table I. Properties of Holter Recorders

Model	Weight	No. of Channels	Type	Bandwidth	Cal.
Advancemed 2450	UA	2	Reel	UA	No
Camscan 7300	935	2	Cassette	.4 → 20 Hz	Yes
Del Mar 445B/447	781	2	Reel	.04 → 100*	No
Hitman Compact IV, IV IM	469	2	Cassette	UA	Yes
ICR 7200	940	2	Cassette	.09 → 20	Yes
Medilog 1	400	3	Cassette	.09 → 20	NO
Medilog 2	390	2	Cassette	.07 → 45	Yes

*From manufacturers catalog - others were measured
by independent testing agency

However, the bandwidth and dynamic range of most of the recorders is
adequate for the purpose, particularly if the primary interest is in VPC
detection rather than the identification of ischemic episodes. If the

evaluators of a drug determined to measure the presence of ischemia as reflected by S-T changes in the electrocardiogram - and there is every reason
to believe that they should become increasingly interested - it is important
that they use recorders with good low frequency response - at least to
.1 Hz, preferably to .05 Hz - and at least two channels. Additionally,
timing stability - to permit accurate correlation with drug administration -
and the presence of a marker channel are extremely important.

Although none of the available recorders are ideal, most of them are
adequate.

3. ANALYZERS

Because analyzers are such complex technological devices, the majority
of this discussion must necessarily focus on them. To simplify this task,
it is useful to focus separately on the components of the analyzer - the
playback, the display, the detection and counting capabilities, and the
hardcopy output. Each of these will be discussed, in turn, below:

3.1 Playbacks

Originally, the development of a suitable playback was a major
challenge for the manufacturer of a Holter analyzer. Although tape heads
and electronics suitable for reproducing .05 Hz at 60 times real time are
difficult, they have been within the state-of-the-art for many years. However, the production of a tape head to reproduce these same frequencies in
real time is extraordinarily difficult. In practice, the problem has disappeared during the past few years as more and more scanners have been
built incorporating analog-to-digital conversion and electronic memories.
Using this technique, segments of electrocardiogram can be played back and
"memorized" at high speed - then reproduced, through a digital-to-analog
converter at any desired speed - typically real time. At the present
time, most manufacturers report their bandwidth for the combination of
recorder and real-time to quasi real-time playback.

3.2 Displays

The original Holter playback used with technique of superimposition
of successive complexes with concurrent audio indication of QRS (5).
Most playbacks still use this technique because it highlights the
occurrence of anomalous waveforms. Recent enhancements, using computer
techniques, superimpose sinus beats on one location of the screen, pre-
ported VPCs on a second location, and apparent superventricular premature

90

beats in yet a third location (Figure 1). Using this technique, the primary function of the technician is to assure that the computer is correct rather than to do the counting himself/herself.

FIGURE 1.   Segmented Superimposed Display

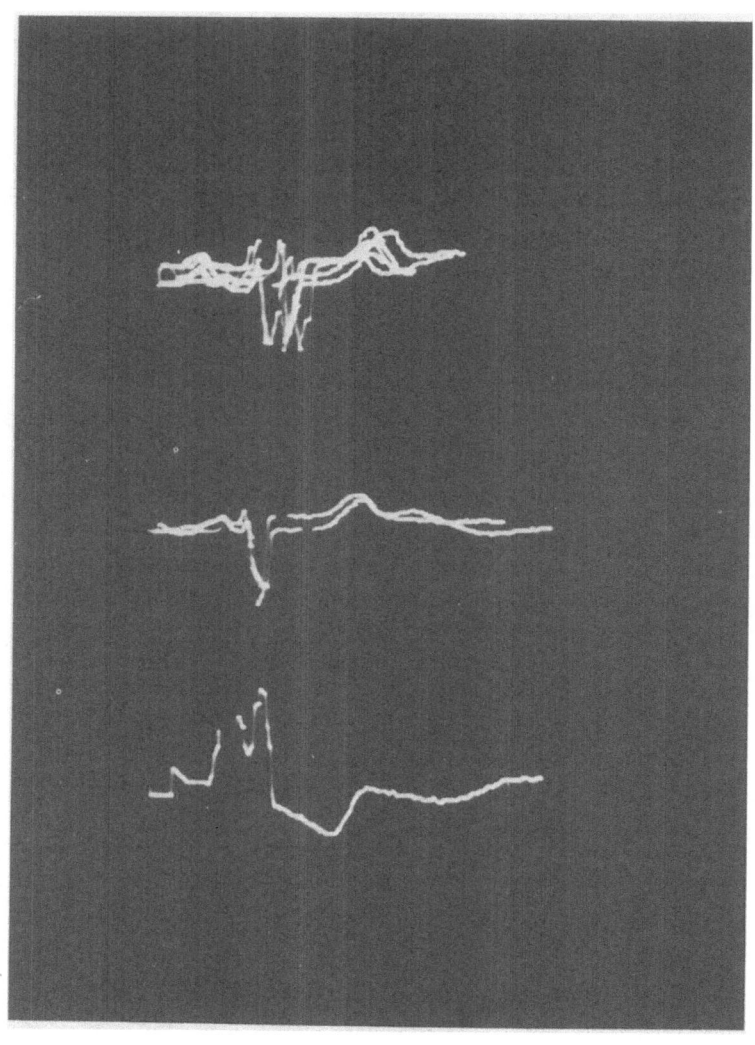

Recently, Stein et al (6) have suggested that the presentation of several minutes of data spread out on the screen give superior results. They have compared their results with those attained using the conventional superimposition technique with a computer-based system but not with any hand-counted results, making it impossible to draw conclusions about absolute accuracy.

3.3 Ectopic Beat Detection

Today, almost all manufacturers of Holter analyzers offer semiautomatic methods for detecting and counting ectopic events. Additionally, there are several computer-based systems that are not generally available for sale, but have been used extensively over the past five to ten years for the evaluation of new anti-arrhythmic agents and in a variety of epidemiologic studies whose goal is to discern more clearly the relationship between the occurrence of ventricular ectopic events and the likelihood of sudden death. Theoretically, there is no reason why either the hardwired detection devices available on commercially available analyzers - some of which have computers attached for counting and report generation - or the central processor-based systems should necessarily be preferred. In practice, the computer-based systems offer greater accuracy for a given level of operator attention at relatively modest increase in capital investment. The reason is that current computer technology using general-purpose processors and stored programs offer a much broader range of logical and arithmetic tasks for a given initial cost than can be done with available combinations of hardwired integrated circuit logic.

If, for reasons of cost or availability, it is desirable to use a hardwired ectopic beat detector/counter the key to its successful use is a very high level of operator training and motivation. The logic of most of the available devices permits interactions by the operator that will "tune" it to the ectopic morphologies exhibited by any given patient. Patience and judgement in tuning these devices together with careful beat-by-beat "walk through" during periods of artifact do permit good results, albeit at the expense of large amounts of operator time. For example, in one recent quality control study of six high activity types analyzed by a commercial scanning service (7) that specializes in drug studies, the intercept regression coefficient and correlation coefficient of a scatter diagram of ectopic beat counts from a superimposition scanner versus physician read results of the same tape were -441, .991 and .966

respectively. Of course, if the analyst simply puts the tape on an analyzer and plays it through with careful, often time-consuming over-reading, the results will be much less good. A sense of the quality obtainable under more conventional circumstances is contained in the following quotation. (4)

"All of the currently available arrhythmia analyzers can be fooled by noise or may misclassify normal and abnormal beats. Serious arrhythmias detected automatically must be verified and documented by the operator. Frequently occurring arrhythmias can be spot-checked to judge the accuracy of any arrhythmia counts.

Performance testing of an analyzer's arrhythmia detection abilities is difficult. A system may perform well on one tape and poorly on another, given the wide spectrum of both normal and abnormal beats, the presence, or absence of noise, and the varying skills of operators."

3.4 Computer-Based Analyzers

A number of computer-based Holter analyzers have been described in the literature in the last five to 10 years. Best known, probably, are the university-based systems at Washington University (8) and Stanford (9). Others that have been fairly well described include those by Feldman,(10) Birman, (11) Lovelace, (12) and Sheppard.(13) From a study of the literature and personal knowledge of most of these systems, it appears that excellent results are obtainable with all of them, although several re-quire extensive technician interaction and are, thus, relatively slow. All of these systems, in addition to being inherently more accurate than the hard-wired systems, offer more convenient interactions, greater flexibility, in adapting to a particular protocol, and a much wider range of hardcopy input formats.

To understand the workings of all of these systems, it is useful to divide the algorithms into separate sections as shown in Figure 2. These sections are artifact detection and suppression, QRS detection, feature extraction, and beat-type classification.

The primary technique for noise suppression is linear bandwidth reduction. Most computer-based systems filter the incoming signal such that they look only at that portion of the energy which is between one

FIGURE 2.   Organization of VPC Detection Algorithms

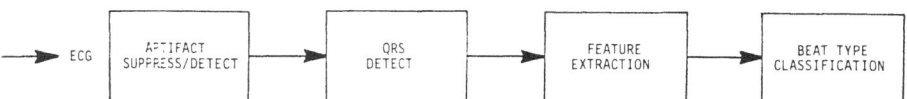

and 20 Hz.   In some cases this filtering is adaptive, depending on the level of artifact.   Additionally, all systems look at the total amount of high frequency energy and signal the other portions of the algorithm to suspend processing when the muscle artifact level exceeds the capabilities of the system.   Some systems also look at low frequency excursions or attempt baseline compensation.

Recently, we reported (14) on a system in which baseline artifact is recorded independently by means of a dual element coaxial electrode.

FIGURE 3.   Artifact Detecting Electrode

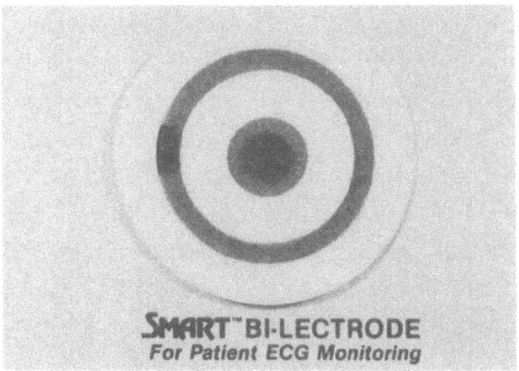

The processor, being able to recognize this artifact independently of the electrocardiogram, is able to suppress processing when the level exceeds tolerable limits.   The results have been demonstrated in real time and in an intensive care setting.   The rate of false positive VPC occurrence has been reduced from a state-of-the-art of five per patient hour to 0.7. The same technique has been successfully demonstrated on Holter tapes.

Its only disadvantage is that the artifact must be recorded on a separate
channel, making nearly mandatory the use of recorders with more than two
data channels.

All modern QRS detectors use a combination of slope and amplitude
criteria, automatically adapted to each subject's own QRS. To compensate
for the usual physiologic variability in waveforms and to detect small
ectopic events, all effective systems have some kind of "look-back"
system in which a long pause (especially one of two R-R intervals)
triggers a second search of the apparently empty region for QRSs which
do not meet the standard detection criteria but do meet a slightly lower
one.

The heart of ectopic beat detection algorithm is the feature extraction section. If nature were always kind, it would be possible to
make a single measurement on each QRS and this measurement would suffice
to permit high sensitivity and specificity in discriminating ventricular
ectopics from beats of supraventricular origin. The measure that comes
to mind, of course, is the QRS width. However, a moment's reflection
upon the occurrence of intraventricular conduction defects which widen
supraventricular beats or of VPCs which are relatively narrow as they
are reflected on one given lead, causes one to realize that width alone
does not permit adequate sensitivity or specificity. Further, anyone
who has attempted to measure width realizes that the measured value is
extremely sensitive to small amounts of artifact. To achieve improved
performance, most systems which depend upon such POINT MEASUREMENTS make
several such measurements as well as some simple INTEGRATIVE MEASURES
and put extensive effort into the beat-type discrimination portion of the
algorithm. Examples of such systems are the ARGUS system (15) which
measures width, height, offset, and area (as shown in Figure 4) and then
discriminates between supraventricular and ventricular in "fourspace"
and the Dynagram system (13) which makes five measurements, allowing
beat-type discrimination in five dimensional hyperspace.

Originally introduced in 1968, (16) INTEGRATIVE MEASURES, particularly
the calculation of correlation coefficient, have been used increasingly
in recent years because new and faster hardware permits these complex
calculations to be done quite rapidly. These techniques depend upon
being able to identify one or more template beats which are believed,
with high probability, to be of known type. Each test beat, then is

FIGURE 4. ARGUS Features

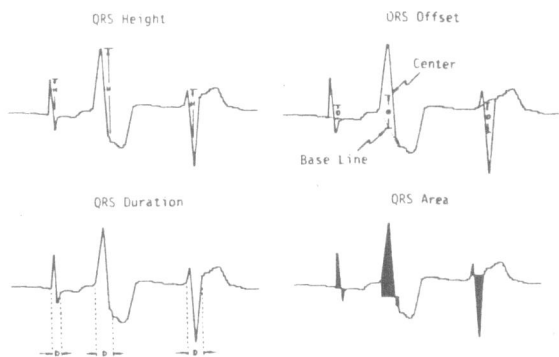

overlayed on top of each of the templates (Figure 5) and a search is made
for the best match. Most current systems which use this technique use
multiple templates which may be classified either automatically or by
the operator, and combine this measurement with the area under the QRS
complex. In general, these correlation-based systems have relatively
simple beat-type discrimination sections. The major advantage of these
systems is that they are relatively insensitive to artifact. A potential
disadvantage is that they are sensitive to "jitter" and QRS detection is
probably no longer relevant since most current systems use multiple
templates - typically two or three "normals" - which correspond to
different fiducial points on difficult to detect QRS complexes.

FIGURE 5. Template Matching

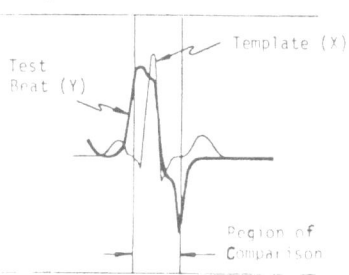

The sine qua non of an analyzer is accuracy. Almost as important is that this accuracy is achievable in a practical manner with minimal dependence upon the technician operating the system. Unfortunately, the measurement of accuracy of any arrhythmia analysis system is extraordinarily difficult and time-consuming. In general, it involves painstaking "eyeball" analysis of large amounts of data - hundreds to thousands of hours - and beat-by-beat comparison with machine produced results. To a greater or lesser extent, most analyzers have been evaluated this way and the results for computer-based systems have generally been reported in the literature.

Prior to this meeting, the most recently published results for our own system were those presented in Table II. That particular test used randomly selected ten-minute segments of randomly selected tapes with independent, duplicated cardiologist visual analysis. Computer readings were taken in order to measure repeatability as well as accuracy. These results, although measured on a specific system, seemed to be representative of published results for the various computer systems.

Table II. Accuracy and Repeatability of Computer VPC Detection Systems
(1977)

	Physician Trial I	Computer Trial I	Physician Trial II	Computer Trial II
Mean Number of VED $\pm$ SEM	92.6 $\pm$ 12.1	86.5 $\pm$ 11.3	91.8 $\pm$ 12.3	86.2 $\pm$ 11.7
Significance of Difference	P < .05		P < .05	
Regression Coefficient	.92		.92	
Correlation Coefficient	.98		.97	
Significance of Correlation	P < .001		P < .001	

Recently we performed some more tests to evaluate changes in the system and in the computer operator interaction. This test consisted of "recycling", in a blinded fashion, 34 separate 12- or 24-hour tapes, each of which had been read beat-by-beat by a cardiologist on a compressed, complete writeout. Because of the random selection process, some tapes were read as many as four times while others were read only once.

A plot of the results for total ectopic count is shown in logarithmic co-ordinate in Figure 6. The results for total ectopic, paired ectopics as beats included in runs of ventricular tachycardia, as evaluated in the usual

FIGURE 6.   Correlation System Test Results - 1980

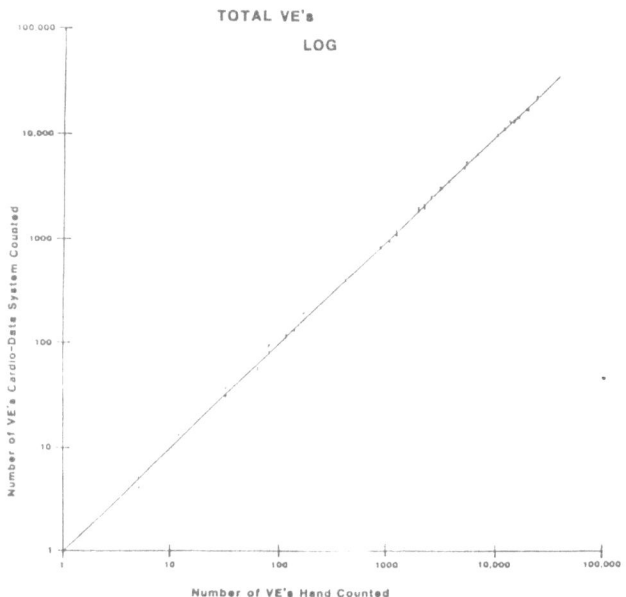

linear fashion, are shown in Table III. Although the slopes of the regression lines and the coefficients are very close to unity, we feel that this linear model is a poor one because tapes with large numbers of VPCs contribute disproportionately to the linear coefficients. Accordingly, we have also analyzed these tapes by a logarithmic model in which we fit a best curve of the form

$$Y = a x^C$$

by finding the best straight line for the curve of log y vs. log x. In this analysis, fractional errors have the same weight irrespective of the number of VPCs in a given test. The result of this analysis are shown in Table IV. The correlation coefficient is the correlation coefficient of the scatter diagram of the logarithms of the data points.

Table III. Accuracy of Computer VPC Detection System (1980) - Linear
Evaluation

	N	b(intercept)	m(slope)	ρ(correlation coefficient)
VPC (total)	55	-45.47	1.018	.9987
Paired VPCs	39	6.75	1.003	.9926
VT Beats	38	- .17	1.030	.9881

Table IV. Accuracy of Computer VPC Detection System (1980) - Logarithmic
Evaluation

	N	a(multiplier)	c(exponent)	ρ_2(correlation coefficient)
VPC (total)	55	.994	1.0019	.9991
Paired VPCs	39	1.014	.9988	.9982
VT Beats	38	.952	1.0043	.9986

BRADYCARDIA PROFILE

TIME ENDING	HEART RATE LO MEAN HI	BRADY EVENTS	BRADY BEATS	BRADY RATE	BRADY TYPE
11:00.0A1	52 53 70	0	0	-	
12:00.0P1	52 58 68	0	0	-	
1:00.0P1	54 61 70	0	0	-	
2:00.0P1	58 64 74	0	0	-	
3:00.0P1	54 61 76	0	0	-	
4:00.0P1	54 60 76	0	0	-	
5:00.0P1	56 60 72	0	0	-	
6:00.0P1	54 65 76	0	0	-	
7:00.0P1	56 61 72	0	0	-	
8:00.0P1	52 62 74	0	0	-	
9:00.0P1	54 57 70	0	0	-	
10:00.0P1	52 56 72	0	0	-	
11:00.0P1	52 55 70	0	0	-	
12:00.0A2	52 55 76	0	0	-	
1:00.0A2	46 53 80	11	1140	46	Sinus
2:00.0A2	48 51 72	2	3368	48	Sinus
3:00.0A2	46 53 70	7	1780	46	Sinus
4:00.0A2	46 52 72	12	2680	46	Sinus
5:00.0A2	46 52 76	7	1508	46	Sinus
6:00.0A2	46 54 76	10	2073	46	Sinus
7:00.0A2	46 55 78	3	1112	46	Sinus
8:00.0A2	46 54 70	7	1019	46	Sinus
9:00.0A2	46 54 66	6	1012	46	Sinus
10:00.0A2	48 56 74	3	216	48	Sinus
10:22.1A2	50 56 68	1	88	50	Sinus
SUMMARY:	46 57 80	69	15991	46	

Figure 7. C.L. Feldman, "How Should Holter Monitoring Analysis be Performed?"

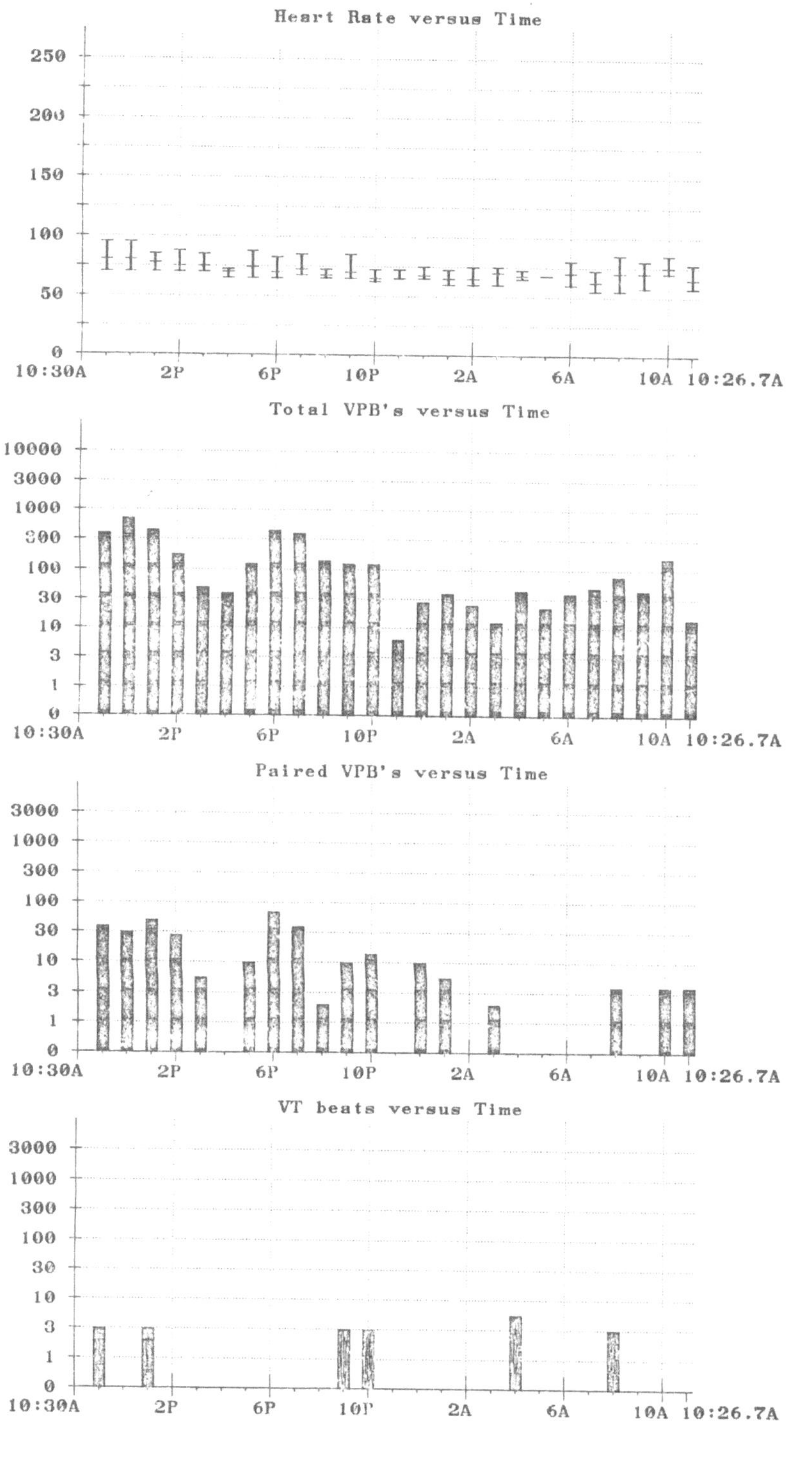

Heart Rate versus Time

```
250

200

150

100

 50

  0
10:30A      2P      6P     10P      2A      6A     10A  10:26.7A
```

Total VPB's versus Time

```
10000
 3000
 1000
  300
  100
   30
   10
    3
    1
    0
10:30A      2P      6P     10P      2A      6A     10A  10:26.7A
```

Paired VPB's versus Time

```
3000
1000
 300
 100
  30
  10
   3
   1
   0
10:30A      2P      6P     10P      2A      6A     10A  10:26.7A
```

VT beats versus Time

```
3000
1000
 300
 100
  30
  10
   3
   1
   0
10:30A      2P      6P     10P      2A      6A     10A  10:26.7A
```

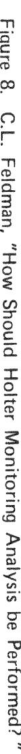

Figure 8. C.L. Feldman, "How Should Holter Monitoring Analysis be Performed?"

4. HARDCOPY OUTPUT

The secondary, but still important, advantage of computer-based systems for arrhythmia analysis is their ability to output results in a wide variety of formats. Although to a casual observer, this might be a merely cosmetic effect, in fact, the practicality of developing special formats results in making measurements that are particularly well suited for the evaluation of any particular drug. An example of the advantages of this kind of flexibility are shown in Figure 7, Bradycardia Profile, which was developed in a manner of a few weeks to help provide a more comprehensive evaluation of a beta blocker. Of course, all systems must be able to present time-related plots of heart rate and ventricular ectopic activity along with sample output strips for subsequent validation. Figure 8 is an example of graphic output.

5. CONCLUSION

In the 20 years since its introduction, Holter monitoring has become the standard technique for the evaluation of anti-arrhythmic agents. At present, several satisfactory recorders are commercially available - both reel-to-reel and cassette type. When selecting one for use in a drug evaluation program, the investigator should satisfy himself that the frequency response and dynamic range are adequate, that it has at least two data channels, and that the recorder has either very high time stability or a timing channel. If a cassette type recorder is used, it is essential that the cassettes be of high quality to minimize mechanical problems.

In selecting an analysis technique, the choice must be made between hard-wired analyzers - with or without computer-aided counting and report generation - and one of several limited-production computer-based systems. The hard-wired systems can give satisfactory results when operated by skilled, highly motivated technicians who are subject to strict quality control standards. At the present state-of-the-art, the computer-based systems seem to offer greater accuracy and repeatability with lower levels of operator interaction. They also offer wider choice of reporting formats. However, no existing computer systems offer adequate accuracy when run unsupervised. For this reason, selection of an analyzer for evaluation of a new anti-arrhythmic agent should consider the entire system - analyzer, technician, and quality control program.

REFERENCES

1. Michelson, EL, Morganroth, J. 1979. Spontaneous variability of complex ventricular arrhythmias detected by long-term electrocardiographic recording. Circulation 61, No. 4., p. 690.
2. Kennedy, HL, Chandra, V, Sayther, KL, Caralis, DG. 1978. Effectiveness of increasing hours of continuous ambulatory electrocardiography in detecting maximal ventricular ectopy. The American Journal of Cardiology, p. 925.
3. Thanavaro, S, Kleiger, RE, Hieb, BR, Krone, RJ, DeMello, VR, Oliver, GC. 1980. Effect of electrocardiographic recording duration on ventricular dysrhythmia detection after myocardial infarction. Circulation 62,No.2, p. 262.
4. Ambulatory ecg recording systems. 1980, vol. 9, Heath Devices, pp. 215-243.
5. Holter, NJ. 1961. New methods for heart studies, Science 134. pp. 1214-1220.
6. Stein, IM, Plunkett, J, Troy, M. 1980. Comparison of techniques for examining long-term ECG recordings. Medical Instrumentation, Vol. 14, No. 1, p. 69.

7. Loring, R. 1980. Personal communication.
8. Clark, KW, Hitchens, RE, Moore, SM, Potter, SJ, Ritter, JA, Mead, CN, Thomas, Jr., LJ. 1978. ARGUS/2H. Proceedings of the IEEE conference on computers in cardiology. IEEE Catalog No. 78CH1391-2C, Standford, California, pp. 397-398.
9. Lopes, MG, Fitzgerald, J, Harrison, DC, Schroeder, JS. 1975. Diagnosis and quantification of arrhythmias in ambulatory patients using an improved R-R interval plotting system. The American Journal of Cardiology, Vol. 35, p. 816.
10. Hubelbank, M, Feldman, CL, Lane, B, Singer, P. 1975. An improved computer system for processing long-term electrocardiograms. Proc., Computers in Cardiology, pp. 15-19.
11. Birman, KP, Rolnitzky, LM, Bigger, Jr., JT. 1978. A shape oriented system for automated Holter ECG analysis. Computers in Cardiology, p. 217.
12. Lovelace, DE, Knoebel, SB. 1978. Operator assisted/automated review system for ambulatory ECG recordings. Computers in Cardiology, p. 215.
13. Sheppard, JJ, Hansmann, DR. 1977. Applications of the Dyna-Gram 111B Holter ECG analysis system. Computers in Cardiology, p. 211-219.
14. Feldman, CL, Hubelbank, M, Haffajee, CI, and Kotilainen, P. 1979. A new electrode system for automated ECG monitoring. Computers in Cardiology, p. 285.
15. Oliver, GC, Nolle, FM, Wolff, GA, Cox, Jr., JR, Ambos, HD. 1971. Detection of premature ventricular contractions with a clinical system for monitoring electrocardiographic rhythms. Computers and Biomedical Research 4, pp. 523-541.
16. Feldman, CL, Hubelbank, M. and Amazeen, P. 1968. A real-time ectopic heart beat detection system. Proc., Conference on Engineering in Medicine and Biology.
17. Klein, MD, Baker, S, Feldman, CL, Hubelbank, M, Lane, B. 1977. A validation technique for computerized Holter tape processing system used in drug efficacy testing. Computers in Cardiology, pp. 199-201.

LONG-TERM AMBULATORY ELECTROCARDIOGRAPHIC RECORDING IN THE
DETERMINATION OF EFFICACY OF NEW ANTIARRHYTHMIC AGENTS

JOEL MORGANROTH, M.D.

Quality Control Measures in Long-Term Ambulatory Recordings

The adequacy of quality control is a basic tennant of
any research endeavor. The definition of antiarrhythmic
drug efficacy is based on quantitative data obtained by
long-term electrocardiographic recordings. Three important
elements of the quality control of such monitoring data
include: 1) the adequacy of the recording instruments and
the analyzer, 2) the quality of the data tape itself, and
3) the accuracy and repeatability of the analysis method.
Quality control of the recorder and the analysis system
requires careful attention to several technical components
to ensure adequate recorder speed, frequency response of
the instruments, synchronization of the ECG stylus, and
linearity of the amplifiers. The data tape itself must be
carefully scrutinized to determine that proper electrode
application was performed to avoid excessive motion artifact
and to ensure that the recorder was not faulty and that the
battery had adequate power.

Quality control in the analysis of quantitative data
is critically important in new antiarrhythmic drug research.
This begins with the proper analyst training and certifica-
tion. Details of the types of systems available for analysis
are covered elsewhere in the Symposium. To maintain quality
control one must be certain that known data tapes are employed
to 1) evaluate wave form analysis routines on the instrument
before data analysis commences, 2) that several 15-minute
real-time analyses of each data tape are performed to test
the software devices, 3) that the final data are verified

by a cardiologist for algebraeic and physiologic correctness, and 4) that repeatability and accuracy of the system be frequently measured. Repeatability is determined by re-introducing into the analysis system data tapes that have been previously analyzed. We recommend at least 2% of such tapes be reintroduced per month to determine adequate repeatability. Accuracy of the information must be obtained by introducing into the system "gold standard" data tapes which we define as those tapes analyzed in real-time in which the arrhythmia type and frequency have been verified by a cardiologist. Two percent of such tapes should be introduced into the analysis system every month to ensure data accuracy.

A standard quality control program for long-term ECG monitoring must be insured in new antiarrhythmic drug evalu-ation. Before a standard quality control system is developed and can be widely applied using a library of standardized long-term electrocardiographic data tapes, central dedicated research-oriented analysis services for long-term ECG moni-toring data should be utilized. These services must demon-strate adequate quality control measures for cooperative clinical research trials. Individual investigator or hospi-tal-oriented laboratory services without an adequate quality control program or a means of demonstrating accuracy and repeatability would be least desirable.

Definition of Antiarrhythmic Drug Efficacy by Long-Term Electrocardiographic Monitoring

The definition of antiarrhythmic drug efficacy in minimally symptomatic or asymptomatic patients has perplexed clinical investigators for many years. Prior determination of antiarrhythmic drug efficacy has used anecdotal judgment or the philosophical approach of Gallen which is embodied in the quote: "All those who drink from this remedy recover in a short time, except those in whom it does not help--who all die--therefore, it is obvious that it fails only in incurable cases". Today, with the availability of quantitative data obtained by long-term electrocardiographic ambulatory recordings and the application of biostatistics, a more precise and logical approach to the definition of antiarrhythmic drug efficacy is possible. One must not only consider how much the frequency of the ventricular premature complexes must change to define efficacy but whether the placebo and drug data are analyzed on an individual or a group basis.

Some[1] have advocated that individual patient drug and placebo control data should each be pooled so that group data form the basis of drug vs. placebo comparison. This process suffers from the fact that patients used in these studies are heterogeneous and, thus, grouping individual data will mask individual patient responses. Thus, recognition of adverse drug reactions (an increase in ventricular ectopic frequencies) and the type of patients or arrhythmias in which the antiarrhythmic drug appears to be most useful can be missed. We believe that the best approach to analysis of new antiarrhythmic drug data is to determine each individual patient's response on the new antiarrhythmic drug compared to placebo and to other antiarrhythmic agents. The percentage of individual patients studied who respond either with a reduction or an increase in the frequency of ventricular ectopy to a particular drug will define that agent's usefulness in terms of efficacy. Such an analysis of a new antiarrhythmic drug data will stem from placebo-controlled studies and from comparative efficacy studies using currently released antiarrhythmic agents as the comparison. Most of the currently released drugs for suppressing ventricular premature contractions appear to adequately decrease ventricular premature contractions in 50 to 75% of tested patients while they may increase ventricular premature contractions in as many as 5-20% of such patients.[2,3]

It was only a few years ago that the high frequency of spontaneous variability in ventricular premature contractions was documented in clinically stable patients. In 1978, we[4] studied 15 patients with unifocal ventricular premature complexes using serial 24-hour long-term electrocardiographic

monitoring over three successive days. In 1980, 21 patients
with complex ventricular arrhythmias (ventricular couplets
and tachycardia) who had undergone four 24-hour daily ambulatory ECG monitoring sessions were also reported.[5] The
age range of these 36 patients was 38-71 years and 83% were
men. They had a variety of clinical cardiac diagnoses, and
all had non-hemodynamically significant ventricular ectopy
even though many did have mild symptoms. This data was
subjected to an analysis of variance (ANOVA), a statistical
approach that allows for the isolation of the contribution
of each of many components to the variation in a complex
model. The raw data were transformed to natural logarithms
to attempt normality of homogeneous variance since the para-
metric ANOVA statistical approach was employed. A four-
factored nested ANOVA was used evaluating the extent of
variability "between" patients, days, 8-hour periods, and
hours. Initially, in this ANOVA analysis a pure model II
(random effects) approach was assumed accepting all factors
as independent and random. The sources of variation
determined in these individual patients between days, 8-hour
periods, and hours as shown in Table 1 demonstrates that
for unifocal ventricular premature contractions the "between
hour" variable was the primary source of variation. For
ventricular couplets and for ventricular tachycardia similar
results were obtained. When pooled data from all study
patients was used, the primary source of variance was the
patients themselves (Table 2), thus showing that the marked
degree of spontaneous variability not only was accounted
for by differences from hour to hour in premature complex
frequency but that the between individual patients source
of variation was also extremely large. We also determined
that patients with more frequent ventricular premature
complexes have less spontaneous variability that those with
a less frequency. Using this data we suggested quantitative
efficacy guidelines useful in comparing various durations of
ECG monitoring periods in patients with simple and complex
ventricular ectopy which would account for spontaneous

variability. Table 3 shows the percent reductions in ventricular premature complexes using various durations of ECG monitoring which would be required to overcome spontaneous variability in defining antiarrhythmic drug efficacy. Others [2,6,7] using pooled population data with different protocols in terms of statistical data analysis and time spacing of the Holter monitors have found similar results. The range of percent reduction required in ventricular premature beat frequency to define efficacy was from 73 to 90%.

With the realization that the largest source of variation in ventricular premature complex frequency in pooled patient data was between patients, the impact of spontaneous variability on ventricular premature contraction analysis using individual rather than pooled patient data became an important consideration. We have, therefore, conducted another study[8] in which we have evaluated 11 male patients with a mean age of 57 ± 8 years on no antiarrhythmic agents for at least 7 days with frequent but not hemodynamically significant ventricular ectopy who, on placebo, underwent long-term ambulatory ECG monitoring. These individuals had a spectrum of cardiac diagnoses: 6 had coronary artery disease, 2 had valvular heart disease, 1 had cardiomyopathy, and 2 had no structural heart disease. Analyzing individual rather than grouped patient data, the only factors in the ANOVA procedure would be "between" periods and hours. A fixed effects model ANOVA was, therefore, used assuming that the hourly effects should not change from day to day; i.e., they are not random. The hourly ventricular premature complexed frequencies were again transformed to logarithms to achieve normality and homogeneous variances. The ANOVA data demonstrated that the "between" patient variability was extremely large and, thus, the major cause of spontaneous variability in pooled patient data was due to patient heterogeneity. Using individual patient data analysis by a fixed model ANOVA on two or several 24-hour ECG monitorings on placebo, the individual patient's percentage reduction in ventricular ectopy to overcome spontaneous variability can be determined and used

as a definition of antiarrhythmic drug efficacy determined
for each individual (Table 4). Table 4 demonstrates that
some patients may require only a 15% reduction where others
may require up to an 80% reduction in their ventricular
arrhythmia frequencies to define antiarrhythmic drug efficacy. Thus, the use of individual patient data and not
estimates from pooled patient data will not impose a more
rigid standard for antiarrhythmic drug efficacy.

Other statistical methods can be used to determine
differences between treatment and control data such as the
non-parametric tests (e.g., ranked sum wilcoxin), but such
tests are usually less powerful and lack the ability to
separate the sources of variability.

Since the data also demonstrated a large degree of
spontaneous variability between study periods over time,
controlled placebo data should be collected over short
periods of time (less than one week) and at least two-to-
three control ECG recordings are required to determine the
degree of antiarrhythmic spontaneous variability. We
believe that patients should be included in studies who
demonstrate at least an average of 30 premature ventricular
complexes per hour for 24 hours. Both simple and complex
ventricular arrhythmias must be individually analyzed. This
frequency level identifies patients (with structural heart
disease) who have an increased risk of sudden death and a
degree of spontaneous variability in arrhythmia frequency
that is acceptable for statistical management.

In summary, we offer the following recommendations:

1. Individual patient response data should be used to
determine antiarrhythmic drug efficacy rather than pooled
patient data.

2. Efficacy definitions used to overcome the high rate
of spontaneous variability of ventricular premature complexes
should be determined using individual patient data rather
than pooled patient data.

3. New antiarrhythmic efficacy and tolerance studies
should be conducted over a short period of time (days to

weeks) due to the high rate of spontaneous variability in arrhythmia frequency. New antiarrhythmic agents should be compared first to placebo and then to a released antiarrhythmic agent. Subsequent long-term studies (over months) to define antiarrhythmic comparative drug efficacy and safety should consider the reintroduction of placebo periods at three-to-four monthly intervals again because of the high rate of ventricular ectopy spontaneous variability over time.

Table 1. Individual Patients - Sources of Variance

	VPCs	VC	VT
Between Days	23	12	12
Between 8-hour Periods	29	24	17
Between Hours	48	64	70

Table 2. Pooled Patient Data - Sources of Variance

	VPCs	VC	VT
Between Patient	66	65	46
Between Days	10	4	6
Between 8-hour Periods	8	8	10
Between Hours	16	23	38

Table 3. Percent Reduction Using Pooled Patient Data in VPC Frequency Required to Overcome Spontaneous Variability Using the Same Duration of Recording Before and After a New Antiarrhythmic Drug Regimen

Length of Recording	VPCs	VC	VT
12 hours	-89%	-82%	-71%
24 hours	-83%	-75%	-65%
72 hours	-65%	-55%	-45%

Table 4. Percent Reduction in Ventricular Ectopic Frequency Using Individual Not Pooled Data Required to Overcome Spontaneous Variability Comparing Two 24-Hour ECG Recordings Before and After Therapy

Patient #	VPCs	VC	VT
1	-27%	-21%	*
2	-22%	-36%	-59%
3	-39%	-24%	-20%
4	-18%	-35%	-13%
5	-58%	-16%	*
6	-82%	-60%	*
7	-30%	-63%	-73%
8	-22%	-37%	-18%
9	-35%	-46%	*
10	-40%	*	*
11	-27%	-33%	-29%

* = arrhythmia type not present

VPCs = ventricular premature contractions

VC = ventricular couplets

VT = ventricular tachycardia

REFERENCES

1. Winkle RA: Antiarrhythmic drug effect mimicked by spontaneous variability of ventricular ectopy. Circulation 57:1116, 1978.

2. Winkle RA, Gradman AH, Fitzgerald JW: Antiarrhythmic drug effect assessed from ventricular arrhythmia reduction in the ambulatory electrocardiogram and treadmill test: Comparison of propranolol, procainamide and quinidine. Am J Cardiol 42:473, 1978.

3. Velebit V, Podrid PJ, Graboys TB, Lown B: Aggravation of ventricular arrhythmia by antiarrhythmic drugs. Am J Cardiol 43:359, 1979.

4. Morganroth J, Michelson EL, Horowitz LN, Josephson ME, Pearlman AS, Dunkman WB: Limitations of routine long-term electrocardiographic monitoring to assess ventricular ectopic frequency. Circulation 58:408, 1978.

5. Michelson EL, Morganroth J: Spontaneous variability of complex ventricular arrhythmias detected by long-term electrocardiographic recording. Circulation 61:690, 1980.

6. Engler R, Ryan W, LeWinter M, et al: Assessment of long-term antiarrhythmic therapy: studies on the long-term efficacy and toxicity of tocainide. Am J Cardiol 43:612, 1979.

7. Sami M, Kraemer H, Harrison DC, Houston N, Shimasahi C, DeBusk RF: A new method for evaluating antiarrhythmic drug efficacy in individual patients. Circulation (in press) December 1980.

8. Morganroth J, Michelson EL: Precise determination of antiarrhythmic drug efficacy in individual patients based on individual rather than pooled patient data. Circulation 62:III:305, 1980 (abstract)

EVALUATION OF ANTIARRHYTHMIC DRUGS. SHOULD THE LOWN CLASSIFICATION BE USED
AS A MEASURE OF EFFICACY?

R.W.F. CAMPBELL

INTRODUCTION
      Current methods of identifying and developing drugs have provided a
wide range of therapies predominated by those with local anaesthetic activity.
Clinical investigations have shown these drugs to be effective in the control
of an individual patient's ventricular arrhythmias. Confirmation of antiarrhythmic activity of these agents in patient populations has come predominantly from observations of reduced ventricular ectopic complex frequency
with their use. Despite this undisputed efficacy, these drugs have performed
poorly preventing apparently arrhythmic deaths in high risk patient populations. In the management of patients after the acute phase of myocardial
infarction, prophylactic therapy with procainamide (1), diphenylhydantoin (2),
mexiletine (3) and aprindine (4), has usually reduced ventricular ectopic
frequency without affecting mortality. In similar studies, practolol (5)
and alprenolol (6) significantly reduced mortality although neither drug
would be considered as a powerful agent against ventricular arrhythmias.
In survivors of out-of-hospital ventricular fibrillation, a recent report
has suggested reduced mortality with the use of local anaesthetic antiarrhythmic drugs despite a disappointing action on ventricular ectopic complex
frequency (7). These apparent discrepancies may be explained in a variety
of ways. For instance, ventricular arrhythmias may be markers of risk in
some patients but death when it occurs is not arrhythmic. Most evidence
is to the contrary. Any other explanation must question the capabilities
of the drug to prevent fatal arrhythmias. In clinical practice it is rarely
feasible to test antiarrhythmic drugs directly against arrhythmias such
as ventricular fibrillation and we often rely upon their effect against
lesser arrhythmias. What potential flaws can we identify in our methods
of evaluating antiarrhythmic drugs? In clinical research of antiarrhythmic
drugs the Lown Classification of ventricular arrhythmias is the most widely
used system but it was not derived originally for this purpose. Introduced

in 1971 on the basis of ECG observations of patients following acute
myocardial infarction it became the foundation of arrhythmia management in
most coronary care units (8). Even in this context, the validity of the
Classification is now being challenged. Data from analyses of continuous
ECG recordings had suggested that its original premises do not hold
true (9, 10, 11). Whether or not it has a role in the management of patients
with acute myocardial infarction, it remains the only classification of
ventricular arrhythmias in widespread use. Is it justifiable to use this
system in the evaluation of antiarrhythmic therapy? The seductive
simplicity and flexibility of the original classification ensured its
survival, with modifications, to the present (12). These adaptations have
improved the scope and precision of the Classification which can now be
used to describe not only categories of ventricular arrhythmias but also
their incidence and prevalence. Nonetheless, difficulties arise in the
use of this Classification for the evaluation of antiarrhythmic therapy.
The basic problems are the misuse of the Classification and the fundamental
limitations of the Classification.

MISUSE OF THE LOWN CLASSIFICATION
Category Grouping
In many studies categories of the Lown Classification are grouped
together. The most common arrangement is separation of simple ventricular
arrhythmias (grades 0, 1 and 2) from "complex" or "malignant" ventricular
arrhythmias (grades 3, 4, and 5). Reducing the categories of ventricular
arrhythmias from six to two artificially increases the frequency of events
within these two categories. There is no data to support this practice and
indeed it is highly unlikely to be scientifically valid. For instance,
it implies that abolition of multiform ventricular ectopic complexes
(grade 3) has the same significance as abolition of ventricular tachycardia
(grade 4). This is methodologically unsound for antiarrhythmic drug
evaluation.
Hierarchical Use with Single Grade Allocation
A number of investigations have described patient's arrhythmias as
the highest grade achieved in the Lown Classification. Drug effectiveness
has been assessed by reduction of Lown Grades. Whilst acceptable for
Lown Grades 2, 1 and 0 which form part of a continuous spectrum of
frequency of single ventricular ectopic complexes, the practice is not

justified for Grades 5, 4b, 4a and 3. The gradation within the Classification was related originally to a suspected risk of developing ventricular fibrillation in acute myocardial infarction. Even in this context the validity of the grading is questionable. For antiarrhythmic drug evaluation it has no proven scientific basis. If the Lown Classification is used in a hierarchical manner, a patient exhibiting a single R-on-T ventricular ectopic complex beat (grade 5) who has no such early cycle ventricular ectopic complexes following therapy but who has now developed ventricular tachycardia (grade 4b), might be said to be benefited by therapy and therapy viewed as effective, although the deductions are unlikely to be true clinically. Hierarchical use with single grade allocation ignores lesser arrhythmias. Thus, a patient with occasional R-on-T ventricular ectopic complex (grade 5) with frequent ventricular tachycardia (grade 4b), will be accorded grade 5 status when in fact that arrhythmia may not be the one of true importance. The Lown Classification has now been modified to describe the prevalence and incidence of each of the grades as opposed to hierarchical use. Nonetheless, practical use differs in whether a run of ventricular tachycardia which contains multiform complexes and is R-on-T initiated should be entered in each of the categories 3, 4b, and 5.

Arrhythmia Definitions

Whilst some Lown Classification grades are very accurately defined (0, 1a, 1b, 2) other grades are less precise. Perhaps the most important problem concerns inter-ectopic timing to define the rate of ventricular ectopic complex salvos (grade 4b). Unspecified in the Lown Classification, this is left to individual investigators. However, even accredited reference sources fail to agree a universal definition of ventricular tachycardia (13-17). In some studies of drug evaluation, grade 4b encompasses all repetitive ventricular arrhythmias, whilst in others it includes only those above a certain predefined rate. An anomaly can arise if a lower limit is chosen for grade 4b. For example, with a lower rate limit of 120 per minute, a run of consecutive ventricular ectopic complexes of rate 90 per minute would not be accorded grade 4b status. This arrhythmia might be unreported in analysis or feature merely in assessing ventricular ectopic complex frequency (grades 0, 1, 2). By contrast grade 4a (ventricular ectopic complex pairs) status is usually conferred on any two consecutive ventricular ectopic complexes regardless of $R' - R'$ interval as this interval is rarely measured.

Similarly, the highest Lown Class – grade 5 – the early ventricular ectopic complex is imprecisely defined. This important arrhythmias is, perhaps, the most difficult of all to accurately describe and to measure from clinical records. Defined as a ventricular ectopic complex "abutting or interrupting the T wave" of the preceding QRS complex, it is subject to variations of interpretation which make inter-study comparisons difficult.

These potential problems of Lown Classification use can be overcome by: a) analysis of separate arrhythmia categories – a method recommended in the newer versions of the Classification, and

b) by investigators using precise arrhythmia definitions.

LIMITATION OF THE CLASSIFICATION

Ventricular Ectopic Complex Rates

On arbitrary criteria, the Lown Classification defines bands of ventricular ectopic complex frequency. Any ventricular ectopic complex rate greater than 30 per hour occupies the same grade (grade 2) although the total ventricular ectopic complex count for a particular 24 hours can be added as a subscript, the potential importance of ventricular ectopic complex rates greater than 30 per hour is denied. Continuous electrocardiographic analysis with computer assistance now permits accurate ventricular ectopic complex counts even at high rates. The facility of obtaining these data permits statistical definition of antiarrhythmic drug effect against single ventricular ectopic complexes. Continuous recordings also have emphasized the highly variable nature of ventricular ectopic complexes, particularly in patients with relatively low ventricular ectopic complex rates (18, 19). Yet it is at this lower end of the scale that the Lown rate limits are set. A modest reduction of ventricular ectopic rate from 33 per hour to 24 per hour moves the patient from Lown grade 2 to 1, and if a drug had been given, potentially exaggerates a very minor antiarrhythmic effect or reflects natural variation. By contrast, using total ventricular ectopic counts per unit of time, the pattern of natural variation can be statistically evaluated prior to administration of an antiarrhythmic drug. From the characteristics of the natural variation, a minimum level of arrhythmia suppression can be calculated which would define objectively a true antiarrhythmic drug action (20, 21).

Multiform Ventricular Ectopic Complexes

The potential importance of this subjectively defined arrhythmia is difficult to assess. It occupies a mid-place in the Lown Classification but is subject to marked interpretative variations. The ability to detect shape changes of ventricular ectopic complexes depends upon the frequency response in filtering of the ECG recording and play-back system, the sampling rate of a digital signal is being analysed, the number and position of ECG leads available for monitoring and the operator's interpretation. Perhaps in the past, too often a drug's action has been judged successful by its effect against multiform activity. The objective value of this arrhythmia category requires re-evaluation.

Repetitive Ventricular Arrhythmias

The Lown Classification obscures potentially important sub-divisions of repetitive ventricular arrhythmias. Ventricular ectopic pairs are graded as 4a regardless of R' - R' interval. Only the hourly frequency and maximal number of consecutive ventricular ectopic complexes are reported for grade 4b. Features of acceleration and decceleration are not categorized and no rate definition is employed except that used by the investigator. This will usually be a lower limit and no differentiation of ventricular tachycardia rate above this will be made. For example, grade 4b describes equally a ventricular tachyarrhythmia with a rate of 150 per minute and one of 220 per minute. In clinical practice, the rate of ventricular tachycardia is extremely important as faster rates may be more likely to degenerate to ventricular fibrillation, and even without this complication cardiac output is decreased with increasing arrhythmia rate. Repetitive ventricular arrhythmias are clinically important and in the evaluation of antiarrhythmic drugs the initial arrhythmia and its subsequent modification ought to be more clearly defined than is currently possible with the Lown Classification.

R-on-T Ventricular Ectopic Complexes

Although ventricular ectopic complexes may interrupt either sinus or ectopic T waves this grade is conventionally applied to the former. The latter circumstance is a feature of complex ventricular arrhythmia which may prove to be of prognostic importance but at present its significance is unknown. Extension of the concepts of antiarrhythmic drug evaluation might usefully examine the implications and drug modification of this feature.

RECOMMENDATIONS

An arrhythmia classification system, useful for the evaluation of antiarrhythmic drugs, should employ objective definitions, be suitable for statistical analysis, be applicable to continuous long-term ECG recordings and should provide accurate and detailed descriptions of each type of ventricular arrhythmia. It should identify both reduction and aggravation of arrhythmic events. The Lown Classification provides detailed information about some but not all of its grades. Misuse of the system and its limitations have been described already. Design of alternative arrhythmia classification systems is not difficult but each will have its own limitations. Table I presents an alternative system in which ventricular arrhythmias are first classified by their number of consecutive ventricular ectopic complexes. For example, a ventricular arrhythmia with three consecutive ventricular ectopic complexes would be a Class C arrhythmia. Next, the morphological features of each of the Classes is examined to determine "family" characteristics. In this example, single ventricular ectopic complexes (Class **A**), ventricular ectopic complex pairs (Class B – two consecutive complexes), and four consecutive ventricular ectopic complex arrhythmia (Class D) each have only one format.

# Consecutive VECs	# Families	R—T	Frequency /1000 NI QRS	Shortest $R^1 - R^1$
1 = A	A1	A1	$A1^{78-210}$	
2 = B	B1	B1	$B1^{12}$	$B1^{12}$ (720)
3 = C	C3	*C1 C2 C3	$*C1^3\ C2^{21}\ C3^4$	$*C1^3$ (240) $C2^{21}$ (310) $C3^4$ (310)
4 = D	D1	*D1	$*D1^1$	$*D1^1$ (240)
5 = E	E0	E0	E0	

120 mins

$A1^{78-210}$ $B1^{12}$ (720) $*C1^3$ (240) $C2^{21}$ (310) $C3^4$ (310) $*D1^1$ (240)

Table 1.

A proposed Classification of ventricular arrhythmias based on:
a) the number of consecutive VECs in each arrhythmia; b) morphological features; c) sinus – ectopic relationship; d) prevalence;
e) inter-ectopic relationships.

This does not exclude morphological variation within each arrhythmia but rather defines that, for instance, a four complex ventricular arrhythmia, when it occurs, is the same each time with respect to the sequence and shape of its constituent ventricular ectopic complexes. Three consecutive complex ventricular arrhythmias (Class C) in this example, displayed three different families designate C1, C2, and C3. Initiation of arrhythmias C1 and D1 was R' on sinus T and this feature is denoted by the asterisk. The frequency of each of the arrhthmias is presented as the number of occurrences per 1,000 normal QRS complexes. For example, the frequency of arrhythmia A1 is shown as varying between 78 and 210 per 1,000 normal QRS complexes. Finally, the shortest R' – R' interval contained within the arrhythmia is added in brackets. Thus, the shortest R' – R' interval of a ventricular ectopic complex pair (arrhythmia B1) was 720 msec and for arrhythmia C3 was 310 msec. If necessary, the arrhythmia descripters can be written in a way similar to that of the Lown Classification – defining the period of analysis time and the incidence, prevalence, morphologic features, sinus to ectopic relationship and interectopic relationships of each arrhythmia. This system would be as simple and flexible as the Lown Classification and would avoid some of that Classification's limitations. It is applicable to data obtained from computer-assisted analysis of long-term ECG recording. The results are well suited for statistical evaluation and a period of analysis time can be varied as appropriate from mere minutes to many hours.

Nevertheless, this system has faults. Measurement of R-on-T characteristics, accurate measurement of inter-ectopic intervals during rapid repetitive ventricular arrhythmias and the subjective nature of analysis of morphological features of ventricular arrhythmias remain problematic. No easy solution appears likely from conventional surface lead recordings alone but careful choice of monitoring leads can help minimise these difficulties. Moreoever, this system, by basing its major categorisation on the number of consecutive ventricular ectopic complexes reduces the importance of subjective interpretations. Potentially important drug effects such as alteration of sinus to ectopic relationships and inter-ectopic relationships could be addressed employing this system. Despite successful categorisation of ventricular arrhythmias, no classification system incorporates the many clinical indices of importance when assessing the efficacy of an antiarrhythmic drug. Other cardiac effects, on heart rate, conduction, atrial arrhythmias and ventricular performance and non-cardiac side effects and toxicity, must be assessed separately.

It is not the role of a ventricular arrhythmia classification system to assess the relative immediate and prognostic importance of a five consecutive ectopic complex arrhythmia with shortest R' — R' of 480 msec and a three consecutive ventricular ectopic complex arrhythmia with shortest R' — R' of 390 msec. Rather this is a problem for clinical research and for the evaluation of which the current Lown Classification is unsuitable.

The Lown Classification has an important part to play in the continuing evaluation of antiarrhythmic therapy. Recognised internationally, it has evolved and matured to keep place with expansion of knowledge of ventricular arrhythmias. However, it is easily misused and has limitations. It restricts examination of some characteristics of ventricular arrhythmias, hitherto ignored, which may be of major importance in defining drugs effective against one of our major health problems — arrhythmic death.

REFERENCES

1. Kosowsky BD, Taylor J, Lown B, Ritchie RF. 1973. Long term use of procainamide following acute myocardial infarction. Circulation, 47: 1204–10.
2. Collaborative Group. 1971. Phenytoin after recovery from myocardial infarction. Lancet, 2: 1055–7.
3. Chamberlain DA, Jewitt DE, Julian DG, Campbell RWF, Boyce DMcC, Shanks RG. 1980. Oral mexiletine in high risk patients following acute myocardial infarction. Lancet (in press).
4. Hugenholtz PG, Hagemeijer F, Lubsen J, Glazer B, Van Durme JP, Bogaert MG. 1978. One year follow-up in patients with persistent ventricular dysrhythmias after myocardial infarction treated with aprindine and placebo. In: Sandoe E, Julian DG, Bell J. eds. Management of Ventricular Tachycardia — Role of Mexiletine. Amsterdam, Excerpta Medica, pp 572–8.
5. A Multicentre International Study. 1978. Improvement in prognosis of myocardial infarction by long term adrenoreceptor blockade using practolol. Br Med J, 3: 735–40.
6. Wilhelmsson C, Vedin JA, Wilhelmsen L, Tibblin G, Werko L. 1974. Reduction of sudden deaths after myocardial infarction by treatment with alprenolol. Lancet, 2: 1157–9.
7. Myerburg RJ, Conde C, Sheps DS, Appel RA, Kiem I, Sung RJ, Castellanos A. 1979. Antiarrhythmic drug therapy in survivors of pre-hospital cardiac arrest: comparison of effects on chronic ventricular arrhythmias and recurrent cardiac arrest. Circulation, 59: 855–63.
8. Lown B, Wolf M. 1971. Approaches to sudden death from coronary heart disease. Circulation, 44: 130–42.
9. El-Sherif N, Myerburg RJ, Scherlag BJ, Befeler B, Aranda JM, Castellanos A, Lazzara R. 1976. Electrocardiographic antecedents of primary ventricular fibrillation. Br Heart J, 38: 415–22.

10. Lie KI, Wellens HJJ, Downar E, Durrer D. 1975. Observations on patients with primary ventricular fibrillation complicating acute myocardial infarction. Circulation, 52: 755-9.

11. Campbell RWF. 1980. Relation of ventricular arrhythmias to primary ventricular fibrillation. Br. Heart J, 43: 100.

12. Lown B, Podrid PJ, DeSilva RA, Graboys TB. 1980. Sudden cardiac death - management of the patient at risk. Curr Probl Cardiol, 12: 7-62.

13. Marriott HJL, Myerburg RJ. 1978. Recognition and treatment of cardiac arrhythmias and conduction disturbances. In: Hurst JW, Logue RB, Schlant RC, Wenger NK. eds. The Heart. New York, McGraw Hill Book Co. 4: 637-94.

14. Julian DG. 1978. Disorders of rate rhythm and conduction. In: Julian DG ed. Cardiology, 3rd ed. London, Bailliere Tindall.

15. Goldman MJ. 1976. The ventricular arrhythmias. In: Goldman MJ, ed. Principles of clinical electrocardiography. 9th ed. Los Altos, Lange Medical Publications.pp 244-60.

16. Fowler NO. 1977. Treatment of ventricular tachycardia. In: Fowler ND. ed. Cardiac Arrhythmias. 2nd ed. Hagestown, Harper and Row. pp 87-98.

17. Schamroth L. 1976. Ventricular rhythms. In: Schamroth L, ed. An introduction to electrocardiography, 5th ed. Oxford, Blackwell Scientific Publications, pp 145-61.

18. Winkle RA. 1978. Antiarrhythmic drug effect mimicked by spontaneous variability of ventricular ectopy. Circulation, 57: 1116-21.

19. Michelson EL, Morganroth J. 1980. Spontaneous variability of complex ventricular arrhythmias by long term electrocardiographic recordings. Circulation, 61: 690-95.

20. Sami M, Debusk R, Kraemer H, Houston N, Harrison DC. 1979. Assessment of antiarrhythmic drug effect: a new model to distinguish drug effect from spontaneous variations in premature ventricular contraction frequency. Circulation, 59/60: (Supple 2), 188 (abstract).

21. Morganroth J, Michelson EL, Horowitz LN, Josephson ME, Pearlman AS, Dunkman WB. 1978. Limitations of routine long term ambulatory electrocardiographic monitoring to assess ventricular ectopic frequency. Circulation, 58: 408-14.

GENERAL GROUP DISCUSSION: HOLTER MONITORING

Dr. Herling: We haven't addressed the question of what is the sudden death risk in individuals of VPC's. As you point out we've seen that you can suppress ectopy and still have the individual sustain sudden death. On the same token, we can prevent in the electrophysiology laboratory recurrent sustained ventricular tachycardia and still the patient may manifest VPC's and sudden death. Why are we spending so much time defining the arrhythmia on Holter monitoring?

Dr. Morganroth: Unfortunately, we can not address the question in this symposium of: what are the precise factors that predict sudden death and how do we prevent it. Before we are able to answer this question we will have to have effective antiarrhythmic agents that are well tolerated. The purpose of this symposium is to define the most efficient method to make available to investigators such new antiarrhythmic agents. Unfortunately that means using the definition for drug efficacy as the statistical elimination of VPC's. How much must they be suppressed and what the study design should be would be much more easily stated if we knew exactly the pathophysiology of sudden death and its inciting factors.

Dr. Herling: I apologize, I missed that point. There is one other question. In relation to the use of real time computerized telemetry arrhythmic analysis in the in-hospital setting, there is a delay in Holter monitoring whereby the tape has to be removed, processed and results have to come back. In the individual in whom one wants to treat on a daily basis and make adjustments even on an hourly basis, we've turned to this form of computerized analysis at our hospital. What have been your experiences with this and do you feel it is as valuable as Holter monitoring if one includes the recall provision that some of the most recent units now have?

Dr. Morganroth: Dr. Feldman will have more precise information about this system. I think however if you are studying patients with non-hemodynamically significant arrhythmias, the class that we are focusing on this afternoon, these patients are not necessary to hospitalize and I don't think it is a critical issue to know their hour to hour changes. Dr. Feldman, do you have some specific comments on telemetry versus Holter systems?

Dr. Feldman: Sure, my comments are really much more technical than medical, but I think it is certainly possible to obtain data either way. The parameters are easy to look at. The present state of the art of real time in hospital systems varies from system to system, but they are roughly comparable in that you can achieve with good technique approximately 95% sensitivity with roughly one false positive per 1000 beats. Recall features don't pick up the false negatives but they do give you the opportunity with a certain amount of effort to edit out and select out the false positives. From my point of view it may be worth giving away the 5% or so in the Holter system. You are trading away the time lag which may or may not be significant against a certain amount of precision.

Dr. Sami: If I heard you right you mentioned that in studying individual variability in patients we should discard those patients who have a tremendous degree of spontaneous variability and focus on those who tend to be more constant. Isn't the whole point of studying spontaneous variability to give advice to the clinician to what standard he can use for any patient he is going to select. If you don't make conclusions on all patients, then how can you tell the clinician to use a drug in that group.

Dr. Morganroth: Let me clarify the point that you are addressing. I did not mean to infer that patients who have a very high frequency of spontaneous variability in VPC's should not be studied. A patient for example with a high variability requiring a -82% depression efficacy is a perfectly appropriate patient for study. Here are occasional patients with which we have had experience that have a very high variability of arrhythmias and the arrhythmias will be gone for a week or two and then they will be back a month later with no clear change in their clinical condition. Patients in whom statistics cannot be performed are ones I would obviously exclude. My suggestion of using individual patients' placebo data to determine the definition of efficacy for each patient rather than for a group is only practical if you will for research studies. For the clinical cardiologist who uses Holter monitoring I think that the published efficacy criteria using grouped data should be continued to be used because of the necessary expense to be more precise. I think if you want to get

more precise in the definition of efficacy of antiarrhythmic agents one
can go to individual patient data.

Dr. Krikler: I'd like to put two questions, one to Dr. Campbell and one to
the panel generally and to elicit comments from others. To Dr. Campbell
I'd like to put the point that you have presented us with an elegant and
extremely plausible classification. Plausible in the sense that it seems
to offer great promise. Have you a correlation between the variables that
you described and a high incidence of sudden death? That is by using your
classification and expressing things in that way, can we segregate groups
of people and identify those who are likely to run into trouble from those
who are unlikely to run into trouble. This leads me to the question that
I would like to the panel and to people generally. How many lives have
been saved by ambulatory monitoring? To what extent are we being industri-
ous looking at new more interesting and more complex phenomenon and to what
extent can we define benefits that we have achieved and I speak as one who
is as guilty or as innocent as the rest.

Dr. Campbell: I have to say that I have no data about this. Perhaps in
the best traditions I made up that classification specifically to come
here. As I have lived with it, I have begun to wonder if perhaps I should
look formally at it. But, let me say that it was derived for a series of
purposes. First of all to show how relatively easy it is to think about
new arrhythmia classification. It is not that difficult. Finding one
that is as simple and flexible as the Lown classification is rather more
difficult but I think it is important the classification should also be
statistically valid, that you can abstract from it data which allow you
to apply statistics to arrhythmias for antiarrhythmic evaluation. Secondly
that it is easy to fill in from the results of 24 hour analysis. I think
so much of our tape analysis is now looking at arrhythmias graded on lengths
or numbers of ventricular ectopic complexes and on family classifications
of these. I have a little data regarding the definition of ventricular
tachycardia and as you know we have been looking at it very early on in
acute myocardial infarction. It is quite clear that the more stringent
the criteria you place upon the definition of ventricular tachycardia, the
greater are the risks to that individual patient. This is, when I say
risks and greater risks, I am not talking statistically just now, this is
an observation just at the moment. I think there is a lot of work that
needs to be done in refining the definition of ventricular tachycardia

that each one of us would accept at this meeting.

Dr. Kennedy: I wanted to make a comment on Dr. Sami's question before I ask mine. One of the things about the question of variability in individual patient in terms of its relative merit to a clinician is for him to identify the patient with a lot of variability versus the patient with little variability. That becomes a much more important determinant to the clinician out in the field when he has to be careful whether he needs 85% or 20% for efficacy. I want to go back to Dr. Campbell. With regards to the classification, a classification really has two purposes. One is perhaps its descriptive value and the second is its medical value. Its medical value in a diagnostic sense and its medical value in a prognostic sense. Dr. Lown did each of us a favor when he initially introduced his classification. It was in the coronary care unit at a time when we did not have quantitating devices and it gave us some predictive power on a patient with acute myocardial infarction. Then comes along the era of Holter technology, which allows us to quantitate VPC's and immediately we are confronted with a different ball game. The first thing that was apparent was we adopted quantitation and so we quantitated in terms of an hour and all the grades that occurred in an hour were there. I had a difficult choice in 1974, what do I do about unsustained v-tach versus short v-tach. What do I do about different rates. We started adding A' and B' for multiform v-couplets and multiform v-tach. We started looking at all those little features that you mentioned. What happens is there is no predictive power for those and that it overwhelms the reporting system with the technology we have at this time. So we have adopted the attitude that let's have a descriptive classification that at least in the United States is known. Let's present the drug company with data which we think is the state of the art with regards to various classes, classes per hour and give them the quantity. We can actually do just as you mentioned, quantity per class per hour. Now the problem is from a cost effective basis, we have to have an even balance between what we are seeking and what we are recording and that is about where we are. Now if we were to turn to some drug companies, it has only been on recent protocols that they even wanted the classifications quantitated. We provided that for 3 and 4 years and they didn't even look at it. They just looked at total frequency. There really is a problem with descriptive value, regulatory value what they are demanding and prognostic value. I don't know the answer. I agree that we need a more

universal classification, but I would suggest that maybe we should all
take a look at Lown's classification better and I know it can be adapted,
we adapted it internally to meet all the demands that you wanted. But
perhaps that would be an easier logic than trying to re-teach a new
system. I can tell by your talk you see its value universally. I would
like you to comment on that.

Dr. Campbell: Don't prejudge me there with that last remark. I used the
Lown classification as well and I think it does have value and its international acceptability is something important in itself. I think however,
its problems of misuse are very important. I think that the people who
use if fail to define the categories they are using properly. This is not
a reflection on the system itself, it is a reflection on the investigator.
I think it is also important to look at the situation as you think where
this was first introduced in acute myocardial infarction and see whether
it does apply in other disease states. Whatever you say about the Lown
classification we've already heard very eloquently to date the value of
using total ventricular ectopic counts at any unit of time which really
begins to make little sense of category 0, 1A, 1B and 2. My major difficulty with the system is in category 4B, repetitive arrhythmias and I do
sincerely believe that this category does require better definition in a
variety of disease states.

Dr. Kennedy: I accept those limitations, but I would call attention to one
value for class 1. It does reflect density within a unit time. If you
report it with the frequency per unit time, it becomes important.

Dr. Temple: If I understand the origins of your examination of individual
patients, it was because you found the group means unsatisfactory in that
they didn't tell you what heppened to individuals very well and therefore
the point was to learn about them. There is a problem arising, because you
now have your system so refined that you can define a class of patients
with minimal variability and detect drug effects of almost infinitesimal
size so you have no succeeded in being able to tell us that there is a true
10%, 5% or small reduction in VPC's and it is a little troubling to think
of that as the definition of effectiveness. It is the definition of non-
inertness so I guess I am just suggesting that there may be need to distinguish a method whether or not the drug did anything and nevertheless
to keep in mind some inevitably arbitrary measurements of what looks useful. Whether that should be 50% or 90% reduction or anything like that

is any bodies guess, but I think the two ideas need to be separated.

Dr. Morganroth: The real crux of your question I think is, how do we know what the best definition of efficacy should be unless we know whether or not it prevents sudden death. Unfortunately we can't answer that part of the question, so we have dropped back to try to answer how do we know that the drug is actually doing something at all to the patient's VPC frequency. I do not suspect that many patients will meet the -20% definition of efficacy. The 11 patients I mentioned is a very small sample and they are ones that we studied retrospectively having had frequent experience with them. I believe yet we have to test this on new data, is that the patients in whom we would accept an efficacy definition of only -20% would be a samll number because to have such a small percent reduction requires those patients to have quite constant VPC's. The vast majority of patients are still going to require 70-80% reduction.

Dr. Feldman: May I address the question too. I think Dr. Temple that the other answer to that question perhaps is that we are really concerned with ultimately is the effect of the drug on reduction of sudden death not reduction of VPC's. There of course very little information on the relationship of VPC frequency to sudden death and about the biggest is probably the HIP data which suggests that there is probably a break at around 10 per hour. If that is correct, then there is every argument in favor of looking at, of not weighing the data by those patients who might have 2000 or 3000 VPC's per hour just because they are in bigemini but are not at higher risk for sudden death than the patient who is having 10 or 20 per hour.

Dr. Morganroth: It is an experience that patients with 10 to 30 PVC's per hour are going to have a much greater degree of spontaneous variability than those that are over 1000 per hour. I get to in this discussion in terms of guidelines, what should be the minimum percent believe the minimum number of VPC's per hour that should allow patients into studies could be as low as 10 but more practically would be between 30 and 60 per hour per 24 hours.

Dr. Temple: It's pretty easy to determine whether an antiarrhythmic drug is active or inert and group means can give you the answer just as well as looking at individuals although they don't give you information on individuals. I guess I would say that even we don't know what percent reduction is valuable, the best that we may be able to do now is to describe this as precisely as possible and to tell what sort of percent reduction various drugs have and then explore to see whether that is of any use. Now to me the major usefulness of examining a person's individual variability is that it allows you to carry out a more sophisticated test. As you pointed out if you have a very regular patient, you will be able to say yes indeed it did with a very small reduction. You can also test more stringent hypotheses if you have the patient well characterized. You can say did it cause a 50% reduction.

Dr. Winkle: I think that in the discussion today, we probably really missed the true value of Holter monitoring in evaluating new drugs. I think it is because we are hung up on this word efficacy when in effect we would all have to agree we are really measuring pharmacologic effect. I think that the true value of Holter monitoring in the use of evaluating new drugs is in general doing a lot of recordings in a few patients and examining the pharmacologic effects of the drug over a wide range of doses, defining concentration response relationships, looking for evidence that the pharmacologic effect might be due to metabolites in trying to correlate changes in coupling interval of PVC's with suppression and trying to look at relaships between heart rate and arrhythmia frequency and how drugs might affect this. We are one step removed from the ultimate rhythm that we want to treat and I don't think that just by saying we have an 83% reduction will really help us understand what drugs are doing to sudden death. We have all fallen into this trap of the numbers game, but I think that the true value of these things is to look at when is the onset of effect, when is the offset of the effect and sort of view it as a dog lab model, realizing that it is removed from what we really want to study but that it can give us useful information about the pharmacology of the drug and then hope that by understanding that, we'll eventually be able to understand what these drugs do and to have a better insight. I think that to just get hung up on some percent reduction of arrhythmias really side steps the true issue which I know you don't want to talk about today. We can't deny the fact that we don't know what PVC suppression means. I have one comment for Dr. Campbell and that is before we are stuck with the Campbell classification, I don't fully understand why we can't have something that is in plain English. It is very simple to say that somebody had 2000 PVC's in 24 hours and there were 22 runs and 4 pairs and R on T beats and every physician can understand that and I don't understand why we have to have all these fancy classification systems. Why can't we just say what is there?

Dr. Campbell: I accept that as well. It comes a little back to Dr. Kennedy's point as well that how far do you go in characterizing these things. If you are happy in talking about there were 22 runs and it didn't matter if one of the runs was 8 consecutive beats at a rate of 150/minute and another was 5 consecutive beats at a rate of 220/minute, then I would agree with you. In plain English it becomes a very unwieldy sort of thing.

Dr. Morganroth: I think Dr. Winkle that you raised an important issue and I want to ask Dr. Temple. Clinical cooperative trials that are instituted for new antiarrhythmic drugs in this country are preformed to define drug efficacy in terms of showing that the drug is not inert, using Dr. Temple's phrasing. In such trials it seems to me that you have to have like in any other clinical trial a statistical protocol and method which includes how many patients are to be studied and what the quantitation of the data is going to be to define "efficacy" since none of us are using sudden death as an endpoint in these initial studies on new antiarrhythmic agents. I agree with you if we could for example use a patient as we use an animal model in the laboratory in that we study him intensively with frequent Holter monitoring that we could detect the onset of action of a new drug, etc. We would learn a tremendous amount about a new drug in an individual patient. I ask Dr. Temple whether he believes it is sufficient to study a few patients well to determine whether a drug is working. We are not talking about safety issues.

Dr. Temple: It doesn't take a great many patients or studies to show that a drug is an effective antiarrhythmic. I think the bulk of the exposure really is to determine what its hazards are and those trials need to be control trials because this is a population that tends to have things happen to them and you won't really know how to interpret adverse events unless you have some sort of control group. I'll be saying this a little more later. It is a little hard for us to define what our criteria for effectiveness are because there really have been only two new drug applications for antiarrhythmic drugs since procainamide so there is not a whole lot of tract record and only one of those has been approved and as I'll described briefly the effectiveness data that there were and there were really two major multicenter studies and that is all. Not a tremendous amount of it. They did use Holter monitoring of the most simple kind

just total VPC's; it was an older day and that was all we could get. It
seems to me that there are some concerns with isolating studies in a very
small number of people and that you won't in that way be able to have at
least some representation from the various kinds of people that exist.
I've heard Don Harrison describe the various subgroups of people with
antiarrhythmias that ought to be included and if you just count up the subgroups alone and have one of each, you have gotten quite a substantial
study, so I do think you have to have some information in various kinds
of arrhythmias of different etiologies and things like that. We certainly
don't know that those things make a whole lot of difference but they might
and you don't know until you look but the number of people in effectiveness
studies doesn't really have to be that large.

Dr. Morganroth: As you point out when you add all the patients together
from different etiologic groups you're going to end up with not just a study
of 10 or 20 patients.

Dr. Temple: People tell us that those are significant things to look at
and in matters like that it is people here who are the experts we have to
listen to.

Dr. Morganroth: Obviously we would not have to discuss this at any length
if we knew what were the important factors in genesis of sudden death,
but we don't so these issues become important.

Dr. Temple: Obviously people have pointed out to us and we know ourselves
we are not asking the right questions about antiarrhythmics. There is
the grossest kind of assumption that drugs that reduce VPC's may in some
cases prevent what is really hurting people.

Dr. Podrid: I obviously have a vested interest in defending somewhat the
Lown system. I think that there are several important things that were
overlooked in Dr. Campbell's presentation. Number 1, the system has been
modified and is flexible enough to have been modified and there has been
one oversight that you have made which does in fact answer the criticisms
of the system in which you incorporated into your hypothetical system and
that is that there is a series of subscripts in the Lown system which you
overlooked and which do in fact deal with number of cycles in a run of
ventricular tachycardia, maximum number of cycles per hour, the rate of
the ventricular tachycardia, whether it is accelerating or de-accelerating
all factors which as you correctly pointed out we feel are also extremely important in categorizing patients at greater or lesser risk for the

end point of sudden death. The other point to be made is that there is
not as much I think concensus of categories as you pointed out because in
fact the one example that you showed of a run of ventricular tachycardia
initiated by an early ventricular premature beat would be both at least in
the way our technicians were trained in reading the Holter monitors and
we would deal with it in both grade 5 and 4B. The other point is that the
system was initially developed and was trying to categorize patients in
terms of who is at greatest risk for sudden death and that was originally
in the setting of the coronary care unit and now more recnelty applied to
Holter monitoring out patients and when looked at that way, I do have the
data to support the fact that when looked at that way, the Lown system is
valid. When you compare before and after drug in an individual patient,
elimination of certain forms of follow-up of patients it does make a difference and therefore when the Lown system is applied in that way it still
does hold up. I think the Lown system when used appropriately and with
subscripts which fit into your model as well does categorize patients at
higher or lesser risk and does point out differences in terms of drug
therapy. I think that you can't escape from the fact that there are certain characteristics of ventricular premature beats whether they be complex, frequent or whatever, that do in fact impart the risk to the patient
and I don't think it is appropriate to ignore that fact when dealing with
the Lown system or any other grading system because the end point is after
all the prevention of sudden death and not just suppression of VPC's.

Dr. Morgranroth: Why a grading system at all, why not just state what the
patient has in a quantitative way instead of arbitrarily defining it by a
system?

Dr. Podrid: From my point of view, the Holter monitor provides the clinician with a magnitude of data which he cannot fathom because it is present-
ing him with a lot of data some of which is important and some isn't and
I don't think he has a conception what is or is not important and that is
one problem. With this magnitude of data I think it has to be categorized
in a way where what is important stands out and where it is a simple short
hand to utilize to evaluate the efficacy of drugs and also to evaluate
what patient requires therapy and what patient does not. I think there
is a need for simple short hand for people to utilize.

Dr. Campbell: I think you probably missed the point that I did allude to
the fact that the Lown classification does use subscripts and superscripts

etc. It may be a factor of the change of this system that you are using a Lown classification system that I don't know about, but of the published series, the only scripts which help us further define ventricular tachycardia are the maximum length of the ventricular tachycardia, the only rate definition is the one that is set by the investigator himself. But clearly you could make modifications and my system was a classification and not a grading system. You yourself have said that we don't know what is important and I think until we do know what is important it is impossible to grade arrhythmias. Whether or not the grading system works in the context of acute myocardial infarction, it may not work when we are investigating patientw with arrhythmia due to cardiomyopathy or in the late ischemic phases.

Dr. Hai: Like Dr. Podrid being a student of Dr. Bernard Lown, I had many of the same remarkes to be made as Dr. Kennedy and Dr. Podrid did. I wondered about one other thing. In the last 5 years because of the deficiencies you pointed out very well in the Lown classification, we made certain changes and we have been using this modified system now for five years. Like Dr. Podrid says a formula is only a short hand, a short way of expressing a large amount of data and we found it so useful that most of our information in our registers regarding the information on patients is recorded in the form of formulas and we have not found it necessary to go back to the original description.

Dr. Campbell: I think it is amazing the amount of energy that goes into further modifying the Lown classification. Can we still call it the Lown classification? It bears little resemblance to what it originally started out. The second point is that there are still problems of the subjective category, multiform ventricular ectopic complexes. It occupies an important part in that classification but I submit to you that it is highly subjective, it depends upon the number of leads being analyzed, the skill of the investigator, the frequency of responses as we have had of the instruments, the sampling rates if it is a computer, etc.

Dr. Hai: This is all true, but subjective information has to be expressed briefly in some way and this is one way to express it.

Dr. Lazzara: I have just two questions. The first for Dr. Morganroth. The variability that you have pointed out to us and we are grateful to you for it, is a nuisance in analyzing Holters, rather than an unwanted nuisance, have you looked at whether it in itself is predictable. That

in those patients who are more variable may not be the more susceptible
to sudden death or has that been looked at in your lab?

Dr. Morganroth: Unfortunately most of the studies that I have shown you
occurred in patients with non-hemodynamic significant ventricular arrhythmias in whom the sudden death prevalence is relatively low being at most
a few percent per year so we don't have any prospective data to answer your
question.

Dr. Lazzara: My question takes off an a point made by Dr. Feldman and that
is, do you think the relationship between PVC frequency and incidence of
sudden death is a direct continuous one or do you think it is a step relationship on or off at a break point of 10 or 20. Is there a finite low
incidence below a certain rate and a finite incidence above a certain
rate. The second part is if there is a direct continuous relationship
that you feel the data indicates, what do you think is a possible predictive power added on to correct for frequency of subclassification
features we are discussing.

Dr. Feldman: I guess it is not so much a matter of opinion, there is some
data the predictive power of any of these VPC type measures is greater
than 0 and less than 1. I don't know what the data are really. There are
none of these measures that are perfect, none that are inconsequential,
whether it is frequency or complexity or multiformity or R on T.

Dr. Lazzara: But are the others corrected for frequency is really my
question. Do you think there is a direct relationship between frequency
and the incidence of sudden death and secondly, corrected for frequency,
what do the others add in your estimation roughly.

Dr. Feldman: No to the first question and apparently if the HIP data and
some of the other data is to be believed, quite a lot.

Dr. Campbell: The predictive power of changes depending upon what condition
we are talking about for a normal individuals VEC's rate mean nothing, in
acute ischemia they are different and so I think the answer to that is it
depends upon the situation.

Dr. Lazzara: Is it a direct one or a step?

Dr. Campbell: In conditions in which VEC's have a predictive aspect for
sudden death, I believe that the quality of the VEC's means more than just
the rate of the VEC's that are occurring.

Dr. Morganroth: I also agree with these comments.

Dr. Wenger: I do have some concern that the comments that have been made

here today by the investigators have been inappropriately transmitted to
the clinical community and it does relate to the grading system. Because
we talk about grade and severity as if it were uniform for all persons and
have not emphasized as has only been done once or twice that our predictive
power is indeed for the ischemic or cardiomyopathic ventricle and I think
some of the concern with the details of the grading system may be inapproriate
in other disease states and I think it is incumbant upon the investigators
to identify that the grading in many disease states or normals may be totally irrelevant as far as prognosis is concerned.

Dr. Morganroth: I think that is correct. I would like to conclude this
session by the same comments that were used to conclude the morning session. This afternoon we again see we have a great deal to learn. Obviously
if we knew more from basic science about the predictors and specific mechanisms
of sudden cardiac death, a lot of these questions wouldn't arise. Hopefully
we will be able to get agetns in which clinical cardiologists will be
able to test whether or not they do affect the problem of sudden cardiac
death but until then we are going to be left with defining a mechanism that
is going to allow for release of new agents to test the basic hypothesis.

D.M. KRIKLER

My introductory comments must trespass on aspects of the
subsequent session, and points to be made by Dr Zipes.
Though the British regulatory authorities appear to be
somewhat more flexible than the Food and Drug Administration,
this is certainly not at the cost of quality in trials, and
permission to investigate an antiarrhythmic agent requires
full justification with sound documentation. If one can make
out a case, assessment of response electrophysiologically to
single intravenous injections is naturally easiest to obtain;
and this can be done before long-term data on toxicity by
the oral route has been obtained. This brings us immediately
face to face with the question of extrapolation from what is
seen with intravenous studies, in terms of termination of
episodes and prevention of reinitiation, and the likelihood
that this will point to oral efficacy or not. But this is
by no means the whole story; for we may well encounter a
preparation introduced for a different reason, that seems
to have antiarrhythmic activity, and where the action of the
agent given orally differs conspicuously from that seen when
it is administered intravenously. While in the case of
verapamil, with which we are amply experienced, some
correlation between oral and intravenous use is indeed
feasible, this seems by no means to be the case with
amiodarone. This latter agent, given intravenously,
appears to have membrane stabilizing properties, but orally
it acts slowly, by prolonging refractoriness. Indeed its

slow onset and protracted duration of action, even after
discontinuation of therapy, plays havoc with the best-
designed crossover trials. It may even interfere with a
double-blind study; characteristic electrocardiographic
changes may occur with this and other agents, and give the
observer a strong clue to the nature of the agent being
tested. QT prolongation with amiodarone and slowing of the
sinus rate with beta-adrenergic blockers are but two
examples. Unless the investigator is provided with very
full information, he may run into unexpected pitfalls on
this account; and in any case, certain drug actions will
prohibit complete objectivity: we would all like our trials
to be carried out in the best scientific fashion but we have
to balance the limits that may be imposed in design by
recalling the ways in which drug responses may confound us.

My final point does, as I indicated at the start of
these brief comments, impinge on the next session but I
must once again stress a difficulty that we have encountered.
While some drug trials may show that intravenous use
confidently enables prediction of oral response, this is by
no means invariable. A broad generalization of the
contrary seems, however, to be appropriate: we rarely find
good response to a product given orally where its use
intravenously has been unsuccessful. We all naturally wish
to avoid the old-fashioned approach of rough and ready trial
and error, but we do ourselves and our patients potential
harm unless we realise the current limitations of the study
designs available to us. We must always remain alert to
the possibility that explanations other than those we start
with may turn out to be correct, and likewise remember that
many of the antiarrhythmic agents that we are now using or
evaluating started their therapeutic life in the treatment
of angina.

PROPOSED NEW MEANS OF EVALUATING ANTI-ARRHYTHMIC DRUGS

ROBERT TEMPLE, M.D., DIRECTOR
DIVISION OF CARDIO-RENAL DRUG PRODUCTS
BUREAU OF DRUGS, FOOD AND DRUG ADMINISTRATION

It is often helpful to a manufacturer hoping to market a new drug to look at what FDA has required in the past. In the case of anti-arrhythmic agents, however, the past is not too helpful, as we have approved only one anti-arrhythmic agent (other than propranolol), disopyramide, in the last decade and that was in 1977, providing relatively little guidance to a manufacturer in 1980.

Our published anti-arrhythmic guidelines provide considerable help for the phase I and II (clinical pharmacology) phases of drug development, emphasizing close monitoring of patients and avoidance of complicated patients (multiple drugs, other diseases) and endangered patients (recent myocardial infarction, digitalis toxicity, life-threatening arrhythmias) until effectiveness in simpler situations is established. For later phase II and phase III studies, the guidelines recommend controlled comparisons, including long-term studies, with placebo or standard agents. Attempts to correlate plasma level with anti-arrhythmic activity are urged. In these guidelines, developed some years ago, there is relatively little discussion of the criteria that should be used to assess effectiveness, although continuous ECG monitoring methods are recommended. This Guideline, like all FDA guidelines, is undergoing a process of revision and updating.

Studies submitted for disopyramide, the only oral anti-arrhythmic, other than propranolol, approved in the last decade, followed the guidelines pretty well, and included the following:

1. A double-blind controlled 8-week comparison of disopyramide 150 mg q.i.d. with quinidine sulfate 325 mg q.i.d. using Holter monitoring. The two drugs had equivalent effects on ventricular premature beats, both reducing them about 90%, on average.

2. A single-blind placebo-drug-placebo study (4-8-4 weeks) of disopyramide 100-200 mg q.i.d., also using Holter monitoring, showing a roughly 75% reduction in ventricular premature beat rate compared to initial placebo period (60% reduction compared to the final placebo period).

3. Nine-month safety study in normal volunteers comparing disopyramide 200 mg q.i.d. and placebo.

We thus had quite satisfactory evidence that disopyramide could reduce the frequency of ventricular premature beats. We did not have, in retrospect, as Harrison has shown, a complete definition of the dose-blood level response. We also did not expect the drug to be as significant a cause of heart failure and shock as it seems to be[1], although we were aware of its negative inotropic effect and recommended against use in poorly compensated heart failure in initial labeling. We had numerous isolated reports of short- and long-term dramatic effectiveness in drug resistant patients with life-threatening arrhythmias, but no controlled trials involving such patients. Under the circumstances of the studies (mainly the limitations then existing on Holter analysis) we had little good data on suppression of couplets, ventricular tachycardia, etc., i.e. the arrhythmias that probably matter most. We had no direct comparison of disopyramide with procainamide and, of course, no comparison with other investigational agents with respect to either safety or effectiveness.

In dealing with subsequent drugs we have asked for similar kinds of studies, improved, naturally, by the better Holter monitoring and analysis now available, and manufacturers, familiar with our Anti-arrhythmic Drugs Guideline, have usually provided the hemodynamic, electrophysiologic, and pharmacokinetic studies that are the groundwork for later trials. It is worth asking, however, whether this is the best we can do. We have been very impressed recently by the large number of patients with severe arrhythmias (presumably the real target population for these agents) who are left out of formal trials and instead are studied under "emergency" protocols.

We have generally allowed anti-arrhythmics to be used under emergency protocols for treatment of life-threatening arrhythmias and, increasingly, have tried to make the emergency protocols reasonably tight. Nonetheless, they have major deficiencies, insofar as providing useful data in support of an NDA or useful information for publication purposes: patient follow-up is often incomplete; the evaluation of drug effect typically varies from investigator to investigator; and, of course, there is no concurrent control group. Our experience so far is that it is difficult to rely to any great extent on data from these emergency drug uses in considering a new drug application.

Nonetheless, emergency uses can constitute most of the patient exposure to the drug. A recent new drug application consisted of over 600 patients given an anti-arrhythmic agent under an emergency protocol and less than 100 treated in controlled studies. Is there some way this huge emergency experience can be made more useful by introducing some elements of a controlled clinical trial? Perhaps there is.

The following proposal is more a prospectus than a protocol, a sketch of a study design that would evaluate anti-arrhythmic agents in a practice setting, utilizing the skill and experience of sophisticated cardiologists to select alternative therapies, and introducing limited random assignment of selected drugs and a standardized follow up. Financial aspects of the proposal have not been considered at all, but as the patients would all be receiving usual medical treatment, it seems possible that most costs could be borne by the usual sources of patient care funding.

Table 1 provides an outline of the proposed overall study plan.

1. STUDY SETTING

There are now many cardiogists who use some systematic means of choosing optimal anti-arrhythmic therapy, such as programmed ventricular stimulation,[2] or repeated exercise testing and continuous ECG monitoring[3]. Often these investigators seek at the outset to find more than one agent that appears acceptable, in case the initial agent chosen induces an adverse effect or proves unsatisfactory. An initial search for more than one agent is an essential feature of the study plan, and the participating investigators must be willing to do this.

Most complex or resistant arrhythmia patients seem to find their way to major referral centers in which an investigator has access to many investigational anti-arrhythmic agents under his own, or drug manufacturers', IND's.

2. PATIENT POPULATION

The patients included in emergency protocols typically have very severe, life-threatening arrhythmias, often involving a history of ventricular tachycardia and/or fibrillation requiring resuscitation or recurrent ventricular tachycardia despite anti-arrhythmic therapy, and

these patients constitute the proposed study population. It is these
patients who are most likely to be subjected to the rigors, and sometimes
dangers, of rigorous screening of anti-arrhythmic agents by means of
programmed stimulation or repeated exercise studies.

It seems possible that other criteria could be used to identify
high-risk patients (e.g., patient without a history of ventricular
tachycardia or fibrillation but who seem to be in a high risk group
because of hemodynamic abnormalities, multi-focal ectopy, etc.) but the
above seem most obvious. Patients should probably be stratified into
higher and lower risk patients as well as possible.

3. INVESTIGATIONAL AGENTS

All marketed drugs and a specified group of investigational agents
would be candidate drugs. The investigational drugs would include all
those with reasonably well-defined clinical pharmacology and some evidence
of anti-arrhythmic activity in a short-term controlled trial, e.g., the
sort of trial currently being carried out by Oates, Woosley and coworkers at Vanderbilt[4], in which an open titration period is used to
select apparent drug responders, the response is verified in a short
randomized, crossover trial, and finally long-term treatment of responders
is begun.

4. PROCEDURE

After patients are identified and documented as eligible, they
would be put through an anti-arrhythmic drug assessment procedure
selected by the investigator on the basis of his clinical judgement.
This could be programmed ventricular stimulation, exercise stimulation,
or some other acceptable method. The objective of the assessment would

be to identify at least two drugs that the clinician would be willing to use in long-term therapy because they appear to suppress the arrhythmia adequately. Some investigators might proceed beyond this and find additional acceptable choices. The order of screening various drugs probably need not be specified, but if there were drugs of particular interest, and if most investigators tended to stop after finding two acceptable drugs, the drugs of interest could be evaluated faster if they were used at the beginning of the screening process. If screening of single drugs did not lead to successful suppression, it might be necessary also to screen promising combinations.

Some drugs might be reserved for non-responders to other agents because of toxicity (e.g. aprindine) and some drugs would not be screened in particular patients (e.g., disopyramide would not be given to patients with heart failure or prostatic disease). This could be left to investigators or defined in the protocol.

When at least two agents were identified, the investigator would contact the study center and the drug assignment would be made randomly at that time. The center could randomize in a balanced or unbalanced fashion, depending on whether there were particular drugs of interest.

Patients would then be placed on therapy and monitored in a defined way.

5. ENDPOINTS

Therapy would be assessed with respect to at least the following:

a. Survival

b. Recurrence of non-fatal arrhythmias

c. Tolerability of therapy, i.e., do patients continue on the regimen.

d. Side effects of treatment.

6. STUDY CENTER AND ORGANIZATION

The organizing center must be defined, as must its funding. Its duties would be to develop a complete protocol, including acceptable screening procedures, minimum needed follow-up, and reporting forms, and to choose the investigational drugs that would be randomized. It would also have to consider the ultimate analysis of the data, obviously a formidable task under the study conditions defined, and decide whether and to what extent stratification should be used (As noted above, stratification according to severity seems warranted).

Presumably all willing drug manufacturers would include the common emergency protocol in their IND's and list the participating investigators.

7. WHY BOTHER?

This suggested protocol is designed to interfere as little as possible with current practices in treating life-threatening arrhythmias. It therefore makes use of screening procedures in common, and growing, use and leaves to the investigator the choice of drugs, asking only that he find at least two acceptable drugs.

Unlike the current emergency protocols, however, the proposed one will provide a controlled comparison regimen for each drug, so that the events that follow drug use can be interpreted. At present, we simply have no way of knowing whether to attribute to drugs such events as death, apparent worsening of the arrhythmia, development of acute myocardial infarction, new laboratory abnormalities, or the host of symptoms that occur in such sick patients, because we do not know what the background rate of the events is in this population.

146

Moreover, certain questions are difficult to answer in the usual short-term controlled trial setting, such as how important it is to have a b.i.d. rather than a t.i.d. or q.i.d. regimen or the extent to which symptoms such as dizziness interfere with treatment. The more "natural" setting of the proposed trial may be a better place to assess such questions.

Finally, the study would, by virtue of the large numbers of patients involved, and its multi-drug design, allow comparisons among many drugs simultaneously, the sort of comparison that probably could never be made in any other way if individual drug vs individual drug trials were depended upon.

Obviously, the feasibility of this suggested trial design must be examined closely; so far as I know nothing like it has been tried before. But the anti-arrhythmic field seems unique in having a large variety of agents with different properties under study and in tending to exclude most of the best candidates for therapy from formal controlled trials. Perhaps the suggested approach can define the advantages and disadvantages of the various agents in the patients who need them most.

REFERENCES

1. Podrid PJ, Schoenberger A, Lown B. Congestive heart failure caused by oral disopyramide. N Eng J Med. 1980; 302:614-617.
2. Ruskin JN, DiMarco JP, Garan H. Out of hospital cardiac arrest: electrophysiologic observations and selection of long-term anti-arrhythmic therapy. N Eng J Med. 1980; 303:607-613.
3. Lown B. Sudden cardiac death: the major challenge confronting contemporary cardiology. Am J Cardiol. 1979; 43:315-328.
4. Roden DM, Steel SB, Higgins SB, Mayol RF, Cammans RE, Oates JA, Woosley RL. Total suppression of ventricular arrhythmias by encainide: pharmacodinetic and electrocardiographic characteristics. N Engl J Med. 1980; 302:877-882.

Table I

Study Outline

1. Investigators

   Referral centers/physicians who use some systematic method to select anti-arrhythmic therapy.

2. Patients

   a. People with unequivocally life-threatening arrhythmias, particularly those who have been resuscitated after spontaneous ventricular tachycardia or ventricular fibrillation.

   b. Lesser arrhythmias if there is evidence of potential for VT, VF (e.g., development on programmed stimulation).

3. Investigational Agents

   All marketed anti-arrhythmic agents and selected investigational drugs, i.e., those with sufficient clinical pharmacologic and early effectiveness data.

4. Procedure

   a. Evaluate qualification for entry

   b. Use clinical assessment (e.g., programmed ventricular stimulation or exercise tolerance) to choose at least two acceptable drugs.

   c. Randomized assignment among acceptable drugs by study center.

5. Endpoints

   a. Survival

   b. Recurrent non-fatal arrhythmias

   c. Tolerability of therapy

   d. Side effects

PARALLEL OR CROSSOVER DESIGNS IN EVALUATION OF ANTIARRHYTHMIC THERAPY

HELENA CHMURA KRAEMER
STANFORD UNIVERSITY

The crucial considerations in selecting a research design to test drug efficacy include:

1. Validity: If the drug is not effective, is the chance of a false positive finding less than 5% or 1%?

2. Power Efficiency: If the drug is effective, is the chance of a true positive finding reasonably high?

3. Feasibility and Cost: Can the design be reasonably implemented in the research situation for which it is proposed?

4. Clinical Value: Does the design yield information sufficient in extent and quality to serve as a basis for evaluation of the clinical value of the drug?

Obviously, if a design is unfeasible, it cannot be considered. Consequently, for evaluation of the clinical effect of coronary artery bypass grafts one would never consider crossover design. Of the statistical criteria, however, validity is paramount. It is for this reason that controlled, randomized, double-blind clinical trials are uniformly preferred. This is not because clinical trials lacking these characteristics necessarily yield false results, but because experience has shown that the risk of questionable results in such trials is unacceptably high. Since the value of controlled, randomized, double-blind trials is not here in question, this statement may seem obvious and trivial. However, it merits stating since when, in further consideration, this same principle is invoked, it will be in a context less palatable to many researchers.

150

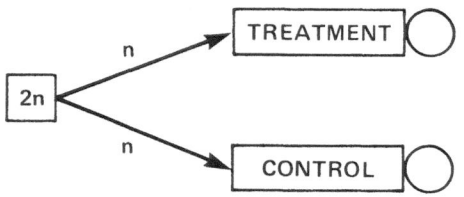

DEGREES OF FREEDOM: 2(n—1)

NONCENTRALITY PARAMETER:

$$\sqrt{\frac{n}{2}} \quad \frac{\Delta}{\sqrt{\sigma_{\alpha}^2 + \sigma_{\beta}^2 + \sigma_{\epsilon}^2}}$$

NUMBER OF OBSERVATIONS: 2n

The Simple Parallel Design is one (Figure 1) in which half the subjects are randomly assigned to the treatment group and half to the control group, with response observed only at the end of the treatment period. For purposes of discussion, it will be assumed that response data is of the kind that a t-test would be appropriate to test group differences. The results, however, apply whatever the test procedure.

The simple parallel design is an easily implemented, valid and very common design in all medical research areas. The power of the test comparing responses of the drug and control groups depends to a minor extent on the degrees of freedom of the test, to a major extent on the so-called non-centrality parameter (Cohen, 1969):

$$NCP = \sqrt{\frac{n}{2}} \quad \sqrt{\frac{\Delta}{\sigma_{\alpha}^2 + \sigma_{\beta}^2 + \sigma_{\epsilon}^2}}$$

where Δ is the true mean response difference in the two groups,
σ_α^2 is variance due to individual differences in baseline response;
σ_β^2 is variance due to individual differences in responsiveness to intervention;
σ_ϵ^2 is spontaneous variability of response and error of treatment.
Since every possible source of variability is here present, this design
generally yields little power: clinically significant differences are
likely to be found statistically significant only when very large sample sizes
are used.

Nevertheless, in some types of clinical trials this design is the only
feasible one: i.e., when observation itself produces a permanent effect
(e.g., surgical biopsy) or when observation of response entails invasive,
risky or costly procedures (e.g., heart catheterization). Neither situation
pertains in evaluating response to antiarrhythmic therapy. Because of the
lack of power of this design and the lack of clinically necessary information
(since this design yields no information on individual response), in this
context, this design has low appeal.

FIGURE 2: **EXTENDED PARALLEL DESIGN**

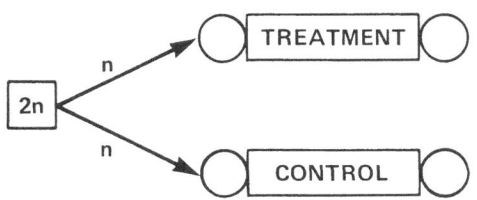

DEGREES OF FREEDOM: 2(n−1)

NONCENTRALITY PARAMETERS:

$$\sqrt{\frac{n}{2}} \ \frac{\Delta}{\sqrt{\sigma_\beta^2 + 2\sigma_\epsilon^2}}$$

NUMBER OF OBSERVATIONS: 4n

The <u>Extended Parallel Design</u> (Figure 2) differs from the simple
parallel design only in that response is observed both before and after
treatment and change is compared between treatment and control groups.

This, too, is a valid design. In arrhythmia research it is easily
implemented since evaluation of response either on exercise tests or using
ambulatory monitors does not entail highly invasive, risky, costly or
uncomfortable procedures. Certainly, it contains more information of clinical
value than does the simple parallel design, since individual as well as group
response can be evaluated. Whether or not this design is more powerful
depends, in general, on the relative size of the variance due to individual
differences at baseline and that due to nonreproducibility of response, since
in this case:

$$NCP = \sqrt{\frac{n}{2}} \, \frac{\Delta}{\sqrt{\sigma_\alpha^2 + 2\sigma_\varepsilon^2}}$$

One, in essence, exchanges the effect of individual differences in baseline
response for an additional effect of inconsistency or error.

There are two drawbacks to this design. First is the fact that
individual response to drug is observed on only half the available subjects.
It is certainly true that clinical value would be enhanced if this information
were available for all the subjects. Second, and more important, is the fact
that informed consent regulations require that patients be told that each
has a 50:50 chance of being a control group subject. Frequently this
exacerbates recruitment problems. Furthermore, if improved response is not
rapidly perceived by the patient, the patient may identify him/herself as a
control group patient (frequently incorrectly), and prematurely drop out of
the study. The net effect is that the power promised by theoretical
considerations often cannot be realized in practice because of such recruitment
and retention problems.

FIGURE 3: **SIMPLE CROSSOVER DESIGN**

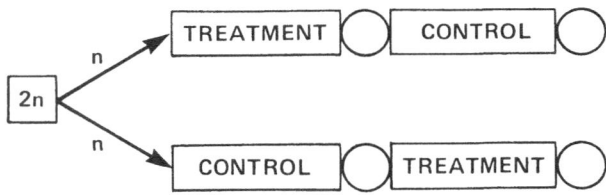

DEGREES OF FREEDOM: 2n−1

NONCENTRALITY PARAMETER:

$$\sqrt{2n}\ \ \frac{\Delta^*}{\sqrt{\sigma_\beta^2 + 2\sigma_\epsilon^2}}$$

NUMBER OF OBSERVATIONS: 4n

With the <u>Simple Crossover Design</u> (Figure 3), many such problems are alleviated. Each subject now is given both drug and placebo in random order, and is so informed in the consent form. Recruitment is eased; drop-out is minimized. Since each patient is now exposed to active treatment, the clinical value of the data is enhanced. The sources of variance are exactly the same as in the extended parallel design, all of which promises that this design should yield more power.

The difficulty is that this design, like non-randomized, uncontrolled or unblinded studies, is very likely to yield invalid results. The basic assumption underlying validity is that after intercourse, virginity is restored. When a patient is exposed to an intervention, the effects of that intervention may persist for some time after the intervention is discontinued. In the case of a drug intervention, this period can far exceed the half-life of the drug, since the effect may persist not only for pharmacological reasons, but for other physiological or psychological reasons as well. Accordingly, many biostatisticians (Brown, 1980) now take the intransigent stand of uniformly recommending against the use of a simple crossover in any clinical trials for the same reason they recommend against non-randomized, non-controlled or non-blinded studies.

EXTENDED CROSSOVER DESIGN

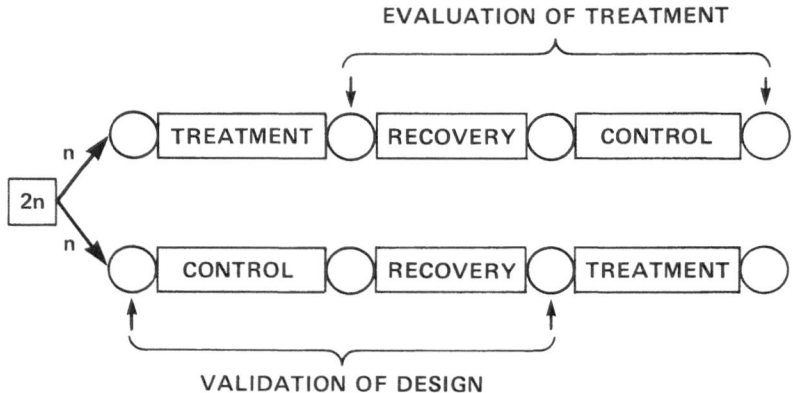

DEGREES OF FREEDOM: 2n−1

NONCENTRALITY PARAMETER:

$$\sqrt{2n}\ \frac{\Delta}{\sqrt{\sigma_\beta^2 + 2\sigma_\epsilon^2}}$$

NUMBER OF OBSERVATIONS: 8n

However, consider the Extended Crossover (Figure 4). Here, an extended period on placebo is interspersed between the first and second treatment period and observations of baseline response error to each period are added here. Before implementing the crossover, it is verified that patients' responses have indeed returned to the baseline level. If this does not occur, the design is simply analyzed as an extended parallel design. It has been our experience in antiarrhythmic drug trials (Sami, et. al., in press) that the patient _does_ return to baseline in short order. Thus, in this design one has all the advantages of the crossover, plus that of assurance of validity.

The power of this procedure is determined by its degrees of freedom (2n − 1) and

$$NCP = \sqrt{2n}\ \sqrt{\frac{\Delta}{\sigma_\alpha^2 + 2\sigma_\epsilon^2}}$$

and is generally greater than that of the extended parallel design, at least in this context.

Specific recommendations were requested and my first applies to all clinical trials: under no circumstances do I recommend use of simple crossover designs.

Since this is undoubtedly the most controversial aspect of this presentation, it deserves some elaboration. A biostatistical consultation is comparable to that with a physician. If a patient 100 pounds overweight, smoking three packs of cigarettes a day, drinking a quart of whiskey, exercising little and in a high pressure job were to consult a competent clinician, the clinician would likely feel it his professional responsibility to warn of the risks incurred in this life style. The patient is free to disregard the warning. If he does so because he feels himself personally immune to such risks whatever the cost may be to others, or on the adivce of another physician who simply ignores the evidence, this is irresponsibility on the part of both the patient and that physician. On the other hand, the patient may ignore the advice on the advice of another physician who is thoroughly knowledgeable of the reported risks and the evidence supporting their identification, but is honestly unconvinced or knows of special circumstances pertinent to this patient which suggests this course. If they choose not to try to amend the patient's life style, they should instead monitor closely for any untoward developments with the intention to coping early and efficiently with any such developments.

Many biostatisticians, including many more experienced and competent than I, disagree with my stance on crossover designs. If researchers by themselves, or on the advice of these biostatisticians, elect to use crossover design, and do so responsibly, taking every precaution in design to minimize the problems, to check their data for the possibility of such problems, and, if necessary, to discard the crossover in order to analyze the first half of the data as a simple parallel design, I can but wish them the best of luck. I myself would not choose this course.

Which of the other designs is to be preferred is context-specific. The following analysis is based on use of Morgenroth's (1978) published data for estimation of variances, and is for a one-tailed 5% level of significance t-test (Kraemer, 1979).

156

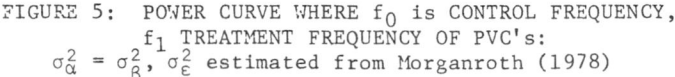

FIGURE 5: POWER CURVE WHERE f_0 is CONTROL FREQUENCY,
f_1 TREATMENT FREQUENCY OF PVC's:
$\sigma_\alpha^2 = \sigma_\beta^2$, σ_ε^2 estimated from Morganroth (1978)

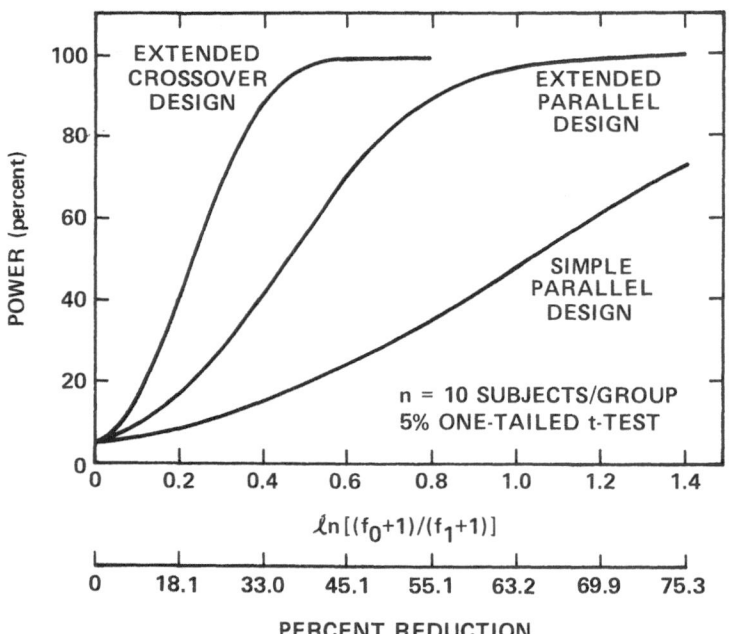

The simple parallel design is the least costly procedure, but it yields very little power and very little clinically useful information. I would view use of this design here as false economy.

The extended parallel design at its best (i.e., with no recruitment or retention difficulty) is little less powerful than the extended crossover design but takes less than half the time and half the number of observations per subject. If the cost or risk of observation were great or if the time necessary to establish drug effect were long, I would recommend this design. In studies of response to antarrhythmic therapy, however, cost or risk of observation is small and response to therapy rapidly established. Therefore, here I would recommend the extended crossover both for its increased power, for its facilitation of recruitment and retention, and for the scope of clinical information it can provide.

REFERENCES

1. Brown, W.B., Jr. The cross-over experiment for clinical trials. Biometrics, 1980, 36, 69-79.
2. Cohen, J. Statistical Power Analysis for the Behavioral Sciences. New York: Academic Press, 1969.
3. Kraemer, H.C. A central t approximation to the noncentral t distribution. Technometrics, 1979, 21(3), 357-360.
4. Morganroth, J., Michelson, E.L., Horowitz, L.N., Josephson, M.E., Pearlman, A.S., and Dunkman, W.B. Limitations of routine long-term electrocardiographic monitoring to assess ventricular ectopic frequency. Circulation, 1978, 58(3), 408-414.
5. Sami, M., DeBusk, R.F., Harrison, D.C., Houston, N. and Shemasaki, C. A new method for evaluating antiarrhythmic drug efficacy in individual patients. Circulation, in press.

GENERAL GROUP DISCUSSION: STUDY DESIGNS: CHRONIC PATIENTS

Dr. Krikler: The approach that Dr. Temple has proposed seems to the
audience to be a reasonable and appropriate one and whether this should
be married with Dr. Kraemer's rather tight method of analyzing and in-
suring validity should be addressed.   Before doing that may I just
utter a couple of words about our own approach to some aspects of antiarrhythmic evaluation and I am referring in particular to evaluation of
agents for paroxysmal reciprocating atrioventricular tachycardias
either reciprocating within the atrioventricular junction or using the
atrioventricular node and an accessory pathway.   We tend to use during
the electrophysiological study, two drugs which we consider appropriate:
one an index drug that we have learned from experience and from acceptance at least on the other side of the Atlantic as being valid and
compare it with another drug, perhaps comparing to calcium antagonists.
Having chosen what we believe to be the most suitable substance, we give
it orally over a period of another three days and repeat the study,
except of course when we are dealing with something like amiodarone
where its intravenous assessment is difficult, we would then tend to
use all treatment on well defined grounds and repeat the testing for
provocation of arrhythmia up to three months later.   The rules are
ideal, but the illnesses and drugs sometimes require us to bend and be
more flexible but we need people like Dr. Kraemer to make sure that we
are not being so flexible that we are being overwhelmed by non-evidence.
In the case of amiodarone I think it would be impossible to carry out a
trial that would respect what you have so clearly laid on.   We do have
a number of other aspects that could be built into the sort of study
that has been proposed by Dr. Temple.   The electrophysiologic study
should involve at that time an assessment of drugs and their likely
benefit so that one has an additional factor.   Indeed, we are comparing

the patients on the drugs to which they did not respond favorably when
these were given intravenously to see whether we can get useful information and we do get surprises from time to time. Can I take the chairman's privilege of handling things in a different fashion in asking
other people toput points to our panel and to the audience. I see
Jean Pierre Van Durme and wonder if he would like to comment on some of
the ways in which antiarrhythmic drugs have been accessed in Europe,
where we have accumulated data that does not necessarily answer the
strict criteria that one may need. Perhaps all that we can say is
that the drugs are now worthy of consideration on this side of the Atlantic. Dr. Van Durme who is from Belgium made just the same sort of
remarks regarding the necessity for proper controlled trials with a
number of agents and I think it might be worthwhile hearing about them.
Dr. Van Durme: The one thing we are more and more puzzled about is
the ideal trial to assess a new drug should be. I am more thinking of
chronic assessment of antiarrhythmic treatment and how to find a design
which mimicks the clinical practice. On one hand we are faced with the
choice of finding a very complicated design implying double blind
cross-over randomized study where we compare different groups and
different treatment periods in the same patients and on the other hand
the use of trials similar to clinical practice. If you ask me to give
my impression right from the start I note that I am still carrying out
the trial in which I am comparing different drugs with the placebo
period in highly selected patients of whom I know for having used them
in other trials that indeed they do have high frequent runs of ectopic
beats that these ectopic beats have an almost ideal small spontaneous
variability. I am almost certain what the trial is going to show but
my major concern actually is how I can extrapolate from the clinical
design of the clinical trial to the clinical practice.
Dr. Krikler: These proceedings are open to the floor and the panel.
Dr. Wyndham: A question to Dr. Kraemer. This question probably
reflects my unfamiliarity with statistical techniques, but what do you
do about two categories of patients? Patients who have to be withdrawn
from study because of unacceptable toxicity and secondly patients who
because of some very real pressing clinical reason have to have added a
specific therapy during study which may effect the parameters that you
are trying to study. For example, somebody who is in a study of an

antiarrhythmic agent who for reasons of heart failure has to have digitalis added to the regimen during the study: how do you handle such
patients?

Dr. Kraemer: That is a very valid question and a difficult one to
answer. It should also include the patient who simply drops out. In
all of these situations, the same principle holds for analyzing all of
the patients whether they drop out for any reason. You cannot just drop
the patient out of the study, because that would be tantemount to
assuming that this is a random selection of patients and particularly
if they drop because they are not random. You have to use as a piece
of information from that subject that is not prejudicial to the validity
of the design so that if you have a good end point, for example, total
suppression of PVC's or 80% suppression of PVC's or a dichotomous end
point, you would assume those patients all failed and it would not
matter in your analysis whether that patient were in the control or in
the treatment period.

Dr. Krikler: I wonder if Dr. Wyndham is satisfied that with answer
because I would like to express a little skepticism. You haven't told
us precisely what you are going to do. Are you going to bring in more
patients? Are you going to put that patient aside and report the information you have obtained? Are you going to say that the addition of
digitalis may have invalidated the results that you have seen? We are
dealing with a type of illness that requires continuing therapeutic and
continuing diagnostic interventions and the longer you go on the
muddier it may become. How can you help us to retain clarity?

Dr. Kraemer: If the patient is removed from the protocol, that includes
the administration of another drug that may be effective it does muddy
the patient's response to the extent that any response that you may see
may be due to the additional drug and not to the original drug. That
patient has to be treated exactly as if he dropped out of the study at
that point. What you actually do with the data, you use in analysis may
make it least favorable to the drug you have under test. You protect
yourself against getting significant findings and so if you have a
success-failure end point, that patient becomes a failure immediately.
I am waffling on one portion of the answer and that is that everything
that I have talked about has the same quantitative response and it is
certainly less clear how you handle quantitative responses. Success-

failure is much easier to handle.

Dr. Krikler: It certainly seems to me that the chances of getting a nice clean result in this particular population is going to become more and more complex because of the design. Perhaps that is one of Dr. Wyndham's concerns.

Dr. Wyndham: This is a fairly common problem in all kinds of clinical trials. It is certainly a problem in the trials that have tried to look at the role of coronary bypass grafting in patients with coronary disease. When patients come out of a medical group and cross over into a surgical group, it is very difficult to know how to deal with those patients. If you throw them out it lessens the beneficial results of surgery, and if you retain them then it lessens the beneficial results of medical therapy. Either way it seems there is a catch 22.

Dr. Kraemer: The only statistical protection I am offering you is that you are not going to report false positive results. You may be reporting false negative results. The scientific approach to this is to protect the significance level and you will lose the power if you don't keep the design clean.

Dr. Krikler: And we may therefore have a better era introduced as a result.

Dr. Temple: If I understand Dr. Kraemer, you are advocating what would certainly be the most conservative possible conclusion. In an intervention study, for example, if you lost 5 patients, you would assume they died?

Dr. Kraemer: That's right.

Dr. Temple: Isn't it possible in at least some situations you will have enough information within the study to know whether certain kinds of concomitant therapy appeared to influence the results and could some way take care of it that way?

Dr. Kraemer: You have opened a door that I would really like to explore. It depends on whether you have designed to protect yourself against this. For example, one of the neat kinds of designs is not one of the ones I have talked about here, the one in which you monitor PVC frequency every second day during the whole treatment period. That gives you partial information on the patient's response and you could use the slope over time to characterize the responsive therapy and if that patient should drop out somewhat earlier than the end of the trial, you

still have a data point for that patient. You will notice that in all
the designs used here, the end point is necessary to define the response.
Regression of slopes analysis is a very protective way of keeping the
power going without losing significance level.

Dr. Copan: I would like to ask Dr. Temple, I think that studies designed
to study antiarrhythmic drugs used for life-threatening arrhythmias need
to be different from the criteria we select to use drugs for prophylaxis
against sudden death or even for treating non-life-threatening arrhythmias. Patients with life-threatening arrhythmias certainly are monitored carefully and are willing to take major risks with using toxic
drugs, even drugs that could make their arrhythmias worse. They're
monitored carefully. If we take those studies and find those drugs
effective, and then put them on the market and they start being used to
prevent sudden death, or to treat non-life-threatening arrhythmias, then
I think we run the risk of making people sicker or causing major toxic
effects which may be riskier than what we are trying to prevent. Several
panelists in the past have alluded to a 5 to 10% incidence of making
arrhythmias worse with some of these drugs. I think in patients who are
not critically ill to start with I think we need some way of being sure
that the risk of a major toxic effect 2 years down the road is not
greater than the risk of sudden cardiac death in somebody with 30 VPB's
per hour.

Dr. Temple: I think I agree with that but I am not sure what the
question is.

Dr. Copan: Does the FDA have any way of dealing with this problem?

Dr. Temple: On the contrary. Drugs are tested principally in control
trials in people who are not all that sick as a general rule. For one
thing, if they are very sick, no one wants to put them on a placebo
for any period of time. That seems reasonable. There is no way that
we now know of determining what the ultimate outcome is going to be.
Even for drugs that we know reduce mortality over a period of time like
anti-hypertensive drugs, we really don't know if some lipid effect of
one or another of them is going to make the curve bend the other way 15
years from now. That is just not known. I'm still not quite sure what
you were asking. Were you worried that if the kind of study I proposed
were done, we would learn that drugs were useful in potentially fatal
arrhythmias and then people would use them for non-fatal arrhythmias?

I think the problem is the other way around. We now know that they suppress things whose significance we don't know and we really know very little about what they do with the really severe arrhythmias.

Dr. Morganroth: I have a question for Dr. Kraemer. The question is if you have a simple cross-over study in which the initial placebo frequency of ventricular arrhythmias is re-established in the intervening period between the treatment and control period it would seem to me that a simple cross-over study with these criteria would be the best design. Do you agree with this thinking?

Dr. Kraemer: There is nothing wrong with your thinking if you have in your design the fact that the VPC's will return to word baseline. There is a statistical test in a cross-over effect. If you go ahead and you do your simple cross-over, run that test and it comes out showing no signs of significance, there are certain rules on determining it you are then in power to go ahead to use the regular analysis. If you find that you do have a significant cross-over effect, your fall back position is to throw out the cross-over and analyze it as a simple parallel design with a very low power. You can of course push the wash-out period until you actually return the patient to baseline.

Dr. Morganroth: We always in fact recommend that one measures more than one Holter monitoring window for each period. Usually we recommend at least a couple or three periods. Clinically patients in these studies are so heterogeneous that one of the problems of using the parallel design is that you would have to use many more patients to match the degree of heterogeneity of each group. This becomes a very difficult protocol.

Dr. Kraemer: You are exactly right. It is not restricted to cardiology. In psychiatry it is much worse.

Dr. Morganroth: My question to Dr. Temple is do you agree that the cross-over design with the safeguards noted is the best design for this sort of studies?

Dr. Kraemer: The worry about it is that you are uncertain when you start the trial exactly what the investment is. This is a planning thing. You are going to have to put in a proposal presumably and cast it out and if you put in a proposal following your logic, you may end up not requesting enough money because you will have to invest far more time and personnel costs.

Dr. Morganroth: That can be dealt with but in terms of the validity of the study designs, Dr. Temple, do you agree with that, or do you see a problem?

Dr. Temple: I thought I understood Dr. Kraemer's distinctions, but if I understand what Dr. Morganroth is saying, he is talking about a good baseline measurement followed by randomization to one treatment, followed by a second as lengthy as necessary baseline period. An intervening period sometimes called a wash out followed by another treatment period. That I thought is what you put up as an extended cross-over.

Dr. Kraemer: That is an extended cross-over.

Dr. Temple: Sure, I don't think anybody thinks that if you can manage that it is a problem. That is a good design. What we are more accustomed to seeing was really a simple cross-over in which there is no extended wash-out and there is just an assumption that the patient hasn't changed and that is often a problem you have to resort to looking for period effects. This design gives you a little more information about each individual patient but with what you are doing during baseline periods to access patient's individual variability, I think a parallel design is probably very close in what it tells you clinically to completing the cross-over.

Dr. Morganroth: What about the problem of heterogeneity of the patient group study?

Dr. Temple: You go and define a patient's inherent variability and you then look to see if the intervention, whether it is drug or placebo moves the patient beyond what would be expected spontaneously. However variable they are, they are not expected in the absence of an active agent to change beyond their predictive variability. If they do, you have shown that the drug is doing something about as well as if you then cross back. The reasons for that are peculiar because you are almost turning that initial baseline period into part of a cross over now. It is a more complex situation than any simple design.

Dr. Kraemer: Your comment about controlling for the heterogeneity of the subjects. If in fact this were a major factor, the difference between the power curves for the extended parallel and for the extended cross-over would be very different, they aren't. It is true that the extended cross over has somewhat more power but not as much as you might expect. My point of view is that you are satisfied with the clinical information that comes from the parallel design, save the money.

Dr. Krikler: On that economic note, shall we move on to Dr. Winkle?

Dr. Winkle: I would like to ask a simple question I guess, except it relates to most of the people in the audience and that is do most investigators of antiarrhythmic drugs in patients who have symptomatic, hemodynamic impairment from their arrhythmias feel it is acceptable to look at two effective drugs, the investigational drug, plus another drug in order to satisfy Dr. Temple's requirements for this organized design in emergency situations?

Dr. Temple: They are all investigational. The two drugs you pick could even be two investigational drugs under the current situation. You need at least two things to compare. They could be one marketed, one non-marketed, two marketed or two non-marketed.

Dr. Winkle: I think that it is actually a noble attempt to encourage a decent evaluation in the sick patient subgroup because this clearly is a subgroup where we can help the patients and there are certainly a lot of these patients out there. I think we have gone astray in assuming that we can't get any useful information out of these patients. I think it is difficult, but certainly the experiences of the past have not led us too far astray, I think an excellent example is the work of Dr. Rosenbaum with amiodarone. A very astute clinician did some very nice observational research in patients and came up with observations that have been verified by any one of a number of other people around the world. I think where we have gone astray in making these drugs available to any doctor in the country who wants to phone in and get them. What we end up with instead of one experienced investigator who has the opportunity to use a drug in 30, 40 or 50 patients is with 40 or 50 physicians who use it in one patient. I think a situation where for example you give Norpace to a patient and he goes into cardiogenic shock is if you only treat one patient, you might say that is just what happened to him. If you treat 30 or 40 and 30% of them go into cardiogenic shock, then it starts to ring a bell. I will be discussing this more tomorrow, but I think that we can do studies in these patients. I don't like your ideal that we find two effective drugs in the same patient. The reason is for instance if you are doing electrophysiologic testing and if you find that drug A works, then you have to do another study of drug A on oral therapy to show that it works and then you might have to study

B, C and D to finally get a drug that worked. Then you have to study drug E with another electrophysiologic study on oral therapy. I think these studies are too psychologically disturbing to both the investigator and the patient and certainly have the potential for great risk. I would be unwilling to go beyond finding the first drug. However, since clearly our choice of drugs is usually random, I would be more than happy to pick out several drugs that I wanted to study and call a center and have them tell me which one to randomly try as the first drug and then you could compare the drugs in that manner, very much to what Dr. Krikler said. I just would like to adopt a philosophy that we can get important information out of this very sick subgroup; it is a group of patients that will benefit from treatment and I would even propose that we don't reserve this treatment for those who failed all standard drugs. I think that once we know a drug works reasonably well then it is appropriate to use that as a first line agent. As Dr. Van Durme said, we want to mimick the clinical situation and we certainly, for instance when Norpace came out physicians started using it right away as the first drug they'd try. I think that if we have a drug that is reasonable decent, we should go ahead and try it in these patients fairly early in their course. Then we could even potentially compare it to a standard drug such as quinidine or procainamide.

Dr. Krikler: Would you like to respond Dr. Temple?

Dr. Temple: Let me make a couple of things clear. First, my suggestion does not require that people fail on other therapy. It requires only that they have a life-threatening arrhythmia as evidenced by a previous cardiac arrest or multiple episodes of ventricular tachycardia. The screening process would include both standard agents and investigational agents so you would have an opportunity to compare the two and there is no suggestion that the standard agent should be tried first. Second, it seems to me there are some good reasons to try to run people through a fair number of drugs until more than one is found. For a start, as you point out, it is unpleasant to be put through these procedures. One of the things you want to know is whether one or another of these drugs is more likely to succeed and it might turn out that drug A is regularly successful at suppressing programmed stimulation whereas drug B is successful only 20% of the time. You won't really learn that unless you have several experiences in each patient because there won't be anything to compare them to. The other reason for finding at least two agents is that it

controls exclusions in a way. One of th things you worry about in
fundamentally uncontrolled trials is whether there are selection criteria
that you really don't know about and that maybe even the investigator doesn't
know about. What requiring a choice of two drugs does is that at least it
says in the direct comparisons that are made, everybody is being thrown in to
the extent that they are being put into a trial in which some randomization
is permitted. I don't think you can actually get comparisons between standard agents, or between marketed agents and new agents or between one new
agent and another unless you have some way of pouring them all into the
same pool from approximately the same setting. If you simply have one
person doing 50 tests under his own rules for selection and then doing
another 30, the two groups can be very different. It is very hard to
control the identity of the patient population under those circumstances.
Dr. Winkle: You may have misunderstood what I said. I am saying that
one investigator randomly selects drugs. We are talking about the
difference between parallel and cross over. You are saying cross over,
I'm saying parallel. The other point is that the only test of efficacy
is what happens to the patient long-term so we can truly only test one
drug per patient, and so for that reason the failure may be death.
Dr. Temple: What will you compare with that?
Dr. Winkle: I'm saying you have a patient with ventricular tachycardia
and you call up a center in Washington and they say quinidine, or they
say encainide or they say amiodarone and whatever they say you put the
patient on and then you'll have a whole series of parallel evaluations
of a drug, rather than requiring that you find two drugs that work in
each patient, which I find unacceptable.
Dr. Temple: Let me explain the origin of that. It is my assumption
that if someone with a patient of this kind were tole put him on amiodarone for example, and the clinician didn't exert some selection over
the drug, he would find that unacceptable. For example, in a center
that does it, the clinician would want to say that this drug suppressed
the response to programmed stimulation and he won't even consider if that
is his method using a drug that doesn't succeed in doing that. The ideal
is that he can use his best judgement to identify a drug that probably
will work by whatever drug he uses and since he is going to do that,
the only way of introducing any randomization or taking the drug assignment
out of his control in any way is to let him use only acceptable drugs so

you can't just tell him just which ones to put the drug on. You can't have an assignment before he has made the selection.

Dr. Winkle: If other physicians have magical powers that I don't I have no way to identify ahead of time which drug will work in any given patient and so I think that most people would find it acceptable to basically within limits to just be randomly assigned a drug. I don't think there is any great magic as to how we decide which drug we want to try first. It may be which ever one we are most interested in at the time or whoever is attending or whatever. Contraindications can influence your choice but generally I think it is a random selection.

Dr. Temple: You would be as happy with procainamide as with mexiletine, amiodarone...

Dr. Winkle: I think in getting the answers to these questions, yes.

Dr. Temple: That surprises me.

Dr. Krikler: We have time for one, possibly two questions.

Dr. Versteegh: I would like to ask Dr. Temple for his thoughts in blinding in antiarrhythmic studies.

Dr. Temple: I think it is worth blinding if you can do it without heroic efforts. There is probably not much reason to blind everybody if the Holter tapes for example are going to be read by someone who won't know the drug assignment. I think you probably will have an adequate measurement there. It is probably worth blinding for purposes of accessing side effects, however, and in general if you can do it I think it should be done. The study I suggested I would not advocate blinding just because of the enormous difficulties of sending out placebos as well as active drugs so I wouldn't propose it there.

Dr. Krikler: With at least two substances, blinding may well be impossible. I am referring to a substance that prolongs the QT interval and those who know the effect will be able to identify as they are looking at the tapes or looking at the routine tracings which drug the patient is taking. This is a difficulty that concerns the best laid statistical plans.

Dr. Kraemer: I thought that I might add a comment that might be useful. This kind of design is used extensively in behavioral research and there are several books that are titled single subject research that have both the distinct advantages for the very reasons that your claiming that it does mimick clinical decision making, systemizes it and produces results in which decision making can be made with some probabilities of errors, but in addition have already identified considerable dangers in doing the research. I realize that this is a technique that is new to arrhythmias, but it might be worthwhile reviewing the experience of clinicians in other field in using these designs.

Dr. Krikler: Last question now from Dr. Campbell.

Dr. Campbell: It is remarkable that we have gathered here the world's elite in management of significant ventricular arrhythmias and that we are all agreeing that the first choice antiarrhythmic drug is often chosen ar random. I think one of the important parts of Dr. Temple's idea is the possibility that we might develop along the road to selecting which drugs might be useful in clinical situations. I think that the reason that we all do use these drugs randomly is that our own personal experience is too small to make out characteristics that if a drug eliminates an arrhythmia then this other range of drugs is inappropriate and we should make a move in another direction. I think one of your more powerful aspects of suggesting that emergency protocols are put on a scientific basis is to ask a little more information about how we are influencing arrhythmias with specific drugs.

Dr. Temple: I would like to add something. Actually thinking about that comment and Dr. Winkle's one group of clinicians might well say I don't have any method of selection. You can give my any one of the following 10 and then they could be randomized to any one of those 10. I think that is perfectly all right; one of the things that you might learn is that it is not as good a way to choose the drug as some other way. I think that is perfectly compatible with that if the clinician is comfortable with that arrangement.

Dr. Krikler: We come to the end of the session and I must summarize during the last few minutes the points that have arisen. Clearly there are many who would like to continue. I think this is a good sign as it is good end before the refractory period has arrived. I am equally sure that as we have come no where near the answers to these problems, this first conference of its type will be the herald of others. I think it is an extremely useful ideal for those of us who have apparently different targets are indeed agreeing that we must find better ways of assessing antiarrhythmic efficacy, under all circumstances including this particular one that has been put to us today: the patient whom we believe to have a

potentially life-threatening but not hemodynamically significant arrhythmia.
I think that the statistical rigor that Dr. Kraemer has provided is essential.
We must not only be aware of it, but we must also be aware of the difficulties
that it may cause us and we need people like Dr. Kraemer to whom we can turn
because our trials tend to for reasons that we have discussed not to come
through as cleanly as one would like, and while our patients may not have
the problems of the psychiatric patients, they nevertheless do need other
medications with all sorts of interactions that we are now learning more
and more about. I think the very progressive ideas that Dr. Temple has
put forward as a means whereby physicians in the United States could
evaluate fruitfully medications that are either brand new or appear to have
worked elsewhere is a progressive one because much of the information that
we have obtained is anecdotal and although we appear to be extremely
satisfied with the results in many cases the fact that we are still
looking further and our patients alas still tend to die suddenly, unexpectedly
without warning us that they were going to do so, indicates that we have
a great need to acquire not only more drugs, but better knowledge of when
to use which drug in which particular patient. I think that we should
look forward to the sort of evaluation Dr. Temple proposes, and Dr. Kraemer
sets the guidelines for, but that we should also think of Dr. Van Durme's
clinical points that in spite of all this, we may still get some answers
without knowing just precisely how we have achieved them until afterwards.
The final analysis must be the clinical one. I think amiodarone has been
able to prove itself despite the fact that it is the sort of substance
resistant to any of these trials and this is by no means a statement of
affection on its behalf. There are other agents for arrhythmias that have
equal problems of assessment and the variability factor is a crucial one
that has to be discussed. Let us now end precisely on time.

J. RICHARD CROUT, M.D.

One of the messages I would like to report to you tonight that I have learned in government is that it is the systems, it is the policies, that we live under that are worth discussing. But basically the people that are administering them are 'come and go.' And it is not the people themselves that are the problem in any sense. It is the systems that we live under that are the greatest interests. Every reform movement has learned this. Reformers move in, and there is a government change, we will clean out the rascals, and things will change. In effect, they don't. And the reason they don't is that we perhaps pay insufficient attention to the 'system.' So I thought I'd comment a little bit on the 'system' in terms of our drug laws.

I think it's impossible to view our drug regulatory system without a sense of ambivalence. One of the things that drug laws have brought is really a revolution in two areas. One is in the area of clinical trials, which if you look back at the New England Journal of Medicine of the JAMA or Annals of Internal Medicine or whatever from the 1950's you will find absolutely nothing in the way of controlled clinical trials. And I believe the drug laws would have triggered our modern interest in that. I think it is now a self-sustaining movement, but the real trigger that brought discipline to science was that far-sighted law of 1962.

The second thing that has happened is an enormous revelation in drug labelling and those of you who don't believe that, go pick up a 1950's PDR and look at it. Unbelievable difference in the amount of information we have got about new drugs. I was astounded to learn when I went to the Food and Drug Administration that a new drug application for a drug in the 1950's was only a small document. And really what was known about the agent was correspondingly thin. The whole of biopharmaceutics, of blood

levels, of mechanisms of action, and of clinical trials for a variety of
indications for the scientific reader is totally different today than it
was then. I believe also, that in spite of all of the public concerns,
there is an increased public confidence as a result of our drug laws.
We think we are under attack in clinical research, and indeed we are, but
I suspect that it would be worse if we didn't have some of the things
like Informed Consent, Review Committees and so on that have developed
since the 1950's. On the debit side, there is also no doubt that we have an
enormously increased cost, enormously increased time and an enormously
increased effort by a variety of people in the development of a new drug
and a new therapy. And that has led to some serious regulatory consequences
and I'd like to comment on this in detail.

One is controlled trials and their necessity and their importance
and their changing character in the United States today. I think one that
is important for all of you to recognize (and it is not widely recognized
by people who engage in drug research and engage in the advancement of
medicine) is that our drug law is (in the United States) unique in one
area. And that is, it is unique in requiring adequate and well-controlled
clinical trials for the establishment of effectiveness. Many countries
have an effectiveness requirement in their laws. None have one that by law,
mandates what are called adequate and well-controlled clinical trials.
This distinguishes U.S. law and practice from other countries and is a
cause of serious contention. What it means is that adequate, expert
opinion, unsupported by the evidentiary base of clinical trials is for
purposes of public decision-making under our drug law is not possible.
And this principle has interestingly gone to the Supreme Court in a case
several years ago. The basic principle espoused is that if experts don't
have an evidentiary base for their opinion, their opinion isn't worth it.
A rather rigorous standard and a bit of a shock to experts who like to
pontificate and I suspect that I am not the only one in the room who has
done that. The most common problem in the past at the Food and Drug
Administration has been to try to reach a decision on a drug that people
thought worked, but the evidentiary base for that was not adequate, it
was incomplete, and the trials were uncontrolled, and it could not be sub-
stantiated. There is a real need to distinguish between an antiarrhythmic
that has some benefit and an antibiotic that has some benefit on the one
hand, and let's say a DMSO on the other hand and a laetrile on the other

hand. And the evidentiary and the scientific base for this has to be
clear. You know there are experts in this world, there are physicians,
there are investigators who will testify to the worthiness of DMSO on
arthritis, a chorionic gonadotropin in obesity, a thyroid for the treatment of obesity. And the only way to separate one from the other is on
the evidentiary base that he can provide to support his point of view.
A very rigorous standard, and that standard is set by law.

So when you view decision-making by the government, you must
realize the legal mandate under which our staff lives and why it is that
we seem to be 'hung-up' about controlled trials. Because that's, so far
as we can tell, the only way to separate out the good things coming down
the pike from some of these strange agents and other things that may have
some value but are less well-supported and are highly promoted.

So 1 of the problems in public life today is to decide whether that
standard should continue to prevail and my only message would be that you
can stick with the adequate, well-controlled trial standard, and we can
provide an evidentiary base for it that costs money and costs effort and
costs time. Or we can think of the alternative, which is to back away
from that standard and go to a standard that is less evidentiary, more
subjective. But you can't do the latter without expecting some of the
more controversial drugs around to be released as new medicines. I am not
advocating one point of view or another to you. I am trying to say simply
that we linve in a world of choices and the choices have costs in either
direction. I doubt that anyone literally wants the effectiveness to be
evaluated solely in the marketplace. On the other end, it's arguable
whether you'd like the perhaps less solid evidence to support effectiveness
or whether it's cost-effective to have control trials in every instance.
You're struggling with that question, you've been struggling today, you'll
struggle tomorrow, and my impression from listening at least to part of
the afternoon session, I heard that that struggle is occurring with great
intellectual honesty, and with innovation and with a good deal of innovating
and thinking. Let me turn then to the issue of one of the things I heard
about control trials today. It's obvious that life would be much easier
if we had placebo-control blinded trials. These are the ones that in all
instances, are easy to interpret scientifically. It's also evident, and I
have to report to you some concern in this regard that that whole principle
is under serious erosion. Some of the people perhaps know, our inter-

national visitors from Germany could report to you, that there is a very
serious movement in Germany. I think it is at the state of actually introducing legislation into their parliament that would prohibit placebo-
controlled trials on ethical grounds. There is a very serious movement
in the United States and other countries that would, in the name of ethics,
have the patient be able to decide whether he or she continued in the trial
based on the progress of the trial itself. The thesis being that informed
consent is not given only at the beginning, but it is a continuous thing,
that must occur through time as the trial proceeds. It is fairly evident
that in order to accomplish that in a practical way, it means that the
results of the trial as it occurs must be made available in a public way
to all of the patients. And I think you can see what would happen to the
conduct of any kind of controlled clinical trial under those circumstances
where the end result would be unlikely to be scientifically interpretable.
So, there are a couple of lessons in this. One is, and I heard a lot of
struggling to this effect, which was good to the extent possible, we're
going to have to design trials that take advantage as much as possible
of the therapeutic situation that have therapeutic goals, and that especially
if this is done in a seriously ill patient. We are going to have to have
and cope with, positively-controlled trials, historically-controlled
trials in those kinds of patients, and somehow find ways to see that
scientifically-valid answers emerge from that kind of research.

The second lesson, I think, is important for us all to recognize.
And that is that there may come a time, indeed it's around and it may get
worse within the next few years. And those of us who are interested in
science have to stand up and be counted on what is scientifically valid,
and what is necessary in order to reach reasonable conclusions for
purposes of public decision-making. I do not believe any of us want to
see in the name of ethics an erosion in our ability to make reasonable
about what valid conclusions can be drawn from the scientific trial. I
think most of us would agree that a worthless trial is totally worthless
both scientifically and ethically. And I believe some or most of us
would agree that there are serious ethical problems with either introducing
into the marketplace, drugs with poor scientific background in their
development. So ethical arguments cut both ways. I'm only pointing out,
I believe, that the medical profession, and particularly those of us who
are clinical investigators, in a very sensitive way are going to have to

participate, in the next few years, in a serious argument. And it would come to the ethics of informed consent on one hand and the ability to make some kind of a scientifically-valid decision on the other. A tough problem, I invite you all to participate in it.

Another controversy has been on at the meeting and is a little bit easier. And that is what is the efficacy of a drug? I think we all recognize that there is in the course of drug development, in the course of use and therapeutics, two kinds of efficacy: One kind is pharmacological mode of action and the other one is whether pharmacology is indeed thera-peutically effective. Does it really benefit the patient? And, I understand that there is a thread of that going through the meeting today, and I would like to tell you just what FDA traditions are in deciding whether the drug ought to come into the marketplace on the basis of its pharmacologic effectiveness, or whether it really ought to have evidence that it treats the disease. For symptomatic remedies, the answer is easy. The two basically are synonymous. The pharmacological effectiveness, that is, pain relief for headache or nasal decongestion. For symptomatic relief, the pharmacological effect and therapeutic effect are the same, and that accounts for a lot of our drugs. But for drugs that alter the course of a disease it is more complicated. And the fundamental principle is that we bury the ground rules depending on the drug class. Sometimes a drug should really cure a disease. Or really, the ultimate therapeutic benefit determines whether it comes into the marketplace. And that is efficacy for purposes of approval of the drug. Examples are: antibiotics, where the Food and Drug Administration has for many years not approved anti-biotics simply on the basis of the fact that they killed bacteria. They are supposed to do something to the disease. Another example that's fairly self-evident, is oral contraceptives. I mean, nobody wants an oral contraceptive which inhibits ovulation or does something only to endocrine mechanisms. They would like to know the ultimate effectiveness in rate in preventing pregnancy. So all oral contraceptives have clinical trials aimed at the effectiveness rate. Sometimes, however, with other classes of drugs, there is a conscious decision to accept pharmacological effectiveness as sufficient. Examples here are the oral hypoglycemic drugs in diabetes and the hypolipidemic drugs in hyperlipidemia. And I would point out the same thing for high blood pressure drugs when they were first introduced, and that is the circumstance today for antiarrhythmic drugs.

Let me cite a third set of drugs which are sometimes ambiguous: steroids. For years we have approved steroids on the basis of their being able to alter the course or provide symptomatic relief. I was never quite sure of whether they cured the disease or not. They certainly improved the quality of life. Another area that is ambiguous is cancer drugs. This is in transition, for many years the approval of cancer drugs was based on their ability to produce what is equivalent to a pharmacological effect for other drugs. That is, they were based on their ability to reduce tumor size and reduce tumor mass on x-rays for example. More recently, there has been an increasing interest that cancer drugs ought to improve the life span or improve the quality of life. We have recnetly reviewed this with our Oncology Advisory Committee and they changed the gound rules a little bit. They said, in our most recent review of guidelines of this area, that the approval of cancer drugs should include -- they didn't say it ought to be solely based on or required, but it ought to include -- an appraisal of those drugs on life span. What I am saying is that the rules vary depending on the drug class and to some extent depending upon the state of the field. Certainly, if we had taken a position years ago, that an effect on life span had to be shown for antihypertensive drugs, no doubt, medicine and the public at large would have been set back enormously. I don't know where the antiarrhythmic field is at this point, that's for you to decide. Because my message is that we vary the ground rules depending upon what experts in the particular field think. For antiarrhythmics today, we're prepared to approve antiarrhythmic drugs on the basis of pharmacologic effect. That is, that they really are anti-arrhythmic, they do suppress arrhythmias; and are not requiring that in addition, they should do something to protect patients or to improve mortality. There may be a time in the future, as these drugs are developed and as the sufficient data are gathered that the ground rules should change. But when that time comes, I will tell you how that will be made. The change will be made by our changing our guidelines, as a result of discussion in front of our advisory committee. And it will be done, because the field itself feels that some kind of a change in standard for effect-iveness ought to occur. And that's how the process works. We try to take advantage of what the particular state of progress is in a particular field and what experts think in front of our advisory committee. So until you come forward or until our advisory committee comes forward or until you present to our advisory committee some change in our guidelines, we will continue to look at antiarrhythmic drugs on the basis of the pharmacological effect as a proper criterion for approval; that is for entering into the marketplace and an appropriate burden that a manufacturer ought to bear. It doesn't mean that that answers all the questions, it simply means that the next set of questions relating to the use of the medicine are more properly born by practitioners, by the NIH, by the VA or whoever supports the kinds of trials that are needed to answer those kinds of questions.

Well, this brings me to the end of this discussion struggling with important issues. It's hard I can tell. You've had a good time today; you've had a good time this evening. Your input to us is welcome. I understand there may be some guidelines for developing drugs that might come out of this symposium. If there are, we'd be delighted to look at them. Our antiarrhythmic drug development guidelines are badly in need of revision, that it would come to our advisory committee, and we would do everything in our power to take advantage of your views, and because our intent is to see that own guidelines, our own approach is up-to-date with modern medicine. I think you've also had a chance to meet Dr. Temple, for those of you who did not know him before as our Division Director in Cardiovascular Medicine. So you know the Food and Drug Administration has made a lot of strides in recent years in attracting good people, and that our government agency is like all institutions. We've had a lot of controversy; we have good people. We have the same gamut of people that you've got in universities, the same gamut of people that you've got in drug industry. You sometimes wish that we had miracles in all the places in the bureaucracy. Then I think we could meet everybody's expectation in government. Lacking that, we are just humans trying to do our job, and I do appreciate having a chance to be here, to let you know a little bit about me. I am glad Dr. Temple is here to carry on with, far better than I, on the scientific side and on scientific communication.

ACUTE DRUG TESTING AS A PART OF A SYSTEMATIC APPROACH TO ANTIARRHYTHMIC
DRUG THERAPY

PHILIP J PODRID

A major challenge of sudden cardiac death is the identification of
the patient at risk (1). The development of the coronary care unit (2)
and widespread use of 24 hour ambulatory monitoring (3) have identified
a large number of patients with frequent and potentially serious ventricular ectopy. CPR programs, such as the Seattle Heart Watch (4), have
saved patients who have experienced malignant ventricular arrhythmia but
who are at high risk for recurrence (5). Once these patients have been
identified the goal of therapy is to suppress ventricular premature beats
(VPBs) (6,7) with drugs and thus prevent a recurrence of malignant
ventricular arrhythmia and sudden cardiac death (8). There are at the
present time 7 antiarrhythmic agents available and many others in various
stages of clinical trials. The ever growing number of patients at risk
for sudden death has resulted in an increased use of these drugs. However,
this has not solved the problem. It is clear that merely placing a patient
on an antiarrhythmic drug is futile (5) and does not guarantee survival.
Neither the characteristic of the arrhythmia nor the electrophysiologic
or pharmacologic properties of the drugs provide useful guidelines for
the selection of an effective agent. If arrhythmia recurs, one cannot be
certain whether this is a result of drug failure, inadequate dose or aggravation of arrhythmia by the drug (9). Frequently, potentially life-
threatening arrhythmia is sporadic and without symptoms. Therefore
recurrence can only be judged by repeated 24 hour ambulatory monitorings
and exercise tolerance tests. This is costly, time consuming and does not
guarantee detection of potentially serious arrhythmia. Most importantly
there is no margin for error when dealing with malignant arrhythmia for
there may not be a second chance.
    The need for certainty of drug efficacy has prompted the development
of new techniques for evaluation of antiarrhythmic drugs. In order to

evaluate therapy we developed a systematic and organized approach which includes four phases (7).

PHASE 0 - DATA ENTRY

Upon admission to the hospital all antiarrhythmic drugs are discontinued. Digoxin is also discontinued unless necessary for treatment of congestive heart failure or rate control of atrial fibrillation. Beta blockers may be continued in patients with moderate angina pectoris. After a period of 24 hours off of all drugs the patient undergoes 48 hours of continuous ambulatory monitoring and a maximal, symptom-limited, exercise tolerance test on a motorized treadmill adhering to a Bruce protocol (10,11). This data serves as a baseline control against which results on drug therapy are compared.

Arrhythmia is graded by the Lown system (6,12) which provides a simple shorthand for categorizing the arrhythmia during a monitoring period or with exercise and permits easy comparison of repeat studies. It is especially useful in evaluating the response to drug (see Table 1).

Table 1. Lown Grading System.

Grade		
0	=	No VPBs
1a	=	<30 VPBs/hour and <1/minute
1b	=	<30 VPBs/hour and occasionally >1/minute
2	=	>30 VPBs/hour
3	=	Multiformity
4a	=	Couplets
4b	=	Ventricular tachycardia
5	=	Early R-on-T VPBs

ACUTE DRUG TEST - PHASE 1

Approximately 80% of patients referred to us have frequent and stable ventricular ectopic activity (VEA) throughout the day. This high density of VEA allows for effective testing of drugs daily utilizing acute drug testing (13,14). Twenty percent of those referred because of malignant ventricular arrhythmia are free of all ambient VEA during phase 0 baseline studies. In these patients there is no way to judge drug effect. Therefore these patients undergo invasive electrophysiologic studies utilizing programmed premature stimulation to provoke multiple repetitive responses (MRVR) (15), defined as 3 or more successive VPBs in response to the premature stimulus. If provoked, a modified acute drug test is performed during electrophysiologic studies. The goal of the acute drug test is to rapidly identify which agents are effective in suppressing VPBs or MRVR.

PHASE 2

At the end of phase 1 studies, the one or more agents judged to be of most benefit are prescribed as part of a program simulating chronic drug management. The aims of this phase are to insure that the drug program is effective and to assess how the drug is tolerated. The dosing schedule is guided by the drug's pharmacokinetic properties. Assessment of drug efficacy is by means of ambulatory monitoring and exercise testing on a motorized treadmill. The results of these studies are compared to those obtained during the phase 0 control period. The criteria for a therapeutic response based on monitoring include:

1. Total elimination of all grade 4B (VT) and 5 (early VPBs).
2. A greater than 90% decrease in frequency of 4A (couplets).
3. A greater than 50% reduction in the number of VPBs per 24 hours and/or a reduction of more than 50% in the number of hours during which grade 2 VPBs occur.

With respect to the exercise test, criteria include:

1. Total elimination of grades 4B and 5
2. A greater than 90% reduction of grade 4A
3. A greater than 50% decrease in the frequency of VPBs during the entire exercise test.

For a drug to be judged effective, criteria for both monitoring and exercise testing must be met.

PHASE 3

After the phase 2 evaluation on an antiarrhythmic program, the patient is continued on the drugs chronically for long term management. Followup is every 3-6 months at which time monitoring and exercise testing are repeated.

The important element of this program is the acute drug test which provides the data necessary to select an effective drug for the individual patient. There are four essential elements of acute drug testing:

1. Administration of a single large oral dose of a selected anti-arrhythmic drug.
2. Programmed trendscription (16) to display the time course of drug action.

3) Exercise on a bicycle ergometer to help define drug action.

4) Sampling of blood for drug concentration to permit correlation with onset and dissipation of antiarrhythmic or toxic effects.

Prior to the test, the patient is monitored for a 30-minute period by telemetry to a trendscriber. This permits observation of the frequency and grade of VPBs present. Low level continuous exercise for 5 minutes on a bicycle ergometer is carried out. This brief exercise is sufficient to achieve an amount of work equivalent to that of routine daily activities and helps define the action of the drug. A complete ECG is recorded, while Lead II and V2 or V3 are obtained at 50 mm/sec to measure PR, QRS and QT intervals. Upon completion of this control period, a single large oral dose of antiarrhythmic agent is given. Generally this amounts to one half of a standard daily dose (Table 2).

Table 2. Drug dose for acute drug test.

Drug	Dose
Quinidine	600 mg
Procainamide	1.5 gms
Disopyramide	300 mg
Propranolol	80 mg
Metoprolol	100 mg
Pindolol	20 mg
Mexiletine	400 mg
Ethmozin	600 mg
Tocainide	800 mg
Levobunolol	2 mg

Trendscription monitoring is continued for 3-5 hours with sampling of one minute every 3 minutes. Each hour the patient repeats the bicycle exercise at the same level as during control. Blood samples for drug concentration are obtained hourly, as well as ECG strips for intervals.

Since trendscription provides on-line data, the results of the acute drug test are apparent by the end of the testing period. The number of VPBs and repetitive forms each minute are counted and grafted for easy visualization (see Fig. 1)

The following criteria at rest and during bicycle exercise constitute a positive response to the drug (see Fig. 2):

1) Total elimination of all 4B (VT).

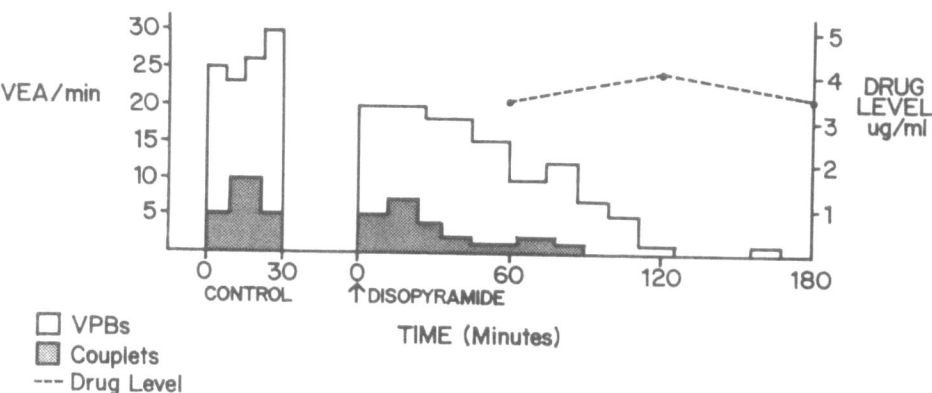

FIGURE 1. Disopyramide acute drug test. The graph of VPB frequency provides easy visualization of response to drug. Disopyramide blood levels
correlate with suppression of arrhythmia.

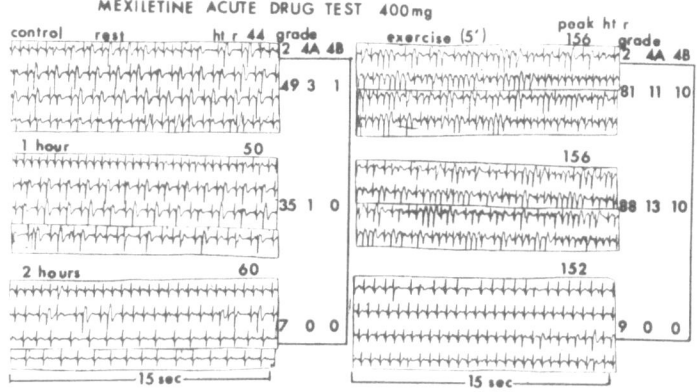

FIGURE 2. Mexiletine acute drug test. Frequent VPBs, couplets, and VT
are present at rest and during exercise. Arrhythmia is still present
one hour after drug, but by 2 hours there is almost total elimination
of arrhythmia.

2)   Greater than 90% reduction in 4A (couplets) compared to control.

3)   Greater than 50% decrease in VPB frequency compared to control.

If criteria are met either at rest or with exercise, the drug is deemed to have only a partial response.

In addition to the above criteria the following are also necessary.

1)   The onset of antiarrhythmic effect must occur between 45 minutes and 2 hours after drug administration.

2)   Antiarrhythmic effects must be maintained for at least 1½ hours. (See Fig. 3a & 3b).

When the acute test is utilized as part of electrophysiologic studies, programmed premature stimulation is performed during ventricular pacing and sinus rhythm prior to and 2 hours after the single large dose of drug. The criterion for response is the inability to provoke MRVR. If MRVR is more difficult to provoke or occurs within a smaller zone of coupling cycles, the drug is considered to be partially effective.

To date, we have carried out 760 acute drug tests as listed below:

Quinidine	140	Pindolol	58
Procainamide	64	Mexiletine	200
Propranolol	49	Ethmozin	42
Disopyramide	113	Tocainide	5
Metoprolol	68	Levobunolol	24

By identifying those drugs that are ineffective, the acute drug test eliminates the need for more time consuming and useless evaluation. Our experience has been that when a drug does not suppress VPBs during the acute drug test, it rarely if ever is effective during maintenance therapy (See Fig. 3a & 3b).

In addition to important information about drug efficacy, the acute drug test offers a rapid and safe technique to identify potentially serious proarrhythmic effects of drugs. We have observed that each of the agents utilized for drug testing has aggravated arrhythmia in a number of patients (9).

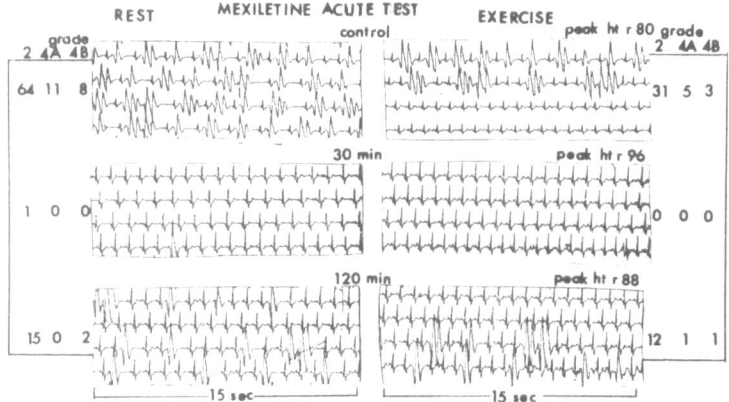

FIGURE 3a. Mexiletine drug test. Ventricular arrhythmia is eliminated at 30 minutes. At 2 hours high grade ventricular arrhythmia has recurred. This drug test did not meet the criteria for efficacy and was considered negative.

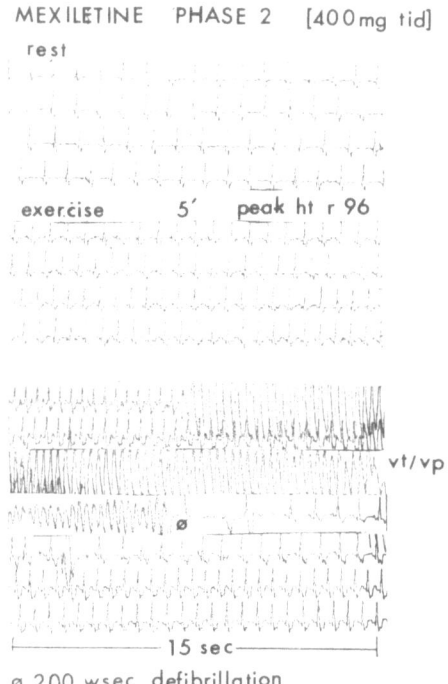

FIGURE 3b. Short term therapy with Mexiletine. After 3 days of therapy, exercise testing provokes VT and VF requiring defibrillation.

Criteria for aggravation of arrhythmia include:

1)   A fourfold increase in VPB frequency.

2)   A tenfold increase in the occurrence of repetitive forms.

3)   The occurrence of VT not observed during control studies.

Additionally this increase has to occur at least 45 minutes after drug administration and the frequency should not have been observed at any time during control phase 0 studies (see Fig. 4). The increase in arrhythmia required is far greater than can be accounted for by random variability in this group of patients. This serious side effect occurred during 11% of all drug studies and was observed in one third of patients tested. The incidence for the different drugs ranged from 5.9% to 15.8%. Generally the worsening in ventricular arrhythmia follows the known time course of drug action that is gradually increasing and abating as the drug level falls. In the case of quinidine, a second pattern was observed wherein

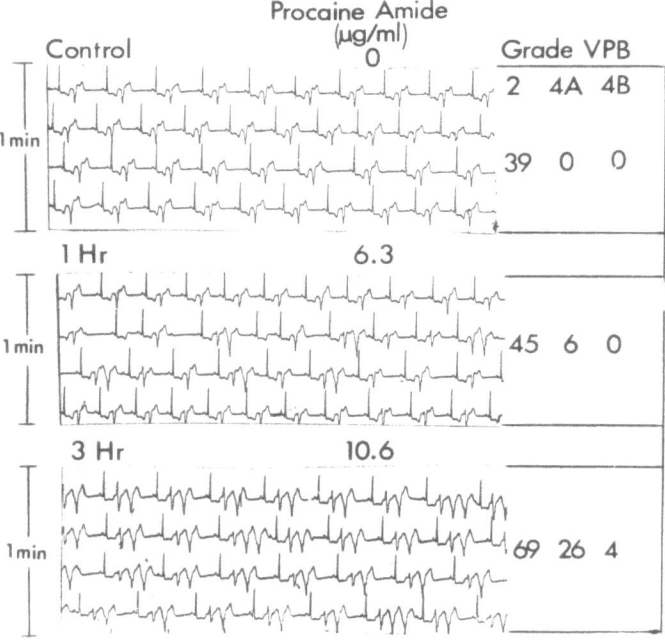

FIGURE 4. Aggravation of arrhythmia by procainamide. As procainamide drug level increases there is a gradual increase in VPB frequency with the development of couplets and VT, not present in control.

arrhythmia was initially suppressed at 1-2 hours, with "rebound" aggravation at 4-5 hours as the drug level was falling yet still in a therapeutic
range.

The major criticism of acute drug testing revolves around the issue
of random variability (17,18). It is argued that patients have spontaneous
variation in the hourly (17) and daily (18) frequency of ventricular
arrhythmia, making comparison to a 30-minute control period, observation
for only 3-5 hours and use of 50% reduction of VPB frequency as drug
response invalid and the results suspect. However, this argument fails
to deal with the following points:

1) The patients in our studies have frequent and chronic ventricular
arrhythmia which is symptomatic. Most have repetitive forms during control
studies. This is a different population than an asymptomatic group wherein variability is high.

2) Although a 30-minute control period was utilized, all patients
underwent 48 hours of ambulatory monitoring which established the frequency,
grade and stability of ventricular arrhythmia. The 30-minute period,
although brief, was representative of the frequency of ectopy and served
as a baseline against which one could make a comparison.

3) The criteria for drug efficacy were stringent and included not
only a reduction in VPB frequency but more importantly the elimination of
repetitive and early forms. It has been well established that the risk
of sudden death lies not in the VPB, regardless of frequency, but in the
repetitive and early VPBs (19,20,21). Therefore, our primary goal is the
suppression of these forms. Moreover, criteria had to be met during
exercise on a bicycle as well as during monitoring at rest. Critics of
acute drug testing have focused only on VPB frequency and have not
addressed the issue of repetitive VPBs or the role of exercise.

4) The criteria for drug effect include time of onset and duration
of action. Thus suppression or aggravation of arrhythmia had to correlate with the known pharmacokinetic action of the drug. This makes random
variability or arrhythmia unlikely as an explanation for drug effect
(see Fig. 2).

Using our criteria for drug response the data reported by Winkle
(17) was re-analyzed. In this study he suggested that random variability
mimicked a drug response in 65% of patients. However, based on our
criteria, only one patient would have been a drug responder. In 5

patients there was no variability of arrhythmia, and in 7 patients VPBs
decreased but grade 4 arrhythmia was present throughout the 5½ hours of
monitoring. Four patients had >50% reduction of VPBs, but this was
transient, lasting for only ½ hour. In 2 patients VPB reduction occurred
during the second half hour period of observation and increased again at
a later time. In one patient VPBs decreased after 3 hours.

  5) Patients underwent multiple drug studies. Prior to each test
a 30-minute period of continuous ECG recording was obtained to confirm
the presence of ectopy. If VEA was suppressed by a drug utilized on one
day, a drug test was performed on the following day only if arrhythmia
recurred.

  In each patient, drugs that were effective or ineffective were identified. If random variability were important, mimicking drug effect, it
might be assumed that criteria for drug response would be met for each
drug. This was not the case (see Fig. 5a & 5b).

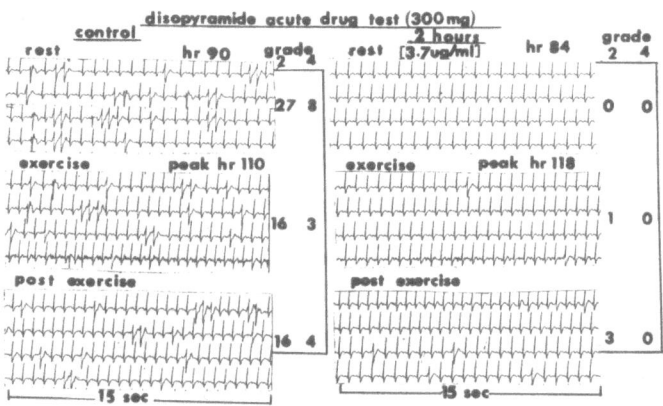

FIGURE 5a. Disopyramide acute drug test. Two hours after administration
of drug there is suppression of arrhythmia.

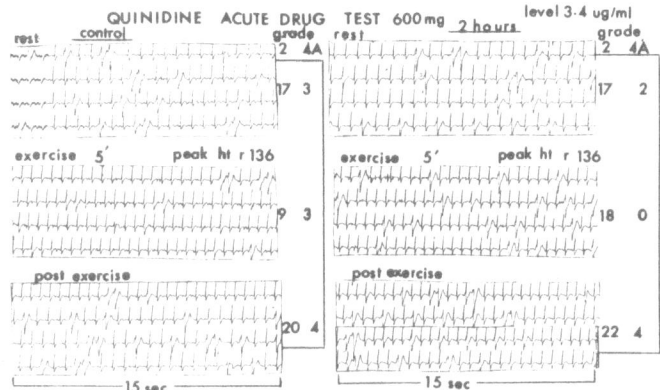

FIGURE 5b. On the following day, arrhythmia had recurred and a quinidine acute drug test was performed. There was no response to this drug.

6) Placebo studies were performed in 20 patients on random days during drug evaluation adhering to the usual procedure for acute drug testing. In none of these were criteria for response achieved. If spontaneous variation in VPB frequency were important, a number of these tests would have been positive.

7) Perhaps the most important factor is the correlation between the results of the acute drug test and the response during phase 2 as evaluated by both monitoring and exercise testing. Indeed, concordancy between phases 1 and 2 is good, ranging from 80-90%. For quinidine the concordancy is 85% (13), for mexiletine, 80% (22), and 88% for pindolol (23). Discordant results have usually been a result of a disparity in blood levels of drug.

We therefore conclude that the acute drug test is a rapid, safe and effective way of evaluating response to antiarrhythmic agents. When integrated as part of a systematic approach to drug therapy, it is an important technique for guiding the selection of an appropriate drug to suppress ventricular arrhythmia and protect against malignant ventricular arrhythmias. It can be adapted for use with invasive electrophysiologic studies to assess drug response and guide therapy in those patients who are at risk for a major arrhythmia, but who have little or no ambient ectopy.

It is thus a useful tool for managing the patient with ventricular arrhythmia, for evaluating efficacy of a drug in a group of patients, and for comparison of different agents.

REFERENCES

1. Lown B. 1979. Sudden cardiac death: the major challenge confronting contemporary cardiology. Am J Cardiol 43: 313
2. Lown B, Fakhro AM, Hood WB, Thorn GW. 1967. The coronary care unit: new perspectives and directions. JAMA 199: 188
3. Lown B, Calvert AF, Armington R, Ryan M. 1975. Monitoring for serious arrhythmias and high risk of sudden death. Circulation 51 & 52: III-189
4. Cobb LA, Conn RD, Samon WE, Philbin JE. 1971. Prehospital coronary care: the role of rapid response mobile intensive coronary care system. Circulation 43: 11
5. Schaffer WA, Cobb LA. 1975. Recurrent ventricular fibrillation and modes of death in survivors of out-of-hospital ventricular fibrillation. N Engl J Med 293: 260
6. Lown B, Graboys TB. 1977. Management of patients with malignant ventricular arrhythmia. Am J Cardiol 39: 910
7. Lown B, Podrid PJ, DeSilva RA, Graboys TB. 1980. Sudden cardiac death - management of the patient at risk. Current Problems in Cardiology, Vol. 4, 1-62, Yearbook Medical Publishers.
8. Graboys TB, Lown B, Podrid PJ, DeSilva RA. 1979. Survival of patients with malignant ventricular arrhythmia treated with antiarrhythmic agents. Circulation 60: II-255
9. Velebit V, Podrid P, Graboys TB, Lown B. 1979. Aggravation of ventricular arrhythmia by antiarrhythmic drugs. Am J Cardiol 43: 359
10. Jelinek MV, Lown B. 1974. Exercise stress testing for exposure of cardiac arrhythmia. Prog Cardiovasc Dis 26: 497
11. Doan AE, Peterson DR, Blackmon JR, Bruce RA. 1965. Myocardial ischemia after maximal exercise in healthy men: a method for detecting potential coronary heart disease. Am Heart J 69: 11
12. Lown B, Wolf M. 1971. Approaches to sudden death for coronary heart disease. Circulation 44: 130
13. Gaughan CE, Lown B, Lanigan J, Voukydis P, Besser W. 1976. Acute oral testing for determining antiarrhythmic drug efficacy. I. Quinidine. Am J Cardiol 36: 677
14. Podrid PJ, Lown B. 1978. Selection of an antiarrhythmic drug to protect against ventricular fibrillation. In: Proceedings of the First US-USSR Symposium on Sudden Death, Yalta, October 3-5, 1977 (US Dept of Health, Education and Welfare, Public Health Service, National Institutes of Health, DHEW Publication No (NIH) 78-1470, p 159, 1978)
15. Matta RJ, Verrier RL, Lown B. 1976. The repetitive extrasystole as an index of vulnerability to ventricular fibrillation. Am J Physiol 230: 1461
16. Lown B, Matta RJ, Besser HW. 1975. Programmed trendscription. A new approach to electrocardiographic monitoring. JAMA 232: 39
17. Winkle RA. 1978. Spontaneous variability of ventricular ectopics frequently mimics antiarrhythmic drug effect. Circulation 57: 1116

18. Morganroth J, Michelson EJ, Horowitz LN, Josephson MC, Pearlman AS, Dunkman WB. 1978. Limitations of routine long-term electrocardiographic monitoring to assess ventricular ectopic frequency. Circulation 58: 408

19. Schultze RA, Strauss HW, Pitt B. 1977. Sudden death in the year following myocardial infarction. Am J Med 62: 192

20. Ruberman W, Weinblatt E, Goldberg JD, Frank CW, Shapiro S. 1977. Ventricular premature beats and mortality after myocardial infarction. N Engl J Med 297: 750

21. Follansbee WP, Michelson EL, Morganroth. 1980. Nonsustained ventricular tachycardia in ambulatory patients: Characteristics and association with sudden cardiac death. Ann Int Med 92: 741

22. Podrid PJ, Lown B. 1979. Mexiletine for refractory ventricular arrhythmia. Circulation 60: II-188

23. Podrid PJ, Matthews K, Lown B. 1980. Pindolol for ventricular arrhythmia. Circulation (in press)

ROLE OF ELECTROPHYSIOLOGY TESTING TO DEFINE DRUG EFFICACY

Douglas P. Zipes, M.D.

Patients we consider as candidates to undergo electrophysiologic testing to define drug therapy are those who have supraventricular tachycardia (SVT) that is drug-resistant, that produces severe symptoms and those patients who have Wolff-Parkinson-White syndrome and a very rapid ventricular response during atrial fibrillation. Regarding patients who have ventricular tachycardia, we would evaluate those patients who are symptomatic during the ventricular tachycardia, and whose ventricular tachycardia is drug-resistant, occurs infrequently, and is more likely to be inducible electrophysiologically, such as those patients who have sustained ventricular tachycardia on the basis of coronary artery disease. Patients who are resuscitated from ventricular fibrillation should also be considered as candidates for an electrophysiologic study.

What does electrophysiologic testing accomplish in these patients? It identifies patients capable of developing tachycardia. Although the frequency of induction of ventricular tachycardia varies somewhat with the zeal of the investigator and the type of electrophysiologic testing done, it seems fairly clear that sustained ventricular tachycardia is induced primarily in those patients who spontaneously develop the tachycardia clinically. Only a very small percent of patients appear to have a false positive response to premature stimulation. Electrophysiologic testing can help identify the electrophysiologic mechanism responsible for a tachycardia and the mechanism by which a drug suppresses or exacerbates the tachyarrhythmia. Electrophysiologic studies help identify potential harmful effects of the drug on the tachycardia or hemodynamic status of the patient. We feel that, whether or not testing after IV administration is done, testing also must be done after oral administration. These studies done by several groups of investigators should be

ROLE OF ELECTROPHYSIOLOGY TESTING TO DEFINE DRUG EFFICACY

Douglas P. Zipes, M.D.

required as part of the evaluation of a new antiarrhythmic drug. We do not think that electrophysiologic testing can be used to identify the high risk patient by the response to single premature ventricular stimulation during sinus rhythm or atrial pacing, if a single repetitive ventricular response is taken as the endpoint.

GENERAL GROUP DISCUSSION: ELECTROPHYSIOLOGY

Dr. Josephson: I agree with every you said Dr. Zipes about sustained VT.
There's a problem when we talk about VT for this audience in that VT isn't
just one thing. Non-sustained VT is different than sustained VT and I'm
not sure we have good natural history data to know whether that's a bad
thing to have or a good thing to have. Nor am I sure what a successful
treatment is. A reduction of 10 complexes of non-sustained VT to three
complexes of non-sustained VT. Does that mean anything? I think that in
sustained VT, particularly in patients with coronary disease, the sensitivity of induction is good. The specificity is also very good. You don't
induce sustained VT in people who don't have it. When we're trying to
figure out why there's a difference between the laboratory and clinical
occurrence of VT, there are several factors that have to be looked at. One
is, you must realize what we're doing in a laboratory is testing the capability of a reentrant circuit, of whatever is in the heart to sustain its
VT, which is different than the Holter monitor which looks at spontaneous
triggers. Part of the problem has to do with drugs which may work by
suppressing the triggers, although it's very hard to suppress all the
triggers all the time. The stress that you use to induce the VT may be
less physiologic. For instance, if after a drug you can still induce VT,
but it takes pacing at 200 beats/min and three extrastimuli, that may be
non-physiologic, or too much of a stress in that patient, so that it
wouldn't have a clinical counterpart. The way the tachycardia is induced
also can influence that, but again, electrophysiologic testing will bring
out some people who would be failurs who you don't think are.
Dr. Rosen: If you induce ventricular tachycardia, it's our experience in
general that predicts the occurrence of clinical tachycardia, be it off
drugs or on drugs. There is a great variable which is called time. Namely
some people have sporadic ventricular tachycardias once or twice a year,
others have it once a month. So that if you induce sustained ventricular

tachycardia in the laboratory, it doesn't predict what the spontaneous frequency is going to be. The other thing is that I don't think any of us have much data on what are the extremes. We may use incremental ventricular pacing at a rate of 250 to induce ventricular tachycardia, and that's the only way we can induce it. And yet the patient has had spontaneous tachycardias a couple of times. Exactly what it is that induces the spontaneous tachycardia and how it relates to what you're doing in the laboratory is a very interesting and difficult question.

Dr. Winkle: I would just like to expand for a second about your comment about the fact that if you can still induce VT in the electrophysiology laboratory after a drug, that the patient might still do well long-term. I would agree with that statement, but I think that you have to put it in a little bit of perspective. You have to realize that the electrophysiologic test is not perfect. And there will be patients in whom you cannot induce VT, who over time, sometimes even the next day on that drug, will have VT; and there are patients, as Dr. Zipes showed, in whom you can still induce VT and over the long term they'll do very well. We feel fairly strongly that the only way to look at this problem is with some sort of an actuarial table over time, and if you do that you'll find that there's quite a marked discrepancy between the curves of the people who have inducible VT and those who still don't have inducible VT. In our experince by about 18 months of follow-up, in people in whom we could not induce VT there was only a 30% recurrence rate of VT, whereas in those cases where we could still induce VT on that drug by, 18 months there was an 89% recurrence rate of VT, so you have to put that in the clinical perspective. if you can still induce VT, then you have to make a clinical decision. If that patient's had a lot of episodes of VT that have been reasonably well tolerated, seems like a poor surgical candidate, then it might be reasonable to use a drug where you could still induce VT. But if that patient has cardiovascular collapse every time he has VT, then I think it would be most logical to go onto surgery or some alternative therapy.

Dr. Ruskin: We've analyzed a group of patients in whom we could not suppress inducible VT and who were not surgical candidates and we found that one of the interesting features is that the grade of stimulation required to induce the VT when you discharge may be highly predictive of how they do. For example, if a patient has VT that's readily inducible with a single premature beat off drugs, but has VT that can only be initiated with

bursts of rapid pacing at a rate of 280 on a particular drug, the likelihood is that that patient will not have spontaneous VT that year. The
other point that I'd like to make is to take Dr. Zipes to task a little
bit for the patient that you showed. I think you point about inducibility
not necessarily predicting recurrence rate is well taken, but it was not
a good example for two reasons. One, amiodarone I think is a drug which
cannot be adequately assessed at 10 days or 2 weeks, and we may have to
retest them at three months before we really know whether the drug is effective. The other point is that the patient died at 11 months and it's not
a very good follow up or a good result. I think Dr. Kraemer would take
you to task for that in the sense that despite the fact that the patient
had chest pain at the time that he collapsed, the fact is that he was
susceptible to VT/VF and you could argue that he really had no protection
from his regimen.

Dr. Zipes: In response to your first comment, I would agree. It's very
difficult to evaluate data on patients receiving amiodarone who were
studied about 2 weeks after onset of therapy, which is roughly when we
studied them, but you just can't keep them in the hospital forever.
Dr. Krikler said he's bring them back in 3 months, which is certainly a
reasonable way to evaluate amiodarone. The problem is you're sending the
patient home without an electrophysiologic test for that 3-month follow-
up. In terms of whether that patient was a success or not, he clearly
died at 11 months. All we can say is that he had recurrent syncope and
out of hospital VT on 6 occasions in the past 6 months prior to starting
therapy. Dr. Kraemer can take me to task, nevertheless the patient had no
VT for 11 months on that regimen.

Participant: We've studied about six patients, several months out on
amiodarone, and they're still inducible. Hein Wellens has the same experience, except with more patients. And he doesn't find, at least with
amiodarone, unlike the others, the correlation between inducibility and
clinical episodes. There are disparate results.

Participant: That's exactly right, and the majority of our patients in
whom we induce the arrhythmia electrophysiologically and subsequently
do well are amiodarone patients.

Dr. Josephson: We thought this was going to be great until three of the
last eight that were like this died.

Participant: But you can't predict which ones will do well.

Dr. Josephson: I understand that, but we felt comfortable with this because it's everyone's experience from Europe that amiodarone is terrific.
Even if you can still induce VT, they're not going to have it spontaneously.
We had three patients die of eight that still had it, so I'm a little
less optimistic that I was initially.

Dr. Wyndham: I would like to disagree with something else that Dr. Zipes
said. I think that what I would like to do is make a plea to the drug
companies for making available more commonly the intravenous form of
various agents that come onto the market in the future. I think it's
clear that we still have a great deal to learn about the pharmacokinetics
of drugs. And I think we should try to learn in the precess of doing
drug studies on patients with electrophysiologic testing what the real
difference is between intravenous and oral medication, since it clearly
is very complex relating to active metabolites. To be able to give an
intravenous form of the drug during acute testing I think has the advantage
of being able to look at that question, and it comes back to Dr. Kraemer's
argument regarding washout periods during chronic electrophysiologic
study. One is frequently concerned that the 24-hour washout period after
an orally administered drug or an intravenously administered drug may
not be sufficient to be able to test intravenous forms of drugs on sub-
seuqnt days. I think that at least partly eliminates the question of
washout period.

Dr. Zipes: First of all, I don't think you're really disagreeing with me,
because I did not say I.V. studies should not be done. What I am stressing
is that oral studies definitely should be done, both to establish the
mechanism of action of the drug, and so on, as well as efficacy; because
particularly in canine, the example I used, what happens in 4 days may
be quite different from that which happens following an I.V. administration of the drug.

Dr. Wyndham: Yest, I think we need both.

Dr. Herling: Based on Myerburg's data and the work that Dr. Josephson and
I've done, suppression of ventricular ectopic activity in sudden death
victims doesn't relate to subsequent survival. Just as a panel opinion,
in people who've sustained one sudden death episode and who have survived,
is there any role for empiric antiarrhythmic therapy or should all these
individuals try to be referred to a center where EP(electrophysiologic)
testing can be done?

Dr. Podrid: I think that some of the data that is now coming out from the Heart Watch program in Washington suggests that there are a strata of patients who are at risk for recurrence, i.e., a patient who has single vessel disease or no heart disease may be at a low risk for recurrence, whereas in a patient who has significant triple vessel disease and a lot of LV dysfunction there is a much higher risk for recurrence. I think that empiric therapy, although I'm not an advocate of empiric therapy, may work in the patient who is at low risk, simply because they're at low risk for recurrence. My feeling is that the type of patient that we're seeing and I think most of the other people here see, who are at high risk for recurrence simply because they have had numerous recurrent episodes before coming to us, I believe should be managed at a center or centers where this type of work is ongoing and is becoming routine. They have the expertise with not only using drugs, but with using techniques to evaluate the patient.

I also would just like to make a comment as to inducibility and non-inducibility if I can. Although we have far fewer patients who have gone through EP studies simply because of who we select to do it on, we have had 35 patients now in whom we've done this. Again, about 20% of our referral practice. Thirty of them have been inducible: five have not been able to be suppressed by any drug or combination of drug, 25 have been. Of the 25 there has only been one recurrence in 15 months followup. That one occurrence was in a young fellow with prolonged QT syndrome and I don't think he fits into the same category as your coronary artery disease patient. Of the other 5 patients who had the arrhythmias still inducible we have had now in less than 1 year followup two recurrences.

Dr. Winkle: I would say yes, if you mean by empiric therapy just taking a patient and slapping him on a drug and not doing anything.

Participant: Or using your Holter monitor to judge efficacy of therapy, or suppression of complex forms.

Dr. Winkle: I just don't think that should be done.

Dr. Rosen: Sudden death is scientifically very difficult as opposed to ventricular tachycardia where you could quantify occurrences. Sudden death only happens once unless you are rescusitated. This leaves very little room for maneuverability. You have very little room for quantification of effectiveness. I think such patients either with or without heart disease ought to be studied in hopes of defining a mechanism and hopefully therapy.

Dr. Josephson: It turns out that the answer is yes, that you ought to study them. It turns out that a vast majority of the people who you find in VF on the street have the VF initiated by V-tach. The V-tach is the same V-tach you can induce in the laboratory. If you look at the anatomy of the patients who are successfully rescusitated, who are already a selected population, it is an identical anatomy to those who have sustained V-tach. An in the laboratory they behave the same. The difference is that they have hemodynamic collapse early or they degenerate to VF after 5 seconds. The protocol proposed to induce V-tach is comparable to this, as Dr. Ruskin has already shown.

Dr. Ruskin: Our findings are similar. We found that somewhere, the series is larger now, it was 31 when published, it's now 50; but between 75 and 80% of the patients have inducible ventricular tachycardia of one type or another; many of them sustained, others non-sustained that may progress to VF, and in others it may not. But the one common feature was that when the VT, the inducible VT, was completely suppressed by drug therapy as assessed by repeat programmed stimulation, that the recurrence rate of symptomatic arrhythmias in sudden death so far in this group has been zero. Obviously there will be some recurrences, but it appears that in one year the survival rate will be very high.

Dr. Woosley: If you ask the people who use the electrodes if people should be studied, and they say yes; and if you ask people who do Holters if they should do Holters, they say yes. There's something that is really basically wrong with the numbers that I've seen with EP testing. You're comparing the outcome of people who respond to your test to people who do not respond to your test. And by that you've possible selected two totally different populations who can't have two totally different outcomes. Your results which show discordance between outcome in some individuals we've seen also, and it raises real doubts in my mind as how do you know if you should be putting someone on chronic therapy based on the results of your test when you can get good results either way you go. I think the people on the panel right now have at their disposal the patient population, the resources to answer the question. If you would do a controlled trial to compare outcome, randomize your patients to go through serial Holter tracings and then follow their outcome on therapy. Have the other population go through programmed stimulation, obtain the best results possible and then follow their outcome. I'm not convinced either method is the way to go. I don't think the data proves it in either case.

Dr. Josephson: I think that the data are available, because most of the patients we see have already been treated empirically as you suggest, by looking at the Holter monitor, evaluating suppressibility of arrhythmias and saying this looks good. Then it's not so good because they have an arrest or they have V-tach. Most of the patients referred to us have been previously treated in such a manner where they get antiarrhythmic therapy, and it's based on Holter monitoring and exercise testing, and if they have recurrences despite the fact that these non-invasive tests prove good, that's when they get referred. Clearly, they've been on anti-arrhythmic agents and in dosages that are commonly accepted as reasonable, but it doesn't work, and then we may or may not be able to de-ise an antiarrhythmic regimen in the laboratory; and there is a very good correla-tion. I don't think Dr. Zipes meant to imply that there's no correlation. I think that if you polled everyone that does these studies, we'd agree, if you can still induce V-tach, the odds are overwhelming that you're going to get V-tach clinically. The odds depending on who's talking are going to be 80-90% that they're going to have V-tach again.

Dr. Rosen: One of the problems is that all of us talk about different patients; some are the same, some are different. When we talk about paroxys-mal sustained ventricular tachycardia, for our laboratory that means several discrete episodes of VT. A patient profile that consists of 2.3 coronaries obstructed, a mean ejection fraction of 35%, 1.7 old in-farctions, two or more confluent areas of wall motion abnormality, half of the time anterior, half of the time posterior. Holter recording, it may or may not show PVC's. Treadmill testing, it almost universally does not provoke V-tach. Now, if you want to ask me, well why don't you treat that patient empirically using Holter and treadmill, I would say I don't know how to do that. There's nothing to quantify.

Dr. Zipes: We may be all prejudiced, but we do agree.

Dr. David: Dr. Podrid showed us the phenomenon of worsening of arrhythmias after drug treatment. To what extent do you think the high dosage of drug that you give is responsible for that? Do we know what amount of drug to give to patients in a one-stage drug study?

Dr. Podrid: Obviously drug dosage for an individual patient is by no means standardized. To answer the question 1) the doses employed by us are one-half of what is generally accepted as a standard daily dosage in patients who are not currently receiving that drug; 2) blood levels measured each hour for 3-5 hours have never in any of those patients been above what is accepted to be a therapeutic range; 3) there are many people who are using dosages chronically at similar levels throughout the day, i.e. 4 times a day doses similar to what we're giving. There are people being placed on a gram and a half of procainamide six times a day or four times a day. There are patients being placed on 300 mg. of disopyramide four times a day so that we don't feel, based on the blood levels we're getting, based on the amount of drug we're using, that these are in fact manifestations of drug toxicity because of high blood levels of the drug.

Dr. Zipes: Could you comment please on such high dose testing and what it's relevance is in understanind pharmacokinetics.

Dr. Kates: I think what they're approaching are probably comparable to what would be seen during chronic administration. In the absence of metabolites, one would expect the effect to be very similar. And I think your monitoring levels suggest that the level is not up to a point of toxicity. Now, in the cases where you are seeing toxicity I think you're in a position to maybe redefine what is a toxic level with respect to currently published guidelines.

Participant: Do you think there's appropriate equilibration between what is measured in plasma or serum and what may be in the myocardium that is presumably producing the electrophysiologic action? It seems to me that's the key issue of acute drug testing.

Dr. Kates: Based on inadequate evidence I can give you an opinion. We have done studies with propranolol and Tom Tengers has done studies with procainamide and I think there have been a few studies with lidocaine. It appears that antiarrhythmics equilibrate very quickly with gross myocardial tissue.

Participant: Some antiarrhythmics.

Dr. Kates: Certainly not amiodarone and perhaps others. But the question is whether gross myocardial ocncentration is what we're talking about because for some durgs the effect doesn't equilibrate as quickly as the biopsy concentration.

Dr. Zipes: Dr. Podrid has clearly thrown out two drugs from such testing, amiodarone and aprindine. Based on our data we would discount Encainide. It appears to have a betabolite or at least something different is

happening at 3-4 days compared to i.v. administration. Unless someone
has critically looked at and compared a gamut of antiarrhythmic agents,
I'm not certain that you can make the statement that they do equilibrate,
necessarily.

Dr. Kates: No, I qualified by saying that I'm basin this on totally inadequate data, it's something that has not been well studied.

Dr. Josephson: I think that the therapuetic level is a level that works.
It's not a magic number. A toxic level is the level that makes someone
sick. Just because the levels is higher, for instance, a procainamide
level of 10 (ug/ml) doesn't make it a toxic level. It's very frequently
therapuetic. So I think that we have to redefine what we mean by toxic
and therapeutic and a plasma level shouldn't be used as a definition of
that.

Dr. Sami: Before we discard Dr. Woosley's comment, shouldn't we define
what we mean by a drug that works on Holter monitoring in precisely those
patients with recurrent VTs and complex PVC's. Dr. Zipes siad that when
there were no runs of VT on the Holter he was satisfied that there was drug
response. That may be inadequate. If you compare that to the electrophysiologic study where you have a very hard, fast simple answer, can we
induce VT or not induce VT, it's not really comparable. Perhaps if you
had more conservative criteria for drug response on Holter, then you
could use that to compare it to electrophysiologic studies.

Dr. Zipes: When one is taking care of these kinds of patients the room
for error is very small. Ther's no question that at times I am less than
a scientist. In taking care of the patients you really don't want to make
a mistake in choosing a drug. In the patients that we do evaluate, they
have all had a 24-hour Holter recording and at least one 24-hour recording
which shows complete suppression of spontaneous V-tach. If they have VT
on that recording they don't come to electrophysiologic study. We feel
it's a wasted study because they're spontaneously having the very arrhythmia
we're trying to prevent. Admittedly, the data that we have are markedly
influenced by the methods that we're using to select the patients. They've
first gong through a 24-hour Holter, showed no VT and then go to electrophysiologic study. Yet, as I showed in 75% of them we could still induce
V-tach. Now if you take what my colleagues here say, which I don't
entirely believe that induction of VT in the laboratory by an EP study
does indicate the patient will develop it spontaneously, it would suggest

then that a 24-hour Holter recording is not an adequate measure of drug efficacy.

Dr. Josephson: I think again we're talking about apples and oranges. You almost don't need a Holter-monitor for sustained VT because they're all very symptomatic. What you see on the Holter monitor are runs of non-sustained VT and that's not an endpoint, that's not what you're shotting for. You're shotting for prevention of sustained VT and sudden death and to see five complexes in a row on a Holter monitor to me is meaningless. We have a number of people who have been treated successfully for sustained VT either medically or surgically. On Holter recordings they can have no arrhythmias, they can have complex arrhythmias, they can have 4 beat runs of non-sustained V-tach, but they don't have sustained V-tach; that's clinically significant. If someone had 4-beat runs of V-tach at a rate of 120, 6 times a day, I'm not sure I'd even treat that if they were asymptomatic.

Participant: In that regard, we have now 5 patients, and I'm sure many of you do too who have VT, one almost continuously. He's had it for 8 years, he's totally asymptomatic, the VT is a rate of 100-120. He gets sicker with the drugs. He's got VT, no organic heart disease that we could measure, and he's perfectly fine. We would not treat that patient.

Participant: I'm talking about a patient who's been resuscitated from V-fib. He comes to the hospital and when you do 24-hour Holter monitoring he's not in sustained VT, but he has many runs of short VT. If this patient is given a drug, so-called empirically, and you see that there is complete abolition of his PVC's and/or couplets or short runs of VT, and you tell yourself I think that the drug has worked in this particular patient, follow him up, how would this patient compare using this approach versus taking him to the lab and inducing VT in him and trying to design effective therapy.

Dr. Josephson: We have that data on people with sustained V-tach. There was an equal number of patients who had virtually 100% abolition of spontaneous ectopy in the group that had recurrences and in the group that didn't have recurrences; so that absence doesn't mean anything. Presence may mean something, but you can't tell. I really believe the best test is the laboratory.

Dr. Kennedy: I want to extend what Dr. Josephson said, but I also want to point out if we went back 10 years and we took Moss's data and Vismara's data and you'd all done Holters, you'd say the ventricular ectopy we see identifies these people that die of sudden death. And that was your first clue as to whom was going to die suddenly. Now, that data over a 10-year period has shown us that most likely that marker, along with a low ejection fraction and myocardial dysfunction picks out the high-risk group. Now, all of you admit that you have a very well based referral practice. My comments are directed at the perspective of total sudden death. Does your group of patients constitute 5% of the sudden deaths, or 25% or 50% or 60%. Anytime a new technique is introduced, such as agioplasty, everybody would like to apply it to everything, but it may only apply to 5% of the cases. Now, I think that it can be answered. I think in fact if we knew that most of the sudden death people did exactly what Dr. Josephson thinks they'd do, and that many of them will be rescusitated and you'll be able to bring them back and induce them, then I think one of the most important questions that came up during the discussion is what are the characteristics of the people with discordancy? In other words, who are the people that the Holter really does predict and who are the people that you know you cannot rely upon ECG-detected arrhythmias. Because it's very hard to apply EP testing, which is invasive, at this point to 400,000 people across the country. You've got to ask yourself is there a better way non-invasively. And if there's not a better way non-invasively, then we'd like to take the invasive method and narrow down the characteristics of the group that really need that invasive test. Now you all have those little subsets falling out where this discordancy lies. I was very pleased to hear Dr. Rosen mention the characteristics of his patients, because there ought to be distinguishing characteristics such as ejection fraction or wall motion. I'd be very interested in that perspective. It may be that 5 years from now someone has a non-invasive way of doing EP testing. Do we go through the same thing all over again. I think this is an issue.

Dr. Rosen: I think we're all in agreement that you've got to talk about particular patients. When we talk about paroxysmal sustained V-tach we mean something very specific: some people who have random sporadic episodes of a sustained arrhythmia that have been carioverted. In our general epxerience, Holters and treadmills are not terribly helpful in looking at that group. Now, if somebody has ectopy all day long, and you decide for better or for worse that that ought to be treated, then the Holter's great once you define how much spontaneous variability there is from say 24 hours to to 24 hours or 8 hours to 8 hours, 10 minutes to 10 minutes. Then you can reliably use the Holter. If it's realiably replicated, the treadmill can also be used. I would like to say another thing about treadmill. If we get somebody with treadmill VT the first thing he gets is 2 more treadmills before we even begin to give him a drug. But then you have a big problem, because you know your steady state is not reliable.

Dr. Kennedy: Dr. Rosen, do you think your population is 5,20 or 50% of sudden death? What do you think that referred population represents?

Dr. Rosen: Oh that's another very complex problem. Sudden death is a hodge podge.

Dr. Josephson: We now have cathed and studied about 75 patients who have presented with sudden death. The ones that are replicated in the lab, which are now about 2/3 of them, have the same anatomy like Dr. Rosen suggested to you. They have 2-3 vessel disease, they have multisegmental abnormalties. The ones who you can't induce have less abnormalities in their ventriculogram and their hemodynamics. I don't know exactly what that means, but I can tell you that that's true. The ones that are non-inducible have less electrophysiologic abnormalities, less hemodynamic and less angiographic abnormalities. So, I think that a reasonable start might be to propose a study where all these people would be studied.

Participant: Dr. Josephson, can you predict who's going to have discordancy between the Holter and the EP study?

Dr. Josephson: To date? No. Since the vast majority are the ones who have V-tach and behave just like Dr. Rosen suggested, the Holter is not of use in that group of people. I think the Holter may be of use in certain groups of people particularly mitral valve prolapse. Yes , I think you have to define groups of people in whom electrical studies are not useful and go that way.

Participant: And I think that's one of the things that we've learned over the past several years, that all V-tachs are not created equal. They're quite different and VT in a patient with coronary disease is quite different from a patient with mitral valve prolapse or who has QT prolongation, etc. The mere difference in our success rate of induction in the lab suggests that there may be EP differences between the VT in the different subgroups of patients according to the etiology of their heart disease. That to me is new knowledge from the past several years that hopefully will be very important as we begin to dissect out more differences or similarities.

Dr. Anderson: Just to follow up on an earlier comment by Dr. Josephson
and also your patient on amiodarone, I think that the Ep studies have demonstrated elegantly that they can predict success with type 1 agents, but in
the use of bretylium which is also a class 3 agent, along with amiodarone
at least, we have not seen success at EP testing with the use of bretylium
in preventing induction of VT in perhaps 10 patients or so. On the other
hand, in many patients, perhaps 10, who responded to i.v. bretylium and
were then placed on oral bretylium, there's been a rather good response
with some dropouts, perhaps 3 of 8 etc. I wonder if this is a general
attribute to type 3 drugs and because they're such a fascinating group
whether any of you have a handle on their use.

Dr. Zipes: They don't respond. We have 8 consecutive patients who have
paroxysmal sustained VT who got dosed with bretylium and were studied 1/2
hour later and they all had, with the exception of one, inducible sustained
V-tach. That one patient was begun on oral bretylium, 2 grams every 6
hours. After 48 hours, although he responded to i.v. he didn't respond
to oral. Now oral bretylium is so painful and unpleasant to take that
it would be very difficult to test the hypothesis of whether the oral
drug prevented the induction of VT. It would be very hard to put these
people on it because they have nausea and hypotension and we've gone onto
other things. Without mentioning names there are two amiodarone abstracts
from the American College that are in the pile that we just reviewed. The
two abstracts in general show that amiodarone doesn't prevent induction and
that event frequetnly presages clinical occurrence of VT or sudden death, not
always but sometimes.

Dr. Podrid: We have used both i.v. and oral bretylium and have not found
it to be particularly effective. I think the comment that not all VT's
are alike is absolutely correct. A VT that is slow and that is less than
220 does not respond to bretylium. When it's more rapid it may. Especially
non-sustained VF might respond appropriately to bretylium. The other
comment is I first of all don't want to be classified an EP zealot, because
I am by no means that. Whenever possible we try to use a non-invasive
technique to evaluate our patients. We're forced into using EP studies when
there are no other guidelines for therapy. It has also become clear that
patients who have more coronary artery disease and who have more contraction
abnormalities on either CAT or nuclear medicine studies, tend to have more
ventricular ectopy of higher grade. This is not universal, but there is

a tendency toward that. The 20% of patients in whom there is no ambient
ectopy in our group unfortunately do not present anything clinically different than the patients who do have frequent couplets and runs of V-tach
on exercise and monitoring. They are a similar group of patients with
similar extent of heart disease and coronary involvement, so although there
is a tendency for patients with more heart disease to have more of the higher
grade froms for which one might use more non-invasive, conventional ways
of evaluating drug therapy, there's really no way to predict this. Our
results at least are that there is a similar response when you use EP
studies vs. more conventional exercise of monitoring. But again, I have
to admit that although they have a similar coronary anatomy and similar
hemodynamic status, they are nevertheless two different groups of patients.
There are patients who have ambient ectopy and patients who do not have
ambient ectopy, despite the fact that they both presented with similar
types of malignant arrhythmias.

Dr. Hai: We've been doing acute drug testing using basically the same
approach that Dr. Lown uses with some modifications and we have had between
150 and 200 patients now, the majority with coronary artery disease and a
very vast percentage with recurrent V-fib. Using these techniques, most
important is not so much that you can even define therapy, but long-term
follo-up has given mortality in the range of about 3%. Slightly higher
than what Dr. Podrid indicated and I think that's probably the most important indication of the validity of the procedure.

Dr. Woosley: I would say that until there are controlled trials comparing
EP and Holter monitoring, I'm afraid that EP testing may not be anything
more than a higher grade of cosmotology.

Dr. Ruskin: I don't think it's as misleading as you're implying, but I
do agree with you entirely that we don't have an answer to the question you
pose, and the only way to get than answer, at least in subsets of patients
who manifest a great deal of spontaneous arrhythmias is to do a prospective
randomized controlled comparison of the two approaches. We wrote a proposal
about 3 years ago to do precisely that, and I had an interesting experience
that will do nothing to illuminate the point, but it does me good to get it
out. We received a great deal of flack from our internal review board
who said, "You actually want to induce arrhythmias in these people. How
can you possible do that?" They held up the proposal for quite a while
and eventually when some additional data from other laboratories came out

they passed it. We then had a site visit from the NIH about 6 months later, and this followed publications by Mason and by Horowitz and Josephson
on the efficacy of programmed stimulation of predicting response to drugs.
And the response that we got from the site visit group was that we couldn't
ethically withhold programmed stimulation so we couldn't do the study.
There you have it. I think it's a serious problem, and I don't know what the
answer is, but I agree with you it ought to be done.

Participant: One of the problems that an investigator will face is taking
the patient on a drug to the lab, inducint VT or VF with programmed stimulation and then sending that patient home on that drug. While the scientist
in all of us says that's the way to do it, I think the clinician at least
in me balks. Now, admittedly, we don't have the controlled data that you're
seeking, but it's very difficult to get.

Dr. Temple: It's possible that it would be really difficult for a single
clinician believing firmly in one method of choosing therapy to carry out
the kind of trial that Dr. Woosley suggests, but it does occur to me that
in Boston there are two different ways of doing drug selection, and it might
be possible for some other party to randomly assign people to Ruskin and
Podrid and let them choose therapy as they believe is right and see if
there's a difference that way.

Dr. Josephson: I think that people are forgetting, that maybe giving drugs
is a bad thing. The third part of that thing is to not give anything, and
the truth is that people who are asymptomatic don't take their medicine.
If someone is asymptomatic the only thing you can do is make them feel
worse. It can cost them alot of money and you make them feel worse. The
only way to know whether you have selected an empiric drug therapy that's
worked to prevent sudden death is to call up the patient, and if he answers
the phone, then you know you've selected the right drug.

Dr. Reid: I'd just like to make a comment on something that perhaps needs
re-emphasis, and that has to do with the sensitivity and specificity and
predictive value of either the Holter or EP testing. I think most agree
that it is extremely important to define your substrate, and that if you
haven't adequately defined that substrate, you're going to find discordancy. For example, we do not find the discordancy which some of the
other people have discussed between the Holter and the EP testing. It goes
along relatively well, but there are certainly false positives and false
negatives. When we have a patient who is admitted with symptomatic VT or

is a survivor of sudden death, routinely that patient gets coronary angiography and left ventriculography, stress testing and Holter monitoring. Now, I would think that if we're talking about the PVC being a harbinger of sudden death, these same tactics should apply to that group of patients and that is exactly what we do. We do these same types of tests in patients who have VT on Holter without symptoms. As an example of what may be coming, I don't know yet how significant it is, we found that when one looks at the ventriculogram, you have to look at more than just ejection fraction. Segmental analysis may play an increasingly important role, and in a series of 80 patients who we have just completed, we found that independent of whether therapy was successful clinically or not, that we could predict deaths with an accuracy of 77% by noting two particular segmental wall motion abnormalities. One was in the distribution of the proximal LAD, and the other was in the posterior basilar segment. I honestly don't know what those mean, but they did fall out quite significantly. And if we were to approach a systematic evaluation of the patients, it might have two additional and very important fallouts. One in terms of the drug therapy. We could rationally allocate it and perhaps come up with something other than random assignment. Two, by doing it in this way, we could also approach the patient from the least to the most invasive techniques, depending on what the results were. But we're not going to get there until we take a systematic approach that people can agree upon.

Dr. Zipes: I think it's important to stress that none of us here are minimizing the importance of PVCs, the HIP study, the Coronary Drug Project, etc. But, it clearly may be a marker of a patient who may have sudden death and not necessarily a precipitor of the final event. That's the point I tried to make earlier this morning that these patients who are walking around ambulatory, asymptomatic, with a lot of ventricular ectopy are very fine models to test whether a drug is going to suppress that kind of arrhythmia, see whether the drug has an active component to it, determine toxicity, etc. But we do not know that suppression of that arrhythmia, or indeed the absence of its suppression is in any way related to the VT/VF that causes the sudden death in these patients. But none of us are disregarding the importance of those kinds of PVCs.

Dr. Wenger: It's often been said about new drugs that you ought to use them quickly while they still work, and I think the same can be applied to new investigative techniques. I think that Dr. Hoffman brought up in the

first talk studying EP parameters of drugs, that there are certain aspects
of a drug such as its frequency dependency or use dependence that might
suggest that a drug would or would not work in an EP study, depending
on what the protocol is for study. That's not to say that the EP testing
doesn't work very well in certain settings that have been defined. But
it may be very difficult to predict with a new drug whether or not the
protocol that was used previously, and was shown to be predictive with another
drug, will accurately predict whether or not the next drug is going to be
effective. And if you redesign the protocol to be tailored for that new
agent, you no longer have knowledge of what its predictive accuracy is in
people who are not on the drug, so that I think there may be some problems
in the future in terms of evaluating new agents that have different EP
properties than the agents that are presently available. And in that
light I think that the older models (patients with chronic PVCs who may
or may not be at high risk for sudden death, but may have real symptoms)
might still represent a tried and true legitimate test of an antiarrhythmic
drug.

Dr. Yoshio Watanabe, Japan: My first comment is on the discrepancy between
Holter and EP studies, especially with programmed stimulation. As a very
simple-minded electrophysiologist, I look at the discrepancy in this way.
If you see a patient in whom you can induce VT in the EP study, but you
don't see any spontaneous PVCs or VT on the Holter, then in the lab you
are actually providing a trigger for an already established mechanism for
sustaining VT. But if you look at the Holter, actually you are looking at
the end result of the accumulation of a spontaneous triggering mechanism
and a sustaining mechanism. So if you see this phenomenon in a patient,
it simply means that although the sustaining mechanism may still be present
with the drug, you may have abolished the triggering PVCs. Of course, I'd
be much happier if you can wipe out both of these mechanisms. But if you
cannot eradicate the sustaining mechanism, I'd still be very happy to see
if we could wipe out the triggering mechanisms. And the second point is,
on the effects of bretylium. As I briefly mentioned yesterday from EP
studies in canine preparations with bretylium, in the presence of hypoxia
bretylium actually reverses the effects of hypoxia by increasing the $\dot{V}$max
and also prolonging the action potential duration. But this apparently
depends on the release of catecholamines. So i.v. bretylium may be expected,
by this release of catecholamines, to reverse the effects of hypoxia on

conduction and refractoriness. But if you give oral bretylium it may
not have this effect.

Dr. Zipes: I certainly would agree with your first comments as an equally
simple-minded electrophysiologist. This is how we explain the observation.
I think all of us that do these kinds of studies appreciate that the EP
study is limited by a number of factors. You only have a patient during
a finite period of time when his autonomic nervous system may be totally
different from when he is up, ambulating and having a fight with his wife,
whatever, that you supply a triggering event with stimulation that may or
may not be similar to his spontaneous triggering event. As Dr. Josephson
alluded to before and a point we've also made is that there probably are
two different kinds of ingredients for an arrhythmia, an initiating
mechanism and a sustaining mechanism, and indeed a drug could suppress the
triggering event, not the maintaining event. You could induce it in the
laboratory, on the drug, but yet the drug could be successful clinically.
Clearly, there are a number of drawbacks with electrophysiologic studies.
But I certainly think, particularly in view of the publications that my
cohorts have made in this area, that it's been a real contribution, and
appropriately used does save lives in these patients who are having malignant arrhythmias.

WHAT SHOULD THE STUDY DESIGN BE TO TEST NEW ANTIARRHYTHMIC DRUGS IN
PATIENTS WITH ACUTE MYOCARDIAL INFARCTION, DIGITALIS TOXICITY AND OTHER
ACUTE PROBLEMS

ROGER A. WINKLE, M.D.
CARDIOLOGY DIVISION
STANFORD UNIVERSITY SCHOOL OF MEDICINE
STANFORD, CALIFORNIA 94305

I. ACUTE MYOCARDIAL INFARCTION

In the setting of acute myocardial infarction the largest single use
of antiarrhythmic drug therapy is for the prevention of ventricular
fibrillation. In this setting drug efficacy cannot be judged in a single
patient and can only be inferred from well controlled clinical trials.
Traditionally lidocaine has been the most widely utilized drug for this
indication. We can learn about the potential flaws to be avoided in
antiarrhythmic drug trials by examining the previously performed clinical
trials of lidocaine in acute myocardial infarction. Table 1 summarizes
some of the larger series evaluating lidocaine efficacy in this setting.
None of these studies were able to show a beneficial effect of lidocaine
in preventing ventricular fibrillation until the study of Lie et al.
The pitfalls of all of these studies (except that of Lie and coworkers)
may be listed as follows:

1. Most studies were based on the assumption that warning arrhythmias
    identified patients at risk of ventricular fibrillation and
    therefore the endpoint of therapy was suppression of warning
    arrhythmias. They permitted placebo treated or control patients
    to crossover to lidocaine therapy once warning arrhythmias occurred.

2. There was inadequate knowledge of the pharmacokinetics of lidocaine.
    This resulted in several problems:

    a. No initial loading bolus.

    b. Inadequate maintenance infusion rate.

    c. Failure to achieve or document therapeutic lidocaine plasma
        concentrations.

3. In many instances there was delay in patient arrival at the
    hospital or in institution of drug therapy so that the period of
    highest risk of ventricular fibrillation had passed.

In recent years the following facts relating to the design of studies for prophylaxis of ventricular arrhythmias following acute myocardial infarction have become apparent.

1. The role of warning arrhythmias is minimal. A large number of subjects have warning arrhythmias who never develop ventricular fibrillation and a number of patients have ventricular fibrillation without ever having significant warning arrhythmias.

2. The highest risk of ventricular fibrillation is in the very earliest hours following the onset of myocardial infarction and diminishes rapidly over the subsequent 24 hours.

3. Withholding all drugs in the Coronary Care Unit setting and treating ventricular fibrillation with defibrillation when it occurs is probably safe. There is, however, tremendous resistance on the part of non-investigative physicians and nursing personnel to take this approach to therapy.

Based on these observations I would propose the following recommendations for studies of antiarrhythmic drugs for ventricular arrhythmias following acute myocardial infarction.

1. The primary endpoint of the study should be the prevention of sustained ventricular tachycardia and ventricular fibrillation. This will require large numbers of patients to be entered into the study.

2. There should be much less emphasis on the reduction of lesser ventricular arrhythmias.

3. Patients must be entered in within a few hours of the onset of chest pain.

4. The study design should carefully consider the drug's pharmacokinetics and be certain that adequate loading and maintenance doses are utilized to rapidly achieve and maintain therapeutic drug concentrations.

5. The study should be a randomized double-blind comparison with placebo.

6. The study should not exclude patients with relative contraindications to antiarrhythmic therapy such as mild congestive heart failure, minor conduction disturbances, etc.

7. The study should carefully monitor clinical hemodynamic status, conduction disturbances, etc., to determine the incidence of adverse reactions in both the drug and placebo group.

8. A major educational process needs to be carried out to convince non-investigative physicians and nursing personnel that placebo therapy is justifiable in the acute myocardial infarction setting.

II. ACUTE SUSTAINED ARRHYTHMIAS

A variety of types of arrhythmias may be considered under this category. These would include new onset atrial fibrillation or atrial flutter with a rapid ventricular response, paroxysmal supraventricular tachycardias of a variety of electrophysiologic mechanisms and sustained ventricular tachycardia. In general, when a drug is efficacious in treating these arrhythmias the beneficial response will be immediately apparent to the investigator and physicians caring for the patient. Major problems in scientifically evaluating an antiarrhythmic drug efficacy and side effects in this setting are the tendency for many of these arrhythmias to terminate spontaneously and for adverse drug reactions to be attributed to the natural course of the underlying disease process. While appropriately designed clinical trials can minimize the chance of attributing drug success to spontaneous termination of arrhythmia and appropriately identify the true incidence of side effects of a drug, in many instances the patient's clinical status and other factors will make it difficult to adhere to strict protocol designs. In our quest for carefully controlled randomized double-blind placebo controlled studies we should not underestimate the value of the opinions of a single experienced clinical investigator using a drug to treat a large number of patients in an unblinded open label manner. As long as careful attention is paid to appropriate dosing regimens and achievement of therapeutic plasma concentrations, such studies, in my opinion, can and should be accepted as evidence of drug efficacy for the treatment of acute sustained arrhythmias.

When controlled trials are to be carried out for acute sustained arrhythmias the study design should depend upon the clinical status of the patient. There are two general situations.

A. Acute sustained arrhythmias occurring in a setting when delay in therapy will not jeopardize the patient's well being.

A typical example of such an arrhythmia might be sustained paroxysmal supraventricular tachycardia in a young healthy adult. In such a setting I would make the following recommendations concerning therapy.

1. Antiarrhythmic drugs should generally be given intravenously with careful attention to giving adequate loading doses and achievement and documentation of therapeutic drug plasma concentrations.

2. A double-blind comparison with placebo is appropriate in this situation.

B. Acute arrhythmias occurring in a situation where a delay in therapy will potentially jeopardize a patient's well being.

A variety of arrhythmias resulting in clinical deterioration or the threat of clinical deterioration will fall under this category. In general, ethical considerations dictate that we not withhold active therapy from the patient. In this setting if one desires to carry out a careful clinical trial:

1. Drugs must be given I.V.

2. The most appropriate design should be a randomized comparison with a standard agent.

3. If the first therapy given fails to terminate the arrhythmia then the patient could be crossed over to the other agent. In this situation, the potential additive effectiveness and/or toxicity of the two drugs must be considered.

III. DIGITALIS INTOXICATION

The design of studies to treat arrhythmias associated with digitalis intoxication is extraordinarily difficult because of the wide spectrum of arrhythmias which can be associated with digitalis intoxication and the difficulty in establishing a definite diagnosis of digitalis intoxication. Factors such as clinical situation, type of arrhythmia, digitalis level and potassium concentration often play a role in making a diagnosis of digitalis toxicity which is often only initially suspected and finally diagnosed in retrospect. Only a few general comments will be made about recommendations for such studies.

1. Studies must give precise definitions of the arrhythmias present, clinical setting, digitalis level, potassium level, etc.

2. Antiarrhythmic drugs should only be given *in* *addition* *to* other standard non-drug treatment of digitalis intoxication including digitalis withdrawal, potassium administration, temporary pacing, etc.

3. In most instances arrhythmias of digitalis intoxication are best treated by observation. When therapy is justified it would not seem ethically appropriate to compare a new drug to placebo and thus randomized comparison with more standard agents would seem to be in order.

REFERENCES

1. Darby S, Cruickshank JC, Bennett MA, et al: Trial of combined intramuscular and intravenous lignocaine in prophylaxis of ventricular tachyarrhythmias. The Lancet 1:817, 1972.

2. Bennett MA, Wilner JM, Pentecost BL: Controlled trial of lignocaine in prophylaxis of ventricular arrhythmias complicating myocardial infarction. The Lancet 2:909, 1970.

3. Kostuk WJ, Beanlands DS: The prophylactic use of lidocaine in the prevention of ventricular arrhythmias in acute myocardial infarction. In Lidocaine in the Treatment of Ventricular Arrhythmias. Ed. Scott DB and Julian DG, Livingstone, Edinburgh and London, 1971, pg. 82.

4. Morgensen L: Ventricular tachyarrhythmias and lignocaine prophylaxis in acute myocardial infarction. A clinical and therapeutic study. Acta Med Scan, Suppl. 513, 1971

5. Pitt A, Lipp H, Anderson ST: Lignocaine given prophylactically to patients with acute myocardial infarction. The Lancet 1:612, 1971.

6. Church G, Biern R: Prophylactic lidocaine in acute myocardial infarction. Circulation 45 & 46 (Suppl II):II-139, 1972 (Abstract).

7. Lie KI, Wellens HJ, van Capelle FJ, Durrer D: Lidocaine in the prevention of primary ventricular fibrillation. A double-blind, randomized study of 212 consecutive patients. N Engl J Med 291:1324, 1974.

Table 1.   Summary of Studies Evaluating In-Hospital Postmyocardial
           Infarction Lidocaine Prophylaxis

	No. pts. C	No. pts. L	Controls treated for warning arrhythmias	Lidocaine Dose Bolus (mg)	Lidocaine Dose Inf. rate (mg/min)	% with VF C	% with VF L
Darby et al. (1)	100	103	yes	200*	2.0	4.0	3.9
Bennett et al. (2)	125	118	yes	60	0.5	5.6	9.3
		131	yes	60	1.0		3.8
Kostuk et al. (3)	44	48	yes	none	1.0	0	0
Morgensen et al. (4)	37	42	yes	75	2.0	2.8	0
Pitt et al. (5)	114	108	yes	none or 75-100	2.5	0	0.9
Church et al. (6)	44	42	yes	50-75	2.0	6.8	9.5
Lie et al. (7)	105	107	no	100	3.0	8.6	0

* intramuscular

GENERAL GROUP DISCUSSION: STUDY DESIGNS: ACUTE PATIENTS

Dr. Campbell: We've done two quite large studies of placebo antiarrhythmic
therapy in acute myocardial infarction, and both of them double blind
studies, one of them using mexiletine as the active agent and the other
tocainide as the active agent. Both of these studies were based on oral
therapy and the reason for this was that in Great Britain we don't have
such a well-organized rescue system as exists in many of the cities in
North America. We rely for primary care on our general physicins and
general practitioners who often find it difficult to put up i.v. therapies
out in a patient's home. So we wanted to evaluate oral antiarrhythmic
therapy in preventing ventricular fibrillation, ventricular arrhythmias,
and sudden death in a hospital situation. I think the biggest problem
we came across was the ethical one: Was it justifiable to have people
in a placebo group at a time when figures from Amsterdam suggested that high
dose intravenous lidocaine did significantly reduce the incidence of
ventricular fibrillation? It has been our contention, and it still is
my contention, that safety of high dose i.v. lidocain given to patients
with suspected acute myocardial infarction is as yet unproven. For
these reasons our ethical committee was easy to pursuade that we should
do the study with placebo therapy and with an active agent. As you
probably know, our studies show a very significant reduction of ventricular
arrhythmias in the first 48 hours of acute infarction. But there were
too few incidences of VF and too little in the way of sudden death to
make any further comments. It was about that time that we looked at the
placebo data from these groups in a prospective manner to gain some
information about the natural history of arrhythmias in acute myocardial
infarction. Neither patients were seen very early, within the first
hour of acute myocardial infarction. We wanted to look at warning arrhythmias
in particular. We've examined patients who had primary ventricular

fibrillation in the placebo group and patients who had no primary
ventricular fibrillation in the placebo group, and there is a striking
division of arrhythmias which occur in the initial phase of acute myocardial
infarction: V-tach, R on T ectopic beats and ventricular ectopic complexes
of any type are relatively frequent in the first three hours. Thereafter,
VF and R on T ectopic beats are almost non-existent; whereas V-tach reaches
its peak incidence about 12 hours out from the onset of symptoms. So at a
time when V-tach is very common, R on T ectopic beats and VF are very
rare. Although we were gratified to show a very significant reduction in
V-tach with drugs, I think V-tach and acute myocardial infarction says
nothing about what the drug may do to ventricular fibrillation.

Dr. Kraemer: I agree with you in principle. You say you don't believe
you can assess efficacy in a single patient. I don't think you can assess
the efficacy of the drug as a property of the drug, making inferences
about the effectiveness of a drug for future patients on the basis of a
single patient's response. But I do believe that a single patient studied
intensively can lead to a conclusion within certain error limits of whether
or not the drug is effective for that particular patient. I do believe
that single subject studies are very possible and might yield very
important information. About the comment that 30 was too small a size
for a study: there was a paper in the New England Journal of Medicine a
few years ago that surveyed medical research reports in certain medical
journals and the median number of subjects per clinical research study was
30. That means half of the studies reported actually fall underneath that
number. I think if your endpoint is survival, a binary endpoint, then
30 is too small a sample size. But for many of the types of measures,
the response that you're using is a quantitative one, and 30 may be quite
adequate. You recommended randomized over blind and placebo control
trials. I think it's terribly important that you have techniques to
control sampling bias in your studies. One technique of controlling
sampling bias is randomization, but there are other techniques. Sometimes
it would be preferable not to have complete randomization, but randomization
within blocks, for example. I would not limit the control of sampling bias
techniques strictly to randomization. Similarly, if the measures that
you have are totally objective, reading a Holter monitor comes readily to
mind, I don't know how observer bias could prejudice reading a Holter
monitor. If in addition, there is no possible way that the subject's

knowledge of how he is being treated could affect response, I think an
argument can be made in those particular circumstances that you do not
have to have double blind trials, that in effect the nature of the response
itself controls the sampling bias. I think it is absolutely necessary that
there be some control condition involved, but I don't know any statistical
reason why it has to be a placebo control. So I think that's a clinical
judgement, rather than a statistical one. I think in particular if you
restrict yourself to randomized double blind placebo trials, it may preclude
the possibility of some very good designs, such as a sequential medical
trial design or adaptive trials. Such trial designs may come much closer
to the processes of clinical decision making. These designs may be
clinically much more satisfactory; they have a great deal of power but are
not the classical randomized double blind placebo design.

The other particular question you pointed out was the question of
crossing over and then worrying about intra-active effects. I don't
know what to say except that yes, you're going to have to worry about them.
The only suggestion that I would have is that if you monitor frequently
the response over time, for example to Holter monitor every second day
during the period of treatment, you may not be able to eliminate the
cross-over interactive kinds of effect, but you may be able to understand
it a great deal better. That's the best I can do.

Participant: I just wonder if Dr. Temple might give us some feel for
the FDA's position now for what might the FDA require of a pharmaceutical
company that wants to test a new drug in the specific situation of acute
myocardial infarction, and would suppression of these so-called warning
arrhythmias be adequate for showing efficacy or would you require prevention
of VF.

Dr. Temple: I think what you said before was actually correct. The
issue that I would put wouldn't be "should prevention of VF or warning
arrhythmias be the proper standard" it would be "should suppression of
VF or death be the proper standard. Back to what Dr. Crout was talking
about. I think what he was saying was our present standard would be that
if you can show that you can prevent VF, that would probably be sufficient
and you don't have to show increased survival. Under the circumstances,
the presumption would be that at least sometime someone wouldn't be
rescusitated from his VF even if you couldn't show it in a study of reasonable size. I just wanted to add one thing about the use of expert observa-

tions and opinion. I think it's very important to distinguish between
what an expert thinks and what an expert thinks on the basis of data he
has. You can't help but be impressed as you wander through a meeting like
this that experts don't even believe each other. I can't tell you the
number of times that I've heard in the last few days, "I don't believe
that," and everybody we're talking about is highly expert, at least as
measured by his ability to get into legitimate journals. So the question
comes down to what kind of data do people have? And it's worth saying,
I think Dr. Kraemer put it very well yesterday, that a formal well-controlled
trial is not the only way to study something, it just reduces the risk
that you won't be believed, or something to that effect. In appropriate
situations we've accepted trials in which the person's initial status
was taken as an appropriate control for what then happened after drug
intervention. If you're studying dobutimine and you're seeing an abrupt
change in cardiac output that's pretty plausible. If you're studying
arrhythmias, one has to ask the experts around if a change is plausible.
You pointed out there can be spontaneous reversion of many of these
arrhythmias. I probably wouldn't be telling too much out of school to
comment on some studies on supraventricular arrhythmias that were recently
done with verapamil. It's worth saying at the outset that initially the
trials were proposed as essentially uncontrolled studies in which the
patient would be seen and then put on the drug and then you'd watch
what happened. After some discussion we proposed a sort of rapid cross-
over trial against placebo with cross-over occurring after I think 20
minutes; very short, because that was felt to be the time in which a
response would be seen. Well, in the case of converting supraventricular
tachycardias, pretty much the expected difference between drug and placebo
was seen. In treating atrial fibrillation, however, it turned out that
although the drug reduced the ventricular rate during fibrillation, the
frequency of conversion to normal sinus rhythm was quite similar in both
the placebo and treated groups. The conclusion that the European literature
has reached on conversion of atrial fibrillation by drugs like verapamil
is that there is a low conversion rate, 10 or 15% or something like that.
I think that's probably not true, and in the setting of the study, a
certain number of people convert for reasons that aren't quite clear. So
I guess my urging would be to try to include a control group unless you
just ethically cannot stomach it and cannot figure out a way to do it.

But it's often possible if you have early escape mechanisms: for example, no response in 10 minutes and you cross over, or whatever's appropriate to the kinetics of the drug.

Dr. Winkle: I think the message that we're saying here is that in a lot of situations we can probably study the drugs better than we are now and there are situations where we can apply controls that we're not. And I think there are situations where we're not even attempting to get data that might be submitted to the FDA to support an NDA, where both the FDA and the biostatisticians are telling us maybe we can make some legitimate conclusions that might support an NDA for a new drug.

Dr. Woosley: I'd like to amplify on what Dr. Kraemer said. I think the randomization within blocks would be especially appropriate and might allow you to study a lot of patients and get good information for comparison. The other comment that I would like to make is I think there probably still is in this country time to do a placebo study in the coronary care unit. I wonder though if it isn't getting very near the time when you can't do that. I'm not sure it's worth it, because one of the things we really want to know in the coronary care unit right now is not only does the drug work, but is it really better than lidocaine, and if it isn't why use it? Lidocaine is not the perfect drug, it is difficult to use, and hopefully there will be better drugs. But I think the ethical aspects of it, plus the fact that we want to compare it eventually anyway, makes me think that perhaps the first trials should be controlled comparisons of the two drugs.

Dr. Temple: Let me just ask Dr. Woosley a couple of questions about that. Certainly that is a point well taken, but if you believe the results of Dr. Lie's study, it's quite obvious that no drug is going to beat lidocaine; you can't do better than zero, if that's going to be a consistent finding. So the question is what will you do and conclude if you have a study of a certain number of people, say 30 per group, and the test drug turns out to be about the same, or let's say indistinguishable from lidocaine, one fibrillation in each, or maybe none for lidocaine and one for the test drug. What do you then conclude? That would correspond to no statistically significant difference and you're then in a position of essentially relying on historical information to determine that either agent worked. Dr. Winkle tripped through the literature and found only one adequate study. Is one entitled at this time to conclude that if

something matches -- is indistinguishable from -- lidocaine, in a study
like that, you should attribute effectiveness to both of the drugs. It's
not a simple question.

Participant: I think we've all learned today from the last panel that
everything's different in every institution, and even if lidocaine worked
in Amsterdam it doesn't mean that it will work necessarily in Philadelphia,
or work as well, so there's a lot of merit to what you say.

Dr. Woosley: Let me follow up with part of an answer to that. I agree,
but I think that if the study is as Dr. Winkle described, there are
adequate historical data that will allow us to make some decisions when
that study is finished. If no one patient dies in either group and the
patient population is well described so that we can use historical
controls, t-en I think we're allowed to ask the question what were the
relative instances of toxicity in the two groups. Lidocaine is a very
difficult drug to use. It's misused in at least 30% of the patients at
least in our institution, and reports from the literature show that it is
underused or overused in about that percentage around the country. So I
think that a drug with better pharmacokinetics that would allow simpler
dose regimens, that would hopefully not have to be reduced in dosage for
heart failure, where people really get in trouble. Physicians often
don't make appropriate reductions in dosage for heart failure. I think
lidocaine is a perfect drug when used perfectly, but that's not the real
world.

Participant: If a non-significant difference in the mean effect between
a drug and lidocaine, for example, is the end of the analysis, I think
you're losing a lot of valuable information. That does not necessarily
mean that the two drugs are indistinguishable, and it would be highly
pertinent to ask the question, for example, as to whether certain types
of people are more responsive to lidocaine and other types of people more
responsive to the other drug, which would certainly be clinically valuable
information.

Dr. Temple: Yes, but the design of this study, we'll take the lidocaine
studies specifically, is most likely to show you very few events. You
really don't expect too many ventricular fibrillations in the lidocaine
group. So you have very little power to distinguish much of anything.
I guess that to raise the question is not necessarily to answer it,
but anyone who designs a positive control study and intends to show no

difference in the end sought should think very carefully about how he
knows whether either drug works in the particular setting that the study
is going on in. And that's not true for only antiarrhythmics, it's true
for any agent.

Dr. Campbell: Can I just take up that point about toxicity again, because
I think in acute myocardial infarction the scenario for seeing drug toxicity
is very widespread, and it is very easy to say that it's the natural
consequences of the infarct, rather than the drug that's being administered.
The Lie et al. study certainly was very highly significant in favor in
use of lidocaine with respect to ventricular fibrillation. But to get
that effect, the drug had to be given very early in the course of acute
myocardial infarction. The drug was given to many more patients who were
suspected of having myocardial infarction, but in whom the diagnosis was
not proven, and we really don't have the data for what happened to these
patients who were given inappropriate drugs. And if we go back to look
historically, earlier investigators reported such a group of patients and
found a very disquieting incidence of asystole and sinus arrest in patients
without infarction but with suspected infarction who were randomized into
study. So I think if we are going totalk about gold standards to match
new therapies up against, lidocaine in my opinion is not a gold standard
yet, although it looks promising in that regard.

Dr. Klein: Dr. Winkle, I'd like to take issue with your proposal for
a double blind randomized study on arrhythmias in acute myocardial infarction with a placebo vs. lidocaine. I'd like to address this as the
administrator of a coronary care unit in a University hospital, as someone
who has had to deal with multiple professionals involved in care of patients
like this, someone who has had considerable experience both with the
benefits and the obvious potential side effects of lidocaine and finally
someone who's had experience with clinical investigation of antiarrhythmic
drugs in the second week following MI. I think your proposal is scientifically sound but clinically unwise and will lead to serious disruption
interprofessionally between doctors and nurses. First of all, on a basis
of some of Dr. Kaplinsky's studies, and reports from yesterday from
Dr. Dreifus, it's clear that the arrhythmia mechanism during the early
hours after MI is changing. Early on it may be reentry and there may
be various forms of reentry. Later on it probably is a form of normal
or abnormal automaticity. So it's hard to apply one drug over the first

8 or 12 hours of myocardial infarction and conclude from either its
success or its failure that it's likely to be successful; that the drug
in fact has either succeeded or not succeeded. This is something that
we already know from considerable empirical experience with the use of
lidocaine, and shifting over in the event that it does not work to a type
I antiarrhythmic agent. Secondly, I think it's extremely difficult and
probably now impossible to double blind these studies; and blind not just
the investigator, but blind all of the nurses involved in the care who
are changing over every 8 hours. I think that it is virtually impossible
and clinically unwarranted. Thirdly, I don't visualize the kind of
studies that Drs. Rosen and Josephson were talking about, in the controlled
setting of an electrophysiology laboratory, dealing with the problem of
recurrent sustained ventricular tachycardia and the need to provoke either
the VT or conceivably VR, as being at all analogous to an individual
coming into a hospital with an MI who's likely to have VF once and
hopefully only once. Nor do I regard the event of VF as being at all
benign either in terms of the individual to whom it's happened or to the
professionals, including the nurses who have to respond to it. It raises
a level of alarm, and I don't know how you would structure a double blind
randomized study involving placebo drugs given these types of complexities.
Dr. Kaplinsky: People might think and people may say I don't believe this
and I don't believe that, but I think that a lot of data has been accumulated
by now. I will call your attention to the famous article by Dr. Lown in
1966 that appeared in JAMA: 135 consecutive acute myocardial infarction
patients in the coronary care unit without a single incidence of VT...
the patients of the first report of lidocaine treatment in the intensive
coronary care unit. Until that time it had been well known that the
incidence of VF in coronary care units before that was between 8-10%;
and here was a report of 136 pateints without a single incidence of VF.
Since then, units give lidocaine to most of their patients, about 80-90%,
with infusion rates above 2 mg/min. The incidence of VF in this set of
patients, with known delay of 2-4 hours, is less than 0.5%. We have
enough data from your study, from this study, from previous history that
without lidocaine the incidence is about 8-10%. Then will somebody tell
me why is it necessary and where's the justification to withhold treatment
in patients with acute MI? I grant you that VF is beautifully rescusitated
in the hospital, but nobody wants to make this round trip up and down. We

are fortunate (or unfortunate) that in our hospital not every patient
gets to the intensive care unit, so about 40% of the patients bypass the
unit. And somebody in our hospital took the pain and the time to
analyze data of about 3 or now almost 4 years, the patients who happen to
not come to the unit and thus who went to regular hospital beds. It seems
that we were interested in this 15 years ago and I think that the disappearance of this interest is causing unjustified study designs because we have
forgotten what we learned 15 years ago. We knew that lidocaine prevented
VF and the issue was settled. Now everybody is talking about study
designs and proof and double blind. It's coming through the back door.
Nobody is paying attention to what has been done 15 years ago, and we are
letting patients go into VF because it has to be a double blind study,
placebo control. So in our hospital we analyzed our data and this
difference was found again very clearly. Patients in the age group of
30-50 or 55 who come into the hospital in good clinical condition die at
the rate of 3 times and 4 times higher than a comparable group entering
the coronary care unit, and the only thing that is different in our unit
is that almost everybody gets lidocaine. If you suspect an MI I think the
patient should be protected. Based on the experience from the emergency
ward is the chest pain patient with no PVC's, because all of our primary
VFs in the emergency wards have not a single PVC in the records. But when
a person comes in with chest pain and has two PVC's on the record he
gets lidocaine.

Dr. Pitt: I'd just like to take a little opposite view. It's a very
difficult problem, but I don't think we know the exact answer. In my
last conversation with Dr. Lie, whom we admit has the only good trial,
they have stopped using prophylactic lidocaine in their coronary care
unit. I can't understand the logic, but they feel in their coronary
care unit where they have excellent nursing that if someone fibrillates,
they don't lose those patients. They're there and defibrillate. I'm
not sure I agree with the logic, but there was the only study that showed
any benefit and those investigators are not convinced enough from their
studies to go on using prophylactic lidocaine in the coronary care unit.
So I think there's only one study and there's still room for some controlled
trials. It's a very complex issue.

Dr. Klein: To respond to that, I don't think it was ever recommended by
anybody, at least in Boston, that people be placed on lidocaine routinely.

Is that what you were suggesting? It was only suggested if there were
certain warning arrhythmias that they would be placed on lidocaine.

Dr. Pitt: Yes, but I think we all know from the data now that the whole
warning arrhythmia concept has a lot of flaws. And that early data from
Lown showing no VF, I think that's the natural history of those particular
patients who come in rather late rather than early.

Dr. Klein: I'm not sure that we know that at all. I think that original
data had some deficiencies in it, but I think the accumulated experience
of that and others over the years quite clearly points out that there are
certain types of warning arrhythmias in the early hours following myocardial
infarction and they tend to coincide very nicely with several of the
animal models.

Participant: I would like to agree that we need to have another drug
other than lidocaine available. I think that we've been using it prophylactically for a while and I think that what we're finding is that
with more and more outpatients coming into the CCU already on beta blockers
the addition of lidocaine has brought out a lot of sinus arrest and asystole,
especially in patients with acute inferior MI's and heart block. I've had
to put several pacemakers in patients with acute inferior MI's who did
not escape, which I never saw 10 years ago prior to the use of prophylactic
lidocaine and beta blockers. And I'd like to make one other point, that
in addition to considering drug efficacy, you've got to consider who's
using the drug. It's OK to say lidocaine works wonderfully in the hands
of an investigator with a protocol and with somebody around day and night
measuring drug levels, looking at the patient carefully and picking the
most appropriate dose of lidocaine. If we find a drug that we think is
effective, we've got to remember that it's going to be used in coronary
care units all over the country where there's not going to be a researcher
interested in the optimal use of the drug. I think it's true that with
somebody who really knows how to use the drug we can prevent VF with lidocaine and reasonably safely. But we need a drug that can be used in coronary
care units and in community hospitals throughout the country, without an
extremely experienced person there all the time, and we don't have one at
the present time.

Dr. Winkle: I'd like to respond to a few of the comments. First of all,
if you look at the data that I have presented summarizing the studies,
mostly from the 1960's, I think that one can't conclude that lidocaine

prevented VF. Virtually all of the studies have a 3-6% or 7% incidence of
VF both in the lidocaine group and in the control group. Now, one can
argue that was because the doses were too low, but I think that just re-
emphasizes the point that to prevent ventricular fibrillation with lidocaine
you have to use high doses, probably higher doses than most physicians
around the country are using. And Dr. Campbell's point and the point that
was just made, we really don't know necessarily what the toxicity is of
this high dose lidocaine. How many patients who didn't even have an MI
are having some serious complication which we're passing off as part of the
natural history of what happened to them. But I agree philosophically
with all of the comments. I think we all agree that it's best to prevent
VF, and it's psychologically disturbing to the patient. The problems
that were brought up about creating antagonism between the nurses and the
doctors are very very real ones. We could not carry out a study like I
proposed in our hospital. We just could not do it. I hope there are
hospitals in this country where it could be done and Dr. Campbell and Dr.
Lie and other people have shown us that it can be carried out. If we
really want to propose what is the best science we have to do a study I
think similar to the one I proposed. That's very difficult and I'm not
minimizing the problems associated with this, but I think we should shoot
for the best possible science and compromise only when we've shown that
we can't do it. I don't know that anybody in this country has really
tried to do it. I mean, if we had 20 people here who said I tried to do
it and I couldn't that would be one thing, but I don't think anybody's
even tried to do this kind of study in this country.

Dr. Woosley: Just to reiterate what I've said before. The therapeutic
index for lidocaine is one of the narrowest of the cardiovascular drugs
that we use. A plasma concentration of 5-9 ug/ml may be required in many
patients, and 9-12 ug/ml is certainly toxic in a lot of patients. Some of
the newer drugs had much wider therapeutic in disease in the studies so far,
but before we can really determine that they are better than lidocaine,
it will have to be in a controlled comparison, so I think that they perhaps
should be done that way first.

Dr. Campbell: I agree with many of the comments that have been made and
I certainly agree with many that Dr. Kaplinsky made as well. There's
a lot of data that's gone on in the past which I think has relevance and
is important to look at again. I don't want to go down on record at this

conference as having dissected all ventricular arrhythmias, but one thing
that has happened over the last few years is a realization that VF in
acute myocardial infarction is not a homogeneous entity. There is a
primary VF occurring in the absence of shock or cardiac failure and out of
the context of drug therapy with lidocaine, beta blockers or whatever.
And I do believe, and we have data to support this, that the characteristics
of this arrhythmia are different from VF which occurs in patients who have
features of cardiac failure or shock, or patients who are pre-treated
with beta-adrenergic blocking drugs. So I think in VF there's a stratification; it may be some of the interventions that we have are more appropriate
for one type of VF than the other.

Participant: How do you study the group of patients who come in from the
ER by the paramedic team who have already been pretreated with lidocaine?
I know in many places in this country it is pretty standard practice when
they pick the patient up at the door. The guy's complaining of chest
pain, the first thing they do is they give him lidocaine. Are you going
to be able to treat that patient and be able to do that?

Participant: Well, you obviously have to have control over that. That
may be one difference between Europe and here. Everybody knows the impact
of socialized medicine and somehow I feel the doctors aren't all fighting
with one another over who's getting the referrals, and maybe they can all
get together at one center and agree to do things the same way. So
maybe it really is impossible to do this kind of study in this country.

Participant: I don't think so. I think the study is very feasible and I
think it can be done in an academic institution where there's a lot of
interaction between the investigators and the clinical faculty, and there's
a team approach to it. I think the study can be done. There are plenty
of places: it's certainly not routine in most cities to give lidocaine
by the paramedics.

Participant: I do think the paramedics are the least of the problems
because they basically will do whatever they're told to do, so I think
that's the least of the obstacles.

Participant: One sure thing: another problem. What type of an informed
consent is the patient going to sign? Are we going to tell him that we
are going to withhold treatment until he develops ventricular fibrillation
and explain to him what ventricular fibrillation is. I mean if you do a
double blind study in the acute phase, withholding treatment, it means

that your endpoint is ventricular fibrillation. Are you going to tell this to the patient?

Dr. Campbell: We have had to tackle this problem, as you'll realize from the two studies. The situation is that what you're proposing would be unthinkable if indeed we were withholding a treatment of proven benefit, efficacy and safety. But if you take the stance that high dose intravenous lidocaine may be effective in those patients with proven infarction, but we only know that group in retrospect, then I don't believe we are withholding from a patient a therapy of proven efficacy and safety, and for these reasons we felt that it was legitimate to randomly allocate patients to an active therapy or to an inactive therapy. This results in a situation where a patient, if they do not come to our hospital, but to another within a very short distance of our hospital will have a completely different management of acute myocardial infarction. And whilst in our country we cannot define a standardized management, I think we're in a stronger position to undertake the studies that we described.

Participant: I think it's important that built into the protocol is the comparison of the two drugs, and when either fails the code be broken and usual treatment be given. Now that means that you have to have a lot of drug interaction data before you set the study up. You have to know that the two aren't lethal when used together, or whatever agent or therapy that you plan to use won't complicate things. I think you can tell a patient that there are two drugs, one that's currently used that's effective and has problems and may not be the best drug, we have a new drug that may be better, but we don't know until we do this comparison; we will flip a coin and see which one you get and follow you carefully. If neither works we'll break the code and give you the best possible medical therapy. That's the type of consent form that it would require.

Participant: I was going to ask a similar question to the last one about consent, but I'll amplify a little more how meaningful is a consent in a patient who is acutely and very seriously ill. In some of these patients we're talking about a matter of life and death, at least how the patient sees it. I know that in some of the European studies the consent was waived by ethics committees where they existed in such studies, particularly when patients were studied within a few hours of an acute MI.

Dr. Winkle: I can tell you when the FDA visits your institution, it's pretty important that you have informed consent. But this is a tremendous ethical consideration that's debated by human subject committees. It's difficult to have true and informed consent in that situation, but at least you have to have a signed piece of paper for the record.

WHAT BASELINE ELECTROPHYSIOLOGIC DATA SHOULD BE OBTAINED IN A PHARMACOLOGIC STUDY OF AN ANTIARRHYTHMIC DRUG?

ROSEN, KENNETH M.; STRASBERG, BORIS; PALILEO, EDWIN.

From the Section of Cardiology, Department of Medicine, Abraham Lincoln School of Medicine of the University of Illinois College of Medicine, Chicago, Illinois.

It is the thesis of this presentation, that electrophysiologic evaluation of proposed antiarrhythmic agents is mandatory. The purposes of this evaluation are as follows: 1) Electrophysiologic study provides part of the pharmacologic profile of an antiarrhythmic drug, which is generally biologically important information necessary about a drug and its properties. 2) Electrophysiologic study may allow prediction of drug toxicity, in regard to the cardiac conduction system. 3) Data arrived from electrophysiologic evaluation, may in part predict sites of action and possible mechanisms of effectiveness of antiarrhythmic drugs. 4) Electrophysiologic study may allow direct demonstration of effectiveness of an antiarrhythmic agent (for example, the demonstration that an antiarrhythmic drug prevents induction of paroxysmal supraventricular tachycardia in a patient with this arrhythmia).

When evaluating antiarrhythmic drugs, it is important to note that diseased tissue may respond differently to normal tissue. Application of this differential in responsiveness, is that electrophysiologic testing must be performed in patients with normal electrophysiologic function, as well as in those with suspected or demonstrated conduction disease. For example, an antiarrhythmic agent may have no effect on the normal His-Purkinje system, but a marked effect on the diseased His-Purkinje system.

Catheters and Recording Sites

Electrophysiologic studies are usually performed utilizing electrode catheters passed percutaneously or via cutdown, into

the venous system, and placed at various sites in the right heart.
The catheters are generally multipolar, allowing bipolar recording
and stimulation within the same chamber. A thorough electrophysiologic evaluation of the conduction system necessitates at
least two catheters. One catheter can frequently be used for recording and stimulation of more than one chamber. For example,
an octapolar catheter passed via a left antecubital vein to the
right ventricular apex, can be used for right ventricular stimulation and recording, with more proximal poles used for right
atrial stimulation and recording.

The usual sites for stimulation and recording are as
follows: 1) The right atrium (usually the high right atrium
close to the sinus node). 2) The left atrium (with access to
the left atrium via the coronary sinus, a right atrial structure).
3) The His bundle (standard recording of His bundle electrograms).
Reliable pacing of the His bundle is difficult to achieve. 4) The
right ventricular apex.

The recording equipment for routine electrophysiologic
studies incorporates a multichannel high fidelity recorder.
There must be a means of appropriate amplification and frequency
filtering, so that adequate and meaningful signals can be achieved.
Electrophysiologic study is greatly aided by coupling the recorder
to a multichannel tape system, which allows further study of
important portions of the electrophysiologic evaluation. The
ability for multiple paper speeds is essential.

Programmed Stimulation

The performance of electrophysiologic study is dependent
upon programmed stimulation. Programmed stimulation refers to
the delivery of controlled impulses to selective chambers, so
that the conduction system may be stressed, allowing assessment
of both normal and abnormal conduction system physiology. The
stimulatory techniques utilized in routine electrophysiologic
evaluation include 1) atrial incremental pacing, generally in
10 beat/minute increments, at least up to an atrial paced rate
of 200 beats/minute. 2) atrial extrastimulus testing to sinus
rhythm and to one or more atrial driven cycle lengths (generally

a cycle length just shorter than sinus rate, and frequently a cycle length of 600 msec or 450 msec). 3) Ventricular incremental pacing, in 10 beat/minute increments, generally up to a maximum paced ventricular rate of 200 beats/minute. 4) Ventricular extrastimulus testing to sinus rhythm, to atrial driven cycle lengths, and to ventricular driven cycle lengths.

The specific modalities of stimulation utilized, will relate to the type of information that is being obtained. If emphasis is on ventricular tachycardia and ventricular electrophysiology, the stimulation protocols will be more heavily weighted towards ventricular extrastimulus technique and ventricular incremental pacing.

Sinus Node Function

The most important function of the sinus node is the generation of impulses. Drugs can thus be characterized by their effect on sinus rate. This is most readily done utilizing 24 hour ambulatory recording, which allows definition of mean waking rate and mean sleeping rate. Minimum and maximum waking and sleeping rates can also be observed. Treadmill testing allows delineation of the sinus response to a measurable level of exercise.

Sinus node function can also be quantified in the electrophysiology laboratory. The most commonly utilized test of sinus node function is the sinus node recovery time. Following a period of rapid atrial stimulation, there is a measurable time period before the first sinus escape takes place. This is the sinus node recovery time, which is generally defined as the escape time at a paced rate of 130 beats/minute. Sinus node recovery time can also be corrected for sinus cycle length, allowing measurement of corrected sinus node recovery time. When multiple atrial paced cycle lengths are utilized, the maximum sinus node recovery time can also be quantified. Drugs that depress sinus node function, may thus produce increases in sinus node recovery time, corrected sinus node recovery time, and maximum sinus node recovery time.

Sino-atrial conduction time, is the time necessary for the impulse to get out of the sinus node to surrounding atrium.

Sino-atrial conduction time is not directly measurable in man, since under ordinary circumstances, sinus node activity cannot be recorded directly. However, sino-atrial conduction time can be calculated utilizing the response to atrial extrastimuli which reset the sinus node. This method of calculating sino-atrial conduction time is rather crude, and assumes that time taken for an extrastimulus to reach the sinus node, is the same as the time taken for the sinus node impulse to return in an antegrade fashion to the atrium. Drugs that prolong sino-atrial conduction time, might have the propensity to produce sino-atrial block.

Atrial Function

The atria are directly accessible for electrophysiologic testing. Atrial conduction times can be measured within the right atria and from right atrium to left atrium. The conduction interval from the high right atrium to the low septal right atrium (recorded from a His bundle electrogram), is a measure of high to low right atrial conduction time. Right to left atrial conduction time can be measured from the high right atrium to the coronary sinus (a posterior left atrial recording site). Drugs depressing atrial conduction, may prolong one or both of these conduction times.

Atrial refractoriness can be measured utilizing atrial extrastimulus technique. Delivery of closely coupled atrial extrastimuli allow measurement of atrial effective and functional refractory periods. If atrial effective and functional refractory periods are measured at several cycle lengths, curves can be drawn relating atrial refractoriness to cycle length. One can also estimate dispersion of atrial refractoriness, which might relate to propensity to atrial fibrillation or flutter. Dispersion of atrial refractoriness relates to the difference in atrial refractory periods measured at different atrial stimulation sites.

Closely coupled atrial stimuli may produce single or multiple reentrant atrial beats. It is not clear whether the occurrence of atrial echoes are a normal or pathologic finding. Drugs may effect whether or not repetitive responses are generated in response to atrial extrastimuli.

Our laboratory believes that direct atrial antifibrillatory effects of drugs can be demonstrated utilizing catheter techniques in man. Utilizing rapid atrial stimulation, it is possible to induce atrial fibrillation, particularly in subjects prone to this arrhythmia. Drugs that prevent the ability to induce atrial fibrillation with rapid atrial stimulation, are presumably anti-fibrillatory. Preliminary observation from our laboratory suggests that demonstration of an antifibrillatory effect of drugs on the atria, relates to prevention of subsequent atrial fibrilla-tion, in patients with spontaneous attacks of this arrhythmia.

A-V Nodal Function

Measurement of AV nodal function necessitates recording of low septal right atrium and His bundle electrogram, all of which can be obtained from the His bundle recording catheter placed at the tricuspid valve. The interval from the low septal right atrial electrogram to the His bundle electrogram is known as A-H, and is a relatively direct measure of AV nodal conduction time. The normal response to incremental atrial pacing is an increase in A-H interval, with development of AV nodal Wenckebach periodicity within the AV node at a critical paced cycle length. This cycle length, is another measurement of AV nodal function, and is designated as the atrial paced cycle length producing Wenckebach periodicity. Evaluating the effects of drugs on AV nodal function, one should thus note A-H interval during sinus rhythm, A-H interval at equivalent paced cycle lengths, and the paced cycle length producing AV nodal Wenckebach periodicity. A drug that depresses AV nodal function, will increase all of the above measurements.

AV nodal function can also be assessed with atrial extra-stimulus technique. AV nodal effective and functional refractory periods (measurements of input and output functions respectively), can be measured from the graph generated by plotting A_1-A_2 coupl-ing intervals, against H_1-H_2 responses. AV nodal refractory periods are dependent upon cycle length, and thus should be measured at several atrial driven cycle lengths.

The usual substrate for paroxysmal tachycardia in man is the presence of dual AV nodal pathways. In patients with dual path-

ways, atrial extrastimulus testing generates a discontinuous
A_1-A_2, H_1-H_2 curve. The AV node may thus be categorized as having
fast and slow AV nodal pathways. Both antegrade fast and slow,
as well as retrograde fast and slow pathway properties may be
scrutinized with atrial programmed stimulation. If a drug is
to be effective against AV nodal reentrant paroxysmal tachycardia,
it will have a quantifiable effect on one or more of these AV
nodal pathways.

Anomalous pathways and their function may also be scrutinized
with atrial extrastimulus technique. In patients with AV reentrant paroxysmal tachycardias utilizing anomalous pathways, the
effects of drugs on circus movements may be directly examined.
If a drug is effective against AV reentrant paroxysmal tachycardia,
it will have a measurable effect on either the antegrade or retrograde limb of the circus movement, allowing the occurrence of this
arrhythmia.

His-Purkinje Function

Recording of His bundle electrograms allows measurement of
His-Purkinje conduction time. The HV interval is the conduction
time from the His bundle electrogram to the onset of ventricular
activation as measured on the surface cardiogram. In patients
without significant intraventricular conduction defect, HV interval measures conduction time in the His bundle and bundle branches,
to the onset of ventricular activation. In patients with bifascicular block, HV interval is a measure of conduction time
in the remaining functioning fascicle. Drugs that depress
conduction in the in His-Purkinje system will prolong HV interval.
His-Purkinje refractoriness may be independent of His-Purkinje
conduction time (discordance of conduction time and refractory
period). The His-Purkinje system is less accessible to measurement of refractoriness, since the AV node protects the His-
Purkinje system against closely coupled atrial extrastimuli.
However, in some patients, effective and functional refractory
periods may be measured for selected portions of the His-Purkinje
system. The measurement of His-Purkinje refractoriness, is
dependent upon recording of His bundle electrograms as well as
electrocardiograms. In selected patients (generally with ex-

cellent AV nodal function), it may be possible to measure the
effective and functional refractory periods of bundle branches,
and sometimes the total ventricular specialized conduction system.
If a drug prolongs refractoriness in portions of the His-Purkinje
system, this may suggest   a propensity of this drug to produce trifascicular block in patients with bifascicular block.

Retrograde conduction properties may be measured in the His-
Purkinje system. In some respects, measurement of retrograde
properties is somewhat easier, since the AV node is not in the
way. Retrograde His-Purkinje refractoriness is measured
utilizing ventricular extrastimulus technique. Detailed discussion of this type of measurment is beyond the scope of the
present paper. However, the macroreentrant V3 phenomena, serves
as an excellent means of assessing retrograde His-Purkinje
function.

Ventricular Function

There is no standard technique for measuring conduction time
within ventricular muscle. One may scrutinize QRS duration, or
perhaps measure conduction times from one ventricular recording
site to another. Ventricular effective and functional refractory
periods may be measured utilizing ventricular extrastimulus
technique, coupled to either sinus rhythm and/or ventricular
driven cycle lengths.

The most clinically relevant ventricular electrophysiology,
regards the response of the ventricles to closely coupled ventricular extrastimuli. A closely coupled ventricular extrastimulus may at times provoke more than one ventricular response
(repetitive ventricular firing). These additional responses may
reflect one or more of the following: 1) Ventricular macroreentry
(the V3 phenomenon), reflecting retrograde block of the ventricular extrastimulus in the right bundle branch, retrograde conduction via the left bundle branch, and return to the ventricle
of origin via the right bundle branch. This is a normal electrophysiologic response. 2) Contralateral ventricular microreentry. This is characterized by one or more ventricular responses, originating in the left ventricle, with closely coupled
right ventricular stimulation. Some evidence suggest that this

response may be pathologic. 3) Ipsilateral microreentry, close to the site of the stimulating electrode. The significance of this response is unknown. All of the above responses are important, because they may relate to whether or not a drug may be effective against ventricular tachycardia.

In patients with ventricular tachycardia, the tachycardia can be frequently replicated in the catheterization laboratory utilizing programmed ventricular stimulation. The use of programmed ventricular stimulation in the evaluation of antiarrhythmic effect on ventricular tachycardia, is discussed elsewhere in this symposium. Effects of a drug against ventricular fibrillation, may also be at least partly scrutinized, by noting the effect of the drug on response of the ventricles to closely coupled stimuli. A detailed description of this evaluation, is also beyond the scope of this presentation.

Electrophysiologic Evaluation of Intravenous and Oral Drugs

Meaningful evaluation of the electrophysiologic properties of antiarrhythmic drugs is impossible without some knowledge of the pharmacokinetics of the drug being administered. One must know the time of peak action, and the elimination kinetics, so that a drug may be studied during a steady state. The evaluation of intravenous drugs is generally easier, since peak action can be achieved in a short period of time. With evaluation of intravenous drugs, control electrophysiologic studies can be accomplished in approximately twenty minutes. The intravenous drug can be administered, and repeat electrophysiologic studies performed (another twenty minutes). The mode of administration, should attempt to provide a steady state, for the performance of electrophysiologic studies. The drug can then be evaluated in a group of patients, so that appropriate statistical testing can be performed.

The evaluation of oral antiarrhythmic drugs is considerably more difficult. If a drug is well absorbed and rapidly acting, a control electrophysiologic study can be performed, the drug can then be administered, and repeat electrophysiologic studies can be performed at the same sitting with the same catheter. If the oral drug, has a slow onset of action and relatively long

half life, then evaluation in the course of a single electrophysiologic study may be impossible.

With evaluation of long acting oral drugs, our laboratory
would suggest that initial electrophysiologic study be performed,
for delineation of control electrophysiologic properties. The
drug should then be administered for a time period long enough
to allow achievement of a study state. Repeat electrophysiologic
studies will then have to be performed (one or more days after
initial study). This will usually necessitate recatheterization
of the patient. Occasionally, it may be possible to leave a
temporary catheter in place, for performance of part of the
electrophysiologic testing, when one is studying an oral agent.

Despite the difficulty of evaluation of oral agents, it is
our opinion that electrophysiologic scrutiny is important for any
agent to be used in the treatment of arrhythmia in man. The data
concerning site of action, efficacy, and potential toxicity, is
crucial to the understanding of a proposed antiarrhythmic agent.

REFERENCES

1. Scherlag BJ, Lau SH, Helfant RH, Berkowitz WD, Stein E,
   Damato AN: Catheter technique for recording His bundle
   activity in man. Circulation 39: 13, 1969.
2. Dhingra RC, Rosen KM, Rahimtoola SH: Normal conduction
   intervals and responses in 61 patients using His bundle
   recording and atrial pacing. Chest 64: 55, 1973.
3. Wit AL, Weiss MB, Berkowitz WD, Rosen KM, Steiner C,
   Damato AN: Patterns of atrioventricular conduction in the
   human heart. Circulation Research 27: 345, 1970.
4. Akhtar M, Damato AN, Batsford WP, Ruskin JN, Ogunkelu JB,
   Vargas G: Demonstration of re-entry within the His-Purkinje
   system in man. Circulation 50: 1150, 1974.
5. Denes P, Wu D, Dhingra R, Pietras RJ, Rosen KM: The effects
   of cycle length on cardiac refractory periods in man.
   Circulation 49: 32, 1974.
6. Dhingra RC, Wyndham C, Amat-y-Leon F, Denes P, Wu D, Rosen
   KM: Sinus node responses to atrial extra-stimuli in patients
   without apparent sinus node disease. Amer J Cardiol 36:
   445, 1975.
7. Wu D, Amat-y-Leon F, Simpson RJ, Latif P, Wyndham CRC, Denes
   P, Rosen KM: Electrophysiologic studies with multiple drugs
   in patients with AV reentrant tachycardias utilizing an
   extra-nodal pathway. Circulation 56: 727, 1977.

242

8. Denes P, Wu D, Amat-y-Leon F, Dhingra R, Rosen KM: The determinants of reentrance in patients with dual AV nodal pathways. Circulation 56: 253, 1977.
9. Wyndham CR, Amat-y-Leon F, Wu D, Denes P, Dhingra RC, Simpson R, Rosen KM: Effects of cycle length on atial vulnerability. Circulation 55: 260, 1977.
10. Bauernfeind RA, Wyndham CR, Dhingra RC, Swiryn S, Palileo E, Strasberg B, Rosen KM: Serial electrophysiologic testing of multiple drugs in patients with AV nodal reentrant paroxysmal tachycardia. Circulation, in press.

GENERAL GROUP DISCUSSION: BASELINE ELECTROPHYSIOLOGY

Dr. Morganroth: Dr Rosen, let me ask you a troublesome question. I
think that basic electrophysiologic data on new drugs if of value for all
the reasons you mention. I have a little trouble in understanding how to
do studies that you have outlined when a new agent has no intravenous
preparation and when the peak action is not known. What electrophysiologic
studies do you recommend under these conditions?

Dr. Rosen: The electrophysiologist can't be any better than the clinical
pharmacologist. If the clinical pharmacology of a drug is not clearly
understood, the electrophysiology can't be very well understood. For
example, if one administered 10 mg of verapamil and 45 minutes later
made a set of post-verapamil observations you would conclude that verapamil
had no effect. The electrophysiological changes are dependent on the concentrations of the drug in the serum and tissues. Evaluation of an
intravenous rapid acting drug is rather easy. After a series of control
measurements the drug is administered. If the time of peak action is
known you set up a repeat set of electrophysiologic measurements and then
everything that we have talked about can be measured probably in 20 minutes
with a well functioning team once the catheters are in place. Electrophysiological measurements are more difficult. I would not personally
want to take a stand right now as to whether every oral drug should be
scrutinized in this fashion, but you would need a control study and leave
several catheters in the heart for subsequent studies unless it was a very
rapidly acting oral drug so that measurements could be obtained at 30
minutes, you would need another study several hours or days later. I guess
you would already say that you were probably getting this kind of information on arrhythmic patients because it doesn't sound feasible to get
volunteers for two invasive electrophysiologic studies neither of which
is indicated. Now if it is an oral drug that is potent and is going to be
potentially widely used I would say that some framework has to be arrived

at so that at least some information can be obtained. There are certain
types of information that can be obtained with a single catheter without
resorting to three catheters. Conduction times, Wenckebach point, atrial
and ventricular refractory periods are possible with one catheter. To
make a long story short, I don't know the answer to the oral drug study.
I feel it can only be obtained by two studies.

Dr. Michelson: Is there certain information that is otherwise occult, that
you would only pick up by electrophysiologic studies such as the atrial
or ventricular refractory periods, or H-V prolongation that would have
any significance whatsoever in the evaluation of a new drug by the FDA?
Secondly, when we evaluate new drugs we usually begin to study these
agents in individuals who are otherwise normal. However, these drugs are
frequently used in patients with sinus node disease, intraventricular
conduction delays, and in patients who are at risk from other medical
problems. Hence, what significance can we attach to small changes in
parameters such as the H-V interval when these patients probably die from
serious arrhythmias other than conduction delay?

Dr. Rosen: In response to your several questions, I will repeat that I
do not anticipate that diseased tissue and normal tissues behave in the
same way. Given the current state of knowledge, it would be fair to
assume that a drug that is not toxic to the sinus node in normal individuals might not be toxic to a sinus node in patients with preclinical
sinus node disease. One would have to look at both the population of
patients with normal sinus function as well as the population of patients
with abnormal sinus nodal function. If the drug is going to be administered to elderly individuals it would probably be important to know
where toxicity will emerge. Certain electrophysiologic parameters cannot
be read from the surface electrocardiogram. Furthermore, there is an
animal-man interface and although a good deal of data can be accumulated
from animals, the question is how close is the correlation between man and
animals and even among species of animals? There are some areas where
animals and man will differ. There is no spontaneous animal model of
bifascicular block nor is there a spontaneous animal model of sinus node
disease. Although the data from animals is interesting, I do not think
it substitutes for human data and I don't think that the surface electrocardiogram substitutes for the invasive electrophysiolgoic study. I am
really not knowledgeable enough to say whether every drug should be

studied in this way.

Dr. Michelson: Dr. Zipes, what is your opinion?

Dr. Zipes: Basically, I would side with Dr. Rosen on the value and indications of electrophysiologic studies. You have heard my personal bias on the relevance of oral studies. I would not feel comfortable to send a patient home popping pills without a knowledge of the electrophysiologic effects just as I must understand the electrophysiologic effects after a bolus or a subsequent intravenous drip. I think there is no question that electrophysiologic studies can provide information that is not available from the surface electrocardiogram. One example is the drug encanide. This agent was originally developed for ventricular arrhythmias. However, we have shown that it affects the AV node, the atrium and indeed it is good for many supraventricular tachyarrhythmias. These latter indications emerge from such electrophysiologic studies. Furthermore, I think every new drug should be studied in such a fashion. I feel a new drug should be studied by selected groups such as four or five cneters that are familiar with these studies and have considerable experience with investigational drugs. This data should be available prior to the general licensing of new agents.

Dr. Rosen: I don't strenuously disagree. The problem rests with the oral agents. In the case of fast acting drugs it is rather easy but for a drug that has to be studied after 3 or 4 days of loading and consequently patients requires two studies. Hopefully, they will accept to be studied on both occasions. Another question is directed to the relative effectiveness of IV versus oral preparations. The only way to test this hypothesis is to scrutinize both the IV and oral preparations for either efficacy or electrophysiologic effects. Once a linear relationship between the IV and oral agent is demonstrated, it may be possible to study only the IV drug more intensely.

Dr. Dreifus: I feel that a consensus has been reached. All agree that electrophysiologic studies are important. Furthermore, the intravenous preparations demonstrate a much cleaner and well defined end point. Problems exist with oral drug testing. Factors of absorption and the disadvantage of requiring patients to undergo at least two invasive electrophysiologic studies, first as a control, and then after we are certain that the drug has been absorbed and is active. This requires either leaving catheters in patients for prolonged periods of time or bringing the patient back for a second study. Furthermore, it should be agreed that information in both normal individuals as well as patients suffering with particular types of conduction disturbances and tachyarrhythmias is probably necessary.

ASSESSMENT OF THE HEMODYNAMIC AND INOTROPIC EFFECTS OF
ANTIARRHYTHMIC DRUGS

R.S. ARONSON, S. SISKIND, AND E.H. SONNENBLICK

1. INTRODUCTION

Assessment of the hemodynamic and inotropic effects of
antiarrhythmic drugs is hampered by the lack of easily obtainable and sufficiently sensitive measures of myocardial function.
This situation arises because antiarrhythmic drugs can have
effects on certain hemodynamic parameters that can either
offset or enhance direct actions that these agents may have
on the contractile performance of the heart itself. In the
following discussion we will consider the physiologic basis
for these complex interactions as well as the known hemodynamic and inotropic effects of commonly used antiarrhythmic
drugs. Based on these considerations, we will propose an
approach to assessing the hemodynamic and inotropic effects
of new antiarrhythmic drugs.

2. PHYSIOLOGIC CONSIDERATION

The purpose of the heart is to deliver on demand adequate
amounts of blood to the metabolizing tissues. Thus, although
various indices of myocardial contractility may reflect alterations in muscle performance, the ultimate performance of the
heart must be evaluated in terms of its function as a pump.
Performance of the intact heart is dependent on four major
variables (1,2): (1) Preload, which is the filling pressure
of the ventricle which sets the diastolic length of the fibers
in the ventricular wall. This influences cardiac performance
by the Frank-Starling mechanism. (2) Afterload, which is the
force the fiber in the wall must generate during development
of systolic pressure. Afterload is determined by the effective resistance to ejection of blood presented by the aorta

and peripheral vasculature. Therefore the mean aortic pressure (MAP) and systemic vascular resistance (SVR) can be taken as measures of afterload. (3) <u>Contractility</u>, which is a measure of the force, speed and shortening capacity of the myocardium. At a given preload and afterload, the contractility of the ventricle can be measured in terms of the stroke volume (SV) that can be ejected by the heart from any end diastolic volume (EDV). It is also reflected in the relative speed with which this ejection occurs. The ratio of SV/EDV is termed the ejection fraction (EF). The EF approximates the slope of the Starling curve and, although it will be somewhat afterload dependent, can be used as a clinical index of cardiac performance. (4) Heart rate (HR), which regulates cardiac pump performance because cardiac output (CO) is the product of heart rate and SV.

Alterations in preload have predictable effects on cardiac performance according to the "ventricular function curve" which relates ventricular stroke work to left ventricular end diastolic pressure (LVEDP). Thus when cardiac work, which is the product of CO and MAP, is plotted against diastolic filling pressure, which sets the length of ventricular muscle fibers, it is found that cardiac work increases as end diastolic filling pressure increases. The cardiac output at any given preload (diastolic fiber length) and level of contractility depends on the extent to which the ventricular muscle fiber are able to shorten during systole. The extent of ventricular muscle fiber shortening depends in turn on the afterload. Thus, cardiac performance can be strongly affected by loading conditions independent of any alteration in myocardial contractility. For this reason, changes in blood pressure may affect this type of index.

Ventricular contraction can be divided into a pre-ejection and ejection phase (1,2). In isolated muscle, the rate of force development before shortening is independent of the afterload carried by the muscle when shortening begins. The rate of force development in isolated muscle dp/dt is similar to the rate of pressure development, dp/dt, in the pre-ejection period of the contracting ventricle. Therefore, peak dp/dt has been used as an index of contractility. Unfortunately, changes in end diastolic volume (fiber length) can alter peak dp/dt thereby reducing its usefulness as a unique measure of myocardial contractility. Furthermore, disease states such as hypertrophy and valvular insufficiency, which are associated with abnormal volumes or shortened pre-ejection period, may further limit the specificity of peak dp/dt as a measure of contractility. Nevertheless, a decrease in dp/dt in the face of no change or a fall in LVEDP indicates a decrease in ventricular contractility. In the same sense, a strain gauge applied to a segment of muscle of the free wall of the ventricle of an experimental animal can be used to show specific changes in myocardial contractility (1,2).

The ejection phase begins when the aortic valve opens. The fibers in the ventricular wall shorten and blood is ejected into the aorta with a velocity that is inversely related to the afterload. The amount of blood ejected is the SV and is related to end diastolic volume in a relatively linear manner (ventricular function curve). Unfortunately, when afterload is reduced, the extent of shortening for any end diastolic fiber length (preload) is augmented and EF tends to rise. This diminishes the specificity of EF as a measure of cardiac contractility. In the acute clinical setting, the use of a Swan-Ganz catheter can allow ventricular filling pressures to be assessed along with cardiac output. However, both impedance changes as well as changes in myocardial contractility will effect the derived results. Chronically, the EF can be measured by non-invasive techniques, but again loading may alter the results.

To include a function that is related to the velocity of contraction, the mean rate of fiber shortening (V_{cf}) has been calculated (1,2). Since the duration of contraction is not greatly altered in disease states, V_{cf} tends to parallel ejection fraction. This is the case because the slope of the ejection curve changes as the degree of ejection changes. As was true for other indices discussed above, the extent of shortening and the slope of the shortening curve are load dependent.

All of the indices of cardiac contractility we have discussed for use in man suffer from a lack of sensitivity or specificity because they are influenced by loading conditions or disease states likely to be seen in patients receiving antiarrhythmic drugs. In addition, these indices assume that the ventricle behaves as a homogeneous structure and do not consider regional abnormalities in wall motion. Inhomogeneity in contractile function can occur in coronary disease and cardiomyopathies. For example, augmented function in normal areas may help to maintain a normal EF despite local abnormalities.

The sensitivity of the indices of myocardial contractility and performance can be enhanced by obtaining these measurements under conditions of stress. Normal and diseased hearts show different responses to stresses such as isotonic exercise, isometric exercise and augmented afterload (1,2). For example, increased afterload leads to a larger reduction in stroke volume in the abnormal than in the normal heart (1,2). Thus, assessment of myocardial performance at rest may fail to identify impaired cardiac function that might predispose some patients to develop further depression of function with the use of antiarrhythmic drugs.

Another factor that must be considered is the possible contribution of alterations in coronary blood flow (CBF). For example, a drug that increases coronary vascular resistance and reduces CBF may produce ischemic depression of cardiac function whereas myocardial performance may be enhanced by a drug that increases CBF.

As we will discuss below, many antiarrhythmic drugs appear to have multiple effects on the circulatory system that make it difficult to predict the net effect these agents will have on overall cardiac function. Thus, an agent that has a direct depressant effect on myocardial contractility may not produce a decrease in overall cardiac function because of a concomitant effect on the peripheral vascular system that results in an

offsetting decrease in afterload. Similarly, a drug that decreases myocardial contractility may not produce an overall
decrease in cardiac output because of an associated increase
in EDV. An otherwise mild negative inotropic effect of an
antiarrhythmic drug can be magnified if the drug also induces
an increase in afterload or a decrease in preload. Further,
in chronic heart failure, catecholamines may be reduced or
absent in the myocardium so that compensatory reflexes which
would offset depressant effects of a drug are reduced. Some
of these drugs may also influence cardiac contractility by
altering coronary blood flow. Lastly, one cannot assess the
effects of a drug to depress the heart in normal hearts alone.
Failing hearts may be more sensitive to these effects either
acutely or chronically. Animal studies will only set a background for such considerations since species differences may
also occur.

3. HEMODYNAMIC AND INOTROPIC EFFECTS OF COMMONLY USED ANTI-
    ARRHYTHMIC DRUGS

    Table 1 summarizes the effects of eight antiarrhythmic
drugs on various hemodynamic parameters and indices of myocardial contractility. The effects shown in Table 1 are summarized from studies in both humans and dogs as well as in
isolated muscle preparations. Many of these studies were
performed under vastly different conditions with respect to
both the rate of infusion and dosage of drug used. In general,
the effects shown in Table 1 were obtained in the most recent
studies available and were reported in two or more studies.
For some drugs, such as procaine amide, very limited data
were available and these were often not in agreement. Finally,
results from isolated muscle studies were only included when
similar directional effects were also reported in at least
one intact animal or human study.

Drug	Preload LVEDP	Afterload MAP	SVR	Reflex Effects / Autonomic Effects	Contractility dP/dT max	LVW	CBF	HR	CO/CI/SV
Quinidine	↓/−	↓	↓	1. Vasodilation by α-Blockade and direct action 2. Anticholinergic	−/↓			−/↓	−
Procaine amide	−	−/↓	↓	? Sympathetic Blockade				−/↓	↓/−
Disopyramide	−/↑	↑	↑	Anticholinergic	↓		↓	−/↑	↓
Verapamil	↑	↓	↓	Vasodilation by direct action	↓		↑	−	−
Lidocaine	−	−	−		−	−	↑	−	−
Phenytoin	↑/↓	↓	↓	Vasodilation	↓	↓	↑	−	−
Bretylium	↓	↑/↓	↓	Catecholamine release then sympathetic blockade	↑			↑/−	↑
Propranolol	↑	−	↑	Possible vasoconstriction by unopposed α-tone	↓	↓	↓	↓	↓

Table 1. Hemodynamic and inotropic effects of selected anti-arrhythmic drugs. LVEDP = left ventricular end diastolic pressure, MAP = mean aortic pressure, SVR = systemic vascular resistance, dp/dt$_{max}$ = maximum rate of left ventricular pressure development, LVW = left ventricular work, CBF = coronary blood flow, HR = heart rate, CO = cardiac output, CI = cardiac index, SV = stroke volume, ↓ = decrease, ↑ = increase, − no significant change. The slash separating two effects indicates either different results obtained in separate studies or different results in the same study under different experimental conditions.

3.1 <u>Quinidine</u>. Quinidine has been shown to produce a wide variety of hemodynamic effects in a number of studies. Thus, reviewing the studies of the effects of quinidine illustrates many of the difficulties that arise in assessing the hemodynamic and inotropic actions of antiarrhythmic drugs. Numerous studies have shown that quinidine depresses myocardial contractility. The peak developed tension, dp/dt, and velocity of fiber shortening have been shown to be depressed during treatment with quinidine. Many of the studies have used doses of quinidine which would be considered toxic in humans. When therapeutic doses of quinidine are used, the major hemodynamic effects of the drug appear to involve the peripheral vasculature either directly or indirectly via interactions with the autonomic nervous system. A few studies have even shown an increase in contractile force.

Recent studies in dogs have shown conflicting results. In one study therapeutic levels of quinidine reduced MAP, aortic flow and left atrial pressure while not significantly affecting dp/dt (3). These effects were attributed to a vasodilatory action of quinidine as well as to its known α-blocking effect. In another study, quinidine was shown to cause not only vasodilation, but also to have a direct myocardial depressant effect as measured by a decrease in dp/dt (4).

In humans, it appears that intravenous doses of quinidine produce hypotension because of the ability of the drug to cause vasodilation rather than because of a significant depressive effect on myocardial contractility. Oral quinidine given to normal persons and patients with congestive cardiomyopathy had no adverse effects on left ventricular performance as measured by M-mode echocardiography (5).

In summary, in high doses, quinidine can produce myocardial depression in animals. Furthermore, because of its vasodilating effect, quinidine can induce a reflex increase in catecholamines which can (1) mask inherent or drug induced reductions in contractility and (2) increase HR and SV which can counteract any reduction in CO that would otherwise occur because of a direct negative inotropic effect.

As far as we know, no cases of overt CHF have been seen
secondary to quinidine. Oral doses probably have no significant myocardial depressant effects. When administered paren-
terally, quinidine can block α-adrenergic vasoconstriction,
dilate peripheral vessels, reduce SVR and MAP while only slightly affecting dp/dt and CO.

3.2. Procaine Amide. Procaine amide has been generally considered to be a myocardial depressant. In man, procaine amide
has been reported to cause a slight increase in HR and a decrease in MAP and CO. These effects were thought to be due
to a combination of depressed contractility and vasodilation
(6,7). Similar myocardial depression and reduced SVR has been
reported in studies in dogs (8). As was the case for other
antiarrhythmic drugs, many studies on the hemodynamic effects
of procaine amide were done with doses that far exceed the
therapeutic range in humans.

Procaine amide, like quinidine, seems to cause vasodilation due to a sympathetic blocking action. This effect can
produce reductions in SVR, MAP and preload. If procaine amide
is given in divided doses, and not in excess of one gram
(acutely), there rarely is clinical evidence of myocardial
depression. Mild reductions in BP do occur at doses in excess
of 600 mg. Again, like quinidine, no cases of CHF have been
clearly precipitated by procaine amide.

One study in isolated papillary muscles indicated that
procaine amide can enhance contractile performance (9). This
effect has not so far been demonstrated in studies of the intact heart.

3.3. Disopyramide. Disopyramide can produce dose-dependent
reductions in CO (7-49%) and in the force of contraction (15-
61%) (10). A myocardial depressant action has been demonstrated
in the intact dog heart. Using Walton-Brody strain gauges
to measure contractile force, the drug reduced contractile
force by 42% while increasing end diastolic muscle segment
length (11). Higher doses of disopyramide produced more severe

depression of contractile force and further lengthening of muscle segments. In addition to these effects, disopyramide caused a reduction in CBF, apparently secondary to direct coronary vasoconstriction.

Studies of the hemodynamic effects of disopyramide in man have shown results similar to those described above in dogs. Thus, disopyramide caused a dose-dependent reduction in CO and dp/dt as measured at cardiac catheterization (12,13). Subsequent studies confirmed the myocardial depression induced by disopyramide (14-16), and also documented the occurrence of a reflex increase in SVR, apparently in response to the diminished CO induced by disopyramide. Disopyramide has also been shown to have apparently negative inotropic effects as measured by non-invasive methods (16).

In recent studies, administration of disopyramide caused a decrease in left ventricular work (LVW) and coronary blood flow (via vasoconstriction). These hemodynamic changes produced a reflex increase in SVR (17). When given orally, disopyramide reduced the EF as determined by M-mode echocardiography (18). Thus, disopyramide seems to be a myocardial depressant as reflected by reductions in CO and dp/dt and a reflex rise in SVR.

Some evidence suggests that these effects are more marked in patients with heart disease than in normal individuals. For example, a recent study of the effects of long term use of oral disopyramide showed that 16 of 100 patients maintained on the drug developed symptoms of congestive heart failure (CHF). Three of the patients developed symptoms of CHF within 48 hours of being started on the drug. Twelve of the remaining 13 patients had previous symptoms of CHF. Of 22 patients who had a history of CHF, 55% developed an exacerbation while on the drug. These results indicate that disopyramide should be given cautiously to patients with cardiomegaly or a history of CHF and that many of these patients may suffer exacerbation of heart failure after being given the drug (19).

3.4. <u>Verapamil</u>. Verapamil is similar to propranolol in many
of its hemodynamic effects. Verapamil has a marked negative
inotropic effect on isolated cardiac muscle (20). In the intact heart of dogs, the drug was shown to decrease HR, peak
developed tension, MVO_2 and to increase the left ventricular
efficiency index (21).

In humans, verapamil depresses myocardial contractility
and causes widespread vasodilation. In a study using a 10 mg
bolus of verapamil, the drug caused reductions in ventricular
systolic pressure (18%), dp/dt (17%), and the velocity of fiber
shortening (15%) (22). Heart rate increased 11% and changes
in CO and SV were not significant. In another study in man,
a 10 mg bolus of verapamil produced a 36% increase in LVEDP
and a 25% reduction in dp/dt. MAP and SVR were reduced due to
vasodilation while HR, CO and SV all increased but not significantly (23). Verapamil also reduced coronary vascular resistance and increased CBF.

Verapamil is a negative inotropic agent based on the findings that it depresses dp/dt and increases LVEDP.

3.5. <u>Lidocaine</u>. Most of the studies of the hemodynamic effects
of lidocaine have used doses comparable to those employed in
man. For example, in man a 50 mg bolus had no significant
effect on CO, LVEDP, SV, LVW or dp/dt (24). In another study,
a 1.5 mg/kg bolus of lidocaine had no adverse hemodynamic effects (25). In fact, when frequent ventricular extrasystoles
were abolished by lidocaine, CO tended to rise. In a study
using an intravenous bolus of 100 mg of lidocaine, no significant changes in hemodynamic variables except for a slight decrease in pulmonary artery pressure were observed (17). In
this study, lidocaine also was shown to reduce coronary vascular resistance and increase CBF. Most studies show that
lidocaine, in standard doses, has little or no significant effect on contractility or BP.

3.6. Phenytoin. Studies on phenytoin have shown it to have
catastrophic effects including cardiorespiratory arrest when
large doses are infused rapidly. Slower administration of
smaller doses have produced various effects in animals but
have proven essentially safe in man.

Studies using high doses of the drug have shown that
phenytoin can produce myocardial depression and negative inotropic actions in dogs and in isolated papillary muscles (26).
In the dog, phenytoin (6 mg/kg) caused a marked reduction in
MAP, SVR, CO and a slight reduction of dp/dt. An increase in
CBF was also demonstrated. The results of this study were
interpreted as showing that the predominant effect of phenytoin
is vasodilation and that direct myocardial depression was
minimal (27). In another study in dogs, phenytoin caused
dose-dependent reductions in MAP, SVR and dp/dt and also ele-
vated LVEDP. A consistent reduction in CO did not occur, presumably the decreases in both contractility and afterload
tended to offset each other (28).

In man, at high doses, phenytoin depresses dp/dt and increases LVEDP. When phenytoin (250 mg) was given intravenously
over 5 min, no significant changes in SV, LVEDP and dp/dt
were seen (29). Another study in which similar doses of phenytoin
were used demonstrated no significant alteration in CO, MAP,
SVR or contractility (30).

In summary, high doses of phenytoin can induce marked
vasodilation resulting in reductions of MAP and SVR and can
have a direct depressive effect on myocardial contractility.
There is also some degree of coronary vasodilation. When
moderate doses are given to humans, e.g., 50 mg/min (not ex-
ceeding one gram), no major hemodynamic effects other than
mild hypotension are observed.

3.7. Bretylium. Bretylium tosylate has varied effects on the
cardiovascular system, due primarily to alterations in catecholamine concentrations. In isolated cat papillary muscle,
bretylium has been shown to augment contractility as measured
by both the speed and degree of tension development (9). For

example, Koch-Weser demonstrated an increase in dp/dt, an increase in peak tension and a shortening of the time to peak tension (31). These effects were similar to those of infused norepinephrine. This observation coupled with the finding that the effects of bretylium were blocked by pretreatment with propranolol indicated that bretylium increased contractility through release of catecholamines. In human studies, this initial release of catecholamines produces a transient rise in BP and HR. These effects are brief and BP and HR returned to baseline within 15 minutes. Two hours after administration of bretylium, both BP and SVR were significantly reduced (32).

This effect is due to the fact that bretylium inhibits the release of adrenergic transmitter from sympathetic nerve ending after the initial release phase of its action. The resulting sympathetic blockade reduces both preload and afterload and therefore usually has little effect on SV or CO. An interesting effect of bretylium is the hypersensitivity it produces to infused catecholamines leading to potentiation of their actions.

In summary, bretylium appears to induce an initial release of catecholamines which in turn produces a mild and clinically insignificant increase in BP and HR. Later, sympathetic blockade occurs and produces a decrease in SVR, MAP and left ventricular end diastolic pressure (LVEDP) while HR is unchanged. The net effect of these hemodynamic alterations in 50-75% of patients is hypotension (MAP reduced > 20 mmHg), without a significant change in CO or SV (33).

3.8. Propranolol. Early studies in dogs showed that propranolol was a potent myocardial depressant. It caused significant reductions in contractile force (32%), SV (16%), and ejection rate (27%) (34). Studies in humans showed similar results in that HR, CO, SV and left ventricular ejection rate were all significantly depressed (35). In addition, propranolol reduces CBF, apparently secondary to decreased myocardial oxygen demands (MVO_2) (36). Most studies on the effects of propranolol have been constant in their findings. Contractility as measured

by dp/dt is reduced, LVW is reduced and CO is depressed because
of a decrease in both HR and SV. In addition, the HR and BP
response to exercise is blunted resulting in reduced exercise
tolerance (37).

Negative inotropic effects of propranolol have been demonstrated during cardiac catheterization in patients with cardiac
disease. Propranolol was shown to reduce the rate of fiber
shortening and the rate of change of ventricular volume with
time. In addition, it induced hypokinesia in 2 of 10 patients,
dyskinesia in 1 patient and worsened existing areas of dyskinesia
in 2 more patients. Thus, propranolol not only depresses indices of global cardiac contractility, but also is capable of
producing or worsening regional pre-existing abnormalities in
contraction (38).

On the other hand, it appears that during chronic oral use,
only 1% of patients develop overt CHF while taking propranolol
(39,40). This may be due to widespread physician avoidance
of propranolol in patients with CHF.

4. AN APPROACH TO ASSESSING THE HEMODYNAMIC AND INOTROPIC
   EFFECTS OF NEW ANTIARRHYTHMIC DRUGS

In the preceding sections we discussed many problems encountered in studying and interpreting the circulatory alterations induced by antiarrhythmic drugs as well as the difficulties involved in measuring cardiac performance. Based on this
information we have formulated what we believe to be a reason-
albe approach to assessing the hemodynamic and inotropic effects
of new antiarrhythmic drugs.

The first step in assessing a new drug should probably
be in vitro studies in isolated cardiac muscle from several
species. Effects on contractility can be evaluated independently of cardiac performance in such experiments because
preload and afterload can be precisely controlled. Studies
in more than one species is of importance because of the wide
variability in the response of different species to a number
of inotropic interventions. Depression of contractility induced by a new antiarrhythmic drug in studies on isolated

muscles from one or more species would indicate that the drug has the potential to impair contractility in humans. Of course, the absence of a negative inotropic action in isolated preparations does not exclude the possibility that such an effect could occur in the human heart. Similarly, demonstration of a negative inotropic effect in vitro does not necessarily mean that such an action will occur in the intact human heart. In any case, the finding that a drug is capable of depressing myocardial contractility in isolated muscles is an important indication that the drug has the potential for negative inotropic activity in patients.

The next step should be evaluation of the hemodynamic effects of the drug on the intact heart in experimental animals. The dog has been the most commonly used animal for this purpose. As we indicated earlier, measuring only CO may be misleading because antiarrhythmic drugs may not induce any net change in this measurement despite having substantial hemodynamic effects. It is necessary therefore to assess both direct effects of the drug on the myocardium and reflex effects on other circulation parameters. For example, afterload and preload can be maintained constant to determine the effect of the drug of myocardial contractility as measured by dp/dt, V_{cf}, or EF. The functional importance of a directly demonstrated effect on contractility can then be determined under conditions where preload and/or afterload are allowed to change. The extent to which direct depression of myocardial contractility can be offset or enhanced by other hemodynamic effects of the drug can thereby be determined. For example, drugs that depress contractility mildly but also produce vasodilation leading to reduced afterload would not be as worrisome as drugs that impair contractility but also increase afterload. In this manner, a total hemodynamic profile of the drug can be obtained that should permit a more accurate means of predicting what the effect of a new drug will be on cardiac performance in patients.

Important factors that must be taken into account in animal studies are the dose and rate of infusion of drug. The circulatory effects of antiarrhythmic drugs should be evaluated at plasma levels that are in the "therapeutic" range for suppression of abnormal electrical activity. Rapid infusions of pharmacologic doses of the drug may produce misleading results.

One limitation of animal experiments is that the hemodynamic and inotropic effects of the drug are evaluated under circumstances in which the heart is presumably normal. This is a very important limitation because the diseased heart has less reserve than the normal heart and responds differently to hemodynamic stress. Thus, the degree of depression of myocardial contractility may be greater in diseased than in normal hearts. Similarly, the capacity of the diseased heart to compensate for depression of contractility induced by the drug may be seriously impaired so that offsetting hemodynamic effects of the drug do not result in maintenance of a normal CO. Therefore, it might be useful to test the hemodynamic and inotropic effects of new drugs in dogs with chronic myocardial infarction or a similar model of cardiac disease.

The effect of the drug on coronary blood flow should also be assessed. A drug that decreases coronary blood flow can indirectly depress contractility by inducing ischemia in addition to any other direct effects on the myocardium. On the other hand, cardiac performance may be improved by a drug that causes coronary vasodilation.

The final step, of course, is to test the drug in humans. This presents the most difficult problem because of the lack of a sufficiently sensitive measure of cardiac function that can be obtained on a serial basis.

An initial approach to assessing the hemodynamic effects of a drug is to study its actions during elective cardiac catheterization in patients. This kind of approach is likely to involve studying patients with a number of cardiac diseases and perhaps some who are not found to have significant disease. Therefore, this kind of patient population is likely to be inhomogeneous and therefore the results may be somewhat limited in their application to individual patients.

During catheterization it is possible to measure CO, SVR, MAP, LVEDP, dp/dt, and ejection phase indices of cardiac performance. These measurements permit complete evaluation of the hemodynamic effects of the drug on the circulatory system. A catheter can also be inserted into the coronary sinus to measure CBF by thermodilution. This is an important consideration, especially in patients with coronary disease. The major limitation of cardiac catheterization studies is that they cannot be used for chronic or serial evaluation of the long term effects of new drugs.

Therefore, a more cirtical problem is to identify non-invasive means of assessing the effects of new durgs on cardiac function on a chronic basis. Methods that have been used for this purpose include systolic time intervals and echocardiography. These methods suffer from a lack of sensitivity and specificity. The M-mode echocardiogram can detect changes in LV internal dimensions, EF, and derived V_{cf}. Two-dimensional echocardiography can provide information about ventricular function that is similar to that obtained by cine-angiography in the RAO projection. These non-invasive methods are limited also by relative insensitivity in detecting regional or segmental impairment of contractility.

The EF as determined by radio-angiography may be the most practical and accurate method for serial assessment of cardiac function. This method can also be used during exercise and can delineate segmental contractile abnormalities. Therefore, nuclear studies may be the most practical approach to assessing the effects of drugs on cardiac performance. Such studies can be obtained in a serial manner before and after drug administration to determine if the agent produces abnormalities of wall motion or EF. Nuclear studies can also be repeated after several months of therapy to assess the effects of chronic use on cardiac function.

A serious limitation of this approach is that it may not be possible to detect potentially significant drug-induced alterations by measurements of basal cardiac performance alone. Therefore, it seems important to be particularly careful to identify those patients whose cardiac function is impaired by subjecting them to stress. Since diseased hearts do not respond to stress the way normal hearts do, patients that may be at significant risk for developing drug induced depression of cardiac function can be identified by evaluating their cardiac performance during exercise. Patients should therfore be stressed by exercise both before and after drug administration to improve the sensitivity of the measurements of myocardial function. This can be accomplished by measuring the double product (HR x BP), exercise capacity, oxygen consumption, and nuclear EF and wall motion during exercise. A reduction in exercise time, EF, oxygen consumption or an increase in HR for the same level of work indicates impaired myocardial reserve.

The importance of using stress to evaluate cardiac function is illustrated by the case of disopyramide. As we described earlier, this drug has been found to produce CHF in patients with a prior history of this problem (19). This indicates that if patients with impaired function can be identified earlier by evaluation of cardiac function during stress, then patients showing evidence impaired myocardial reverse can be followed especially closely and vigorously evaluated during drug therapy.

REFERENCES

1. Braunwald E, Ross J Jr, Sonnenblick ES. 1976. Mechanisms of contraction of the normal and failing heart. 2nd ed. Boston, Little Brown and Co.
2. Sonnenblick EH, Strobeck JE. 1977. Derived indices of ventricular and myocardial function. N Engl J Med 296: 978-982.
3. Markiewicz W, Winkle R, Binetti G, Kernoff R, Harrison DC. 1976. Myocardial contractile state in the presence of quinidine. Circulation 53: 101.
4. Engler RL, LeWinter MM, Karliner JS. 1979. Depressant effects of quinidine gluconate on left ventricular function in conscious dogs with and without volume overload. Circulation 60: 828.
5. Crawford MH, White DH, O'Rourke RA. 1979. Effects of oral quinidine on left ventricular performance in normal subjects and patients with congestive cardiomyopat-y. Am J Cardiol 44: 714.
6. McClendon RL, Hansen WR, Kinsman JM. 1951. Hemodynamic changes following procaine amide administered intravenously. Am J Med Sci 222: 375.

7. Angelakos ET, Hastings EP. 1960. The influence of quinidine and procaine amide on myocardial contractility in vivo. Am J Cardiol 5: 791.
8. Folle LE, Aviado DM. 1966. The cardiopulmonary effects of quinidine and procaine amide. J Pharm Exp Ther 154: 92.
9. Hammermeister KE, Boerth RC, Warbasse JR. 1972. The comparative inotropic effects of six clinically used antiarrhythmic agents. Am Heart J 84: 643.
10. Mokler CM, VanArman CG. 1962. Pharmacology of a new antiarrhythmic agent - Disopyramide. J Pharm Exp Ther 136: 114.
11. Mathur P. 1972. Cardiovascular effects of a new antiarrhythmic agent - Disopyramide Phosphate. Am Heart J 84: 764.
12. Befeler B. 1975. The hemodynamic effects of Norpace (Part I) Angiology 26 (Supp I): 99.
13. Willis PW. 1975. The hemodynamic effects of Norpace (Part II) Angiology 26 (Supp I): 102.
14. Jensen G, Sugurd B, Whrenholt A. 1975. Hemodynamic effects of intravenous Disopyramide in heart failure. Eur J Clin Pharmacol 8: 167.
15. Vismara LA, Demaria A, Miller RR, Amsterdam EA, Mason DT. 1975. Effects of intravenous Disopyramide on cardiac function and peripheral circulation in ischemic heart disease. Clin Res 23: 87A.
16. Hulting J, Rosenhamer G. 1976. Hemodynamic and electrocardiographic effects of Disopyramide in patients with ventricular arrhythmias. Acta Med Scand 199: 41.
17. Kotter V, Linderer T, Schroder R. 1980. Effects of Disopyramide on systemic and coronary hemodynamics and metabolism in patients with coronary artery disease: Comparison with Lidocaine. Am J Cardiol 46: 469.
18. Cathcart-Rake WF, Coker JE, Atkins FL, Huffman DH, Hossanein KM, Shen DD, Azarnoff DL. 1980. The effect of concurrent oral administration of Propranolol and Disopyramide on cardiac function in healthy men. Circulation 61: 938.
19. Podrid PJ, Schoeneberger A, Lown B. 1980. Congestive heart failure caused by oral Disopyramide. N Engl J Med 302: 614.
20. Singh BN, Vaughn Williams EM. 1972. A fourth class of antidysrhythmic action? Effect of Verapamil on Ouabain toxicity, on atrial and ventricular intracellular potentials and on other features of cardiac function. Cardiovasc Res 6: 109.
21. Nayler WG, Szeto J. 1972. Effect of Verapamil on contractility, oxygen utilization and calcium exchangeability in human heart muscle. Cardiovasc Res 6: 120.
22. Lewis BS, Mitha AS, Gotsman MS. 1975. Immediate hemodynamic effects of Verapamil in man. Cardiology 60: 336.
23. Singh BN, Roche AHG. 1977. Effects of intravenous Verapamil on hemodynamics in patients with heart disease. Am Heart J 94: 593.
24. Schumacher RR, Lieberson AD, Childress RH, Williams JF. 1968. Hemodynamic effects of Lidocaine in patients with heart disease. Circulation 37: 965.
25. Grossman JI, Cooper JA, Frieden J. 1969. Cardiovascular effects of infusion of Lidocaine on patients with heart disease. Am J Cardiol 24: 191.

26. Gupta DN, Metin MO, Bashour FA, Webb WR. 1966. Effect of Diphenylhydantoin (Dilantin) on coronary and systemic circulation. Clin Res 14: 81.
27. Puri PS. 1971. The effect of Diphenylhydantoin on myocardial contractility and hemodynamics. Am Heart J 82: 62.
28. Mierzwiak DS, Mitchell JH, Shapiro W. 1967. Effect of Diphenylhydantoin and Quinidine on left ventricular function in dogs. Am Heart J 74: 780.
29. Lieberson AD, Schumacher RR, Childress RH, Boyd DC, Williams JF. 1967. Effect of Diphenylhydantoin on left ventricular function in patients with heart disease. Circulation 36: 692.
30. Conn RD, Kennedy JW, Blackman JR. 1967. The hemodynamic effects of Diphenylhydantoin. Am Heart J 73: 500.
31. Koch-Weser J, Blinks JR. 1963. Bretylium. Pharmacol Rev 15: 601.
32. Chaterjee K, Mandel WJ, Vyden JK, Parmley WW, Forrester JS. 1975. Cardiovascular effects of Bretylium tosylate in acute myocardial infarction. JAMA 223: 757.
33. Koch-Weser J. 1979. Bretylium. NEJM 300: 473.
34. Barrett AM. 1969. A comparison of the effects of (+)-Propranolol and (+)-Propranolol in anesthetized dogs: Beta-receptor blocking and hemodynamic action. J Pharm Pharmac 21: 241.
35. Ulrych M, Frohlich ED, Dustan HP, Page IH. 1968. Immediate hemodynamic effects of beta-adrenergic blockade with Propranolol in normotensive and hypertensive man. Circulation 37: 411.
36. Wolfson S, Gorlin R. 1969. Cardiovascular pharmacology of Propranolol in man. Circulation 40: 501.
37. Parker JO, West RO, DiGiorgi S. 1968. Hemodynamic effects of Propranolol in coronary heart disease. Am J Cardiol 21: 11.
38. Helfant RH, Herman MV, Gorlin R. 1971. Abnormalities of left ventricular contraction induced by beta-adrenergic blockade. Circulation 43: 641.
39. Greenblatt DJ, Koch-Weser J. 1973. Adverse reactions to Propranolol in hospitalized medical patients. Am Heart J 86: 478.
40. Stephen SA. 1966. Unwanted effects of Propranolol. Am J Cardiol 18: 463.

GENERAL GROUP DISCUSSION: BASELINE HEMODYNAMICS

Dr. Dreifus: Obviously from this discussion the difficulties of evaluating the hemodynamic effects of antiarrhythmic drugs are complex. In
fact, the evaluation of the oral preparation is even more difficult than
that of the intravenous preparation. Dr. Aronson would you briefly outline
for us the laboratory approach to hemodynamic assessment of an antiarrhythmic
agent? Obviously, you are more limited in the human, but ideally what
would you like to measure in the animal model?
Dr. Aronson: In the animal model of course you have more flexibility.
You can place a strain gauge on the heart to measure contractile force
and measure so-called ejection phase and pre-ejection phase which are
the indices of myocardial contraction. Furthermore, you can control the
afterload and preload by altering the systemic vascular resistance and
the mean aortic pressure or the left ventricular end diastolic volume.
I feel you have to assess the effect of the drug on each one of the
determinants of myocardial performance keeping the other ones constant
as a first step to determine what potential net effect of the drug will
be when it is given when none of these factors are controlled. Furthermore,
I feel you have to realize that there are peripheral effects of the drug,
quinidine being the prime example where you get very significant vasodilation, probably triggering compensatory mechanisms such as catecholamine
release that might offset any of the direct effects that you might observe.
In short, I feel thatone must measure individually all of the determinants
of myocardial contractility then determine the net effect with all of these
parameters permitted to vary in the absence of any control measures.
Dr. Dreifus: In normal individuals and in patients what studies would
you like to see performed in the catheterization laboratory?
Dr. Aronson: In patients you can do similar things accurately and on an
acute basis. However, you are not given the opportunity to place a strain

gauge on the heart. It is possible to measure the pre-ejection phase
indices of myocardial contractility such as the maximum height of developed
pressure which is probably as good as anything. However, you are always
up against the problem of not being able to control pre-load and afterload. After-load can be varied by using angiotensin or nitrates.
However, this still remains a complex problem because of variability of
autonomic tone which is observed during the course of the study. Consequently, the results of these observations must be carefully evaluated.
Finally, both the results and problems noted during the acute studies may
not have relevance to subsequent chronic use of the oral form.

Dr. Kline: Very often we are compelled to give antiarrhythmic agents to
individuals who have pre-existing left ventricular dysfunction. For
example, in the case of disopyramide there is no question that it is a
valuable antiarrhythmic agent. Unfortunately, we did not understand all
of its hemodynamic parameters before it was certified for use. I would
like to elaborate a little further on the indices of systolic function
of the left ventricle. I feel there is some value to Starling curves.
Certainly, one can measure the data of isometric pressure elevation at a
commonly developed isometric pressure and have some indication of myocardial
contractility when one patient is compared to the next. Dr. Aronson,
would you comment further on two areas, the first relates to diastolic
function of the left ventricle and specifically the measurements of left
ventricular distensibility and the elements of isovolumetric relaxation
which I feel are important because of the new calcium antagonists that are
about to come onto the market. It is clear that these new calcium
antagonists may elevate end diastolic pressure and not reflect left
ventricular failure but rather an alteration in early diastolic pressure
volume relationships. Secondly, I would like you to comment whether it
is sufficient to measure just cardiac output or should one really be
looking at regional blood flow to key organs such as the kidney, liver,
renal, cerebral perfusion and limb blood flow.

Dr. Aronson: In reference to the first question that Dr. Kline raises,
it is really crucial and I probably should have mentioned in the
beginning that the left ventricular end diastolic volume pressure
relationship is going to be a high variable depending on the nature of
the underlying cardiac disease. Ischemia, hypertrophy, cardiac myopathies
will change that relationship in such a way that it does not necessarily

mean that because there is an increase in left ventricular end diastolic pressure that there is a compensatory effect by increasing the fiber length. In order to actually assess the diastolic pressure volume relationship you must know the compliance of the left ventricle and this is not easy to determine since it is difficult to measure diastolic volume. However, it can be approached by measurements with radionucleo- tides or by cineangiography but the pressure volume relationship during diastolie will be very strongly influenced by concurrent diseases. With reference to the second question concerning regional blooc flow, it should be understood that regional blood flow alters afterload. I feel that it is important to know what effect afterload may have on cardiac hemodynamics. Other than that I doubt that it is essential to assess the effect of any particular drug on a specific organ. I am not sure that it is essential if there is no effect on afterload.

Dr. Kaplinsky: Could you further elaborate on the use of radionucleotide studies in evaluating drugs from a hemodynamic standpoint?

Dr. Aronson: Well, as far as I can tell, it is probably the most reasonable means of assessing the ejection fraction on a chronic serial basis because you can actually measure ejection fraction. Furthermore, you can assess segmental motion which is useful because the ejection fraction could be normal and yet segmental abnormalities could be present. In addition, indices of the ejection phase can be obtained by the rate of isotope ejection, hence I feel that it is a very useful way to characterize noninvasively, left ventricular function as long as you bear in mind that it is going to be sensitive to afterload changes as well as heart rate. I don't think there is anything better at the moment other than the information obtained by invasive studies in the catheterization laboratory. However, catheterization studies are not easily obtainable on a serial basis.

Dr. Dreifus: Dr. Morganroth, would you like to comment on the usefulness of M-Mode and two-dimensional echocardiography in evaluating hemodynamic alterations noninvasively?

Dr. Morganroth: I do not feel that two dimensional echocardiography will give you a measure of small changes in left ventricular function that might occur in response to a new antiarrhythmic agent. However, large changes can be identified but these may still be subclinical. As you know, echocardiography has been used as one of the primary techniques in detecting cardio-toxicity following andriamycin therapy.

Dr. Aronson: In all of these instances the change must be rather substantial to affect the ejection fraction. This is really the problem. Studies under stress will enhance the sensitivity.

Dr. Temple: The negative inotrophic effects of disopyramide were known prior to its release and it was also known that it increased peripheral vascular resistance. Hence, it was labeled thatit was not intended for use in patients with heart failure. What actually happened is that patients with very low ejection fractions and severe heart failure were treated with this agent anyhow, resulting in the complications that have been recorded. I feel thte lesson that we learned from the clinical use of this agent that you have really to study the patient with abnormalities under controlled situations to precisely assess how serious these effects may be on other than normal individuals. A similar comment was directed to the electrophysiologic studies in normal versus abnormal individuals.

Dr. Aronson: Although we were warned not to use disopyramide in patients with congestive heart failure, we do not understand the degree of left ventricular dysfunction in ambulatory patients that may be asymptomatic but are walking around with an ejection fraction between 25% and 30%. The use of disopyramide in these situations may just tip them over into congestive heart failure although we have been warned not to use this agent in the presence of overt failure.

Dr. Dreifus: One additional comment. Congestive failure occurred in a number of patients because of the recommended 300 mg loading dose. Perhaps if only a maintenance dose had been used we would not have seen the emergence of acute pulmonary edema in some of these individuals.

EVALUATION OF DRUG TREATMENT IN SUPRAVENTRICULAR ARRHYTHMIAS

Elieser Kaplinsky, M.D. and Lechaim Naggan, M.D., Ph.D.

Ideally, drug research should proceed from basic sciences, through animal models to its final test - the clinical trials. In the field of supraventricular arrhythmias, however, the process has to unfortunately by-pass the animal models as we do not have satisfactory methods to produce the experimental counterpart of the human arrhythmias. In this presentation we will try to outline methodological guidelines for conducting clinical trials necessary to evaluate any new medication for supraventricular arrhythmias.

When preparing a strategy for the clinical trials, one first has to classify the supraventricular arrhythmias and define their natural history. The latter is extremely important for the proper evaluation of drug effect. The second ingredient in planning a clinical trial is the establishment of the objectives of the therapy.

From the point of view of drug evaluation, the supraventricular arrhythmia fall into three simple categories:

A. Supraventricular (atrial or junctional) premature beats.

B. Supraventricular (atrial or junctional) tachycardias.

C. Atrial flutter and fibrillation.

The approach to category A, namely the supraventricular premature beats, should be no different from that to premature beats in general. This aspect has been well dealt with elsewhere at this symposium. In this presentation we will therefore address ourselves to categories B and C.

The supraventricular tachycardia tend to appear in paroxysms which last from minutes to hours, and rarely, even days. The frequency varies tremendously among different patients and many times also within the same patients. A chronic form of such an arrhythmia is a medical rarity. The objectives of treatment are thus twofold. One, to abolish a paroxysm when it appears, and two, to prevent recurrence of attacks.

Atrial flutter usually presents itself as paroxysmal arrhythmias, but may occur in chronic forms. Atrial fibrillation is abundant both in its paroxysmal and its chronic forms. In both atrial flutter and fibrillation (in their paroxysmal form), one may wish to terminate the arrhythmia and prevent recurrences. However, in the paroxysmal bouts, and all the more in the chronic form, one has to also deal with a different aspect of treatment, namely, the control of heart rate. The initial approach to atrial flutter and fibrillation, regardless of etiology and form (acute or chronic), is therefore slowing the heart rate. This is usually achieved by increasing the degree of atrioventricular block with drugs. In the chronic form of the arrhythmias (mainly the chronic atrial fibrillation) this is the only therapeutic objective.

In summary, there are three objectives to be achieved in the management of supraventricular arrhythmias:

    I.   Abolish paroxysms of arrhythmias.

    II.   Prevent recurrences of (or decrease) paroxysms.

    III. Control heart rate in atrial flutter and fibrillation.

Different study designs should be utilized for the investigation of each of these objectives.

ETHICAL PROBLEMS

Two problems should be solved before plunging into any clinical trial in general, and into drug evaluation in supraventricular arrhythmias in particular. Should the patient be treated? Many of the supraventricular tachycardias occur in healthy individuals and their benign and rare appearances may render any preventive drug intervention unnecessary. The second problem deals with the applicability of placebo for a double blind study. The benign feature of many of the supraventricular arrhythmias, we feel, justifies the guarded use of placebo in patients who tolerate the arrhythmias well (for the various protocols, see below). However, instead of placebo as control, one can use an old established drug and compare it to the new medication.

ABOLITION OF TACHYCARDIA

Normal sinus rhythm should be restored in any patient who develops a paroxysm of supraventricular tachycardia. If simple physiological maneuvres (e.g. carotid sinus massage) fail to restore normal rhythm - drug therapy (or cardioversion) is indicated. Best results with drugs are achieved via the intravenous route and, if effective, the medication should restore normal rhythm within minutes. Testing a new medication in this context is relatively simple. Indeed, several new drugs have been introduced in recent years for the abolition of supraventricular tachycardia and the studies were properly performed with convincing results. Most, if not all, were open trials where the percentage of reversion to normal sinus rhythm within minutes of drug administration was determined. The natural history of a paroxysm of supraventricular tachycardia is, however, extremely unpredictable, and sometimes the mere sight of a syringe may suffice to frighten the patient into normal sinus rhythm. It is therefore recommended that the new drug be tested against a placebo in a double blind crossover design. The arrhythmia in most cases is extremely benign, with no danger to the patient, and a delay of ten to fifteen minutes in drug administration may be acceptable. Of course, as mentioned above, one may again compare the new drug against an old and approved one, in the same double blind fashion.

A patient with supraventricular tachycardia will enter the study if his clinical state is unaffected by the arrhythmia. He will be given placebo (or the control drug) and the drug under investigation as drugs "A" and "B" in a double blind fashion. One may expect a quick result from such a study.

PREVENTION OF PAROXYSMAL TACHYCARDIAS

Of the three objectives outlined above, this is by far the most difficult to achieve clinically as well as to evaluate. When aiming at double blind studies, we must first decide whether it will be ethical to withhold the hitherto accepted treatment for the study period and let the patient develop paroxysms (during a placebo phase at least). One therefore, again, may use any of the accepted old modalities as control drugs. However, since paroxysms will be treated promptly, and since in some patients the paroxysms are benign and well toler- ated, it is conceivable that one of the control drugs might be a placebo.

The tremendous variability in the clinical picture of supraventricular tachycardia calls for first assessing the natural history of the arrhythmia in each patient. Obviously, only those patients who display a sufficient number of paroxysms may enter such a study. Thus, a baseline period should be defined and a minimal frequency of paroxysms determined. We feel that only patients who have at least one attack per month should be included, and the minimum duration of each phase should be of a few months (this may of course be changed with the scope of the study). The more centers that are incorporated, the stricter the selection, and the speedier the results that will be provided. The study design is simple:

Phase I: Baseline

Phase II: Open titration (?)

Phase III: Double blind drug A

             drug B

An open phase may have to be included to prevent failure due to insufficient dosage. However, the exclusion of patients who do not react to the drug, may introduce an obvious bias. There- fore, we believe that the open titration phase should determine drug tolerance rather than efficacy. This will ensure that the patients will receive the maximal tolerable dose during the study period.

Success or failure should be evaluated by any change in the following parameters: Frequency, duration and severity of paroxysms. If no paroxysm occurs, success is obviously complete. However, one may be satisfied with a significant reduction in the number of attacks, in their duration, and in their severity (as manifested subjectively by patients' discomfort, and objectively by the rate of the tachycardia). Any one of the three may be sufficient to approve the new drug for prolonged administration.

The evaluation of the objective and subjective results may prove to be a major problem in itself. Obviously, one must use outpatient ambulatory monitoring for the prolonged preventive trial. The episodic nature of the paroxysms and the length of the study period preclude the use of the expensive Holter monitoring systems. An ideal and inexpensive model of monitoring for such a study would be the transtelephone electrocardiographic transmission. The patient may carry the simple and small device and contact the research center both routinely and whenever symptoms develop. Such documentation is mandatory, since it has been clearly demonstrated that in a significant number of patients with paroxysmal tachycardias there may be a clear dissociation between symptoms and arrhythmias.

HEART CONTROL IN ATRIAL FLUTTER AND FIBRILLATION

The third objective in the management of supraventricular arrhythmias is heart rate control in atrial flutter and fibrillation. Wide and documented experience with two large groups of medications, namely, digitalis and beta-blocker, has laid the foundation for the proper way to study any new medication designed only to slow the ventricular rate during these arrhythmias.

Heart rate control in atrial flutter and fibrillation may have to be accomplished quickly and a study of the new medication in such a situation is simple. Although the rapid ventricular rate in the uncontrolled arrhythmias may be irregular, it is generally stable. A double blind study thus may not be indicated. Furthermore, if the tested drug is effective, the double blind code will be promptly decoded.

Heart rate control in the chronic form applies mainly to chronic atrial fibrillation. The natural history of this chronic arrhythmia is well-known and its behaviour under various conditions is well documented. It has thus been shown that heart rate control at least is easy to achieve, as is being classically done with digitalis preparations. The situation under stress, however, calls for better control since digitalis is insufficient in controlling heart rate during stress and exercise. Better heart rate control under such conditions is important clinically, as we have shown while studying the new calcium antagonist verapamil. Patients develop better exercise performance with better rate control. Thus a study of the efficacy of any medication in controlling heart rate in patients with chronic atrial fibrillation should be as follows:

Phase I: Open titration

Phase II: Double blind

Drug A (Rest & Exercise)

Drug B (Rest & Exercise)

Drug efficacy should first be documented openly because of a possible marked individual variation in dosage. Since the therapeutic end point here is easy to define, one may use the open titration phase to achieve a range of effective dosage. This will enable the management of an improved double blind study where both the tested medication and the placebo will undergo double blind titration phases.

The efficacy of the tested drug should be checked at rest, during an exercise tolerance test, and during a period of 24 hours of continuous ambulatory monitoring. The importance of the 24 hour monitoring is twofold: One, verification of the data recorded in the artificial atmosphere of a hospital laboratory, and two, the recording of heart response during sleep. Even with no medication, heart rate is quite adequately controlled during sleep and caution should be exercised not to produce excessive slowing with the addition of drugs. The preferred method here is the 24 hour Holter system, since one or two recording sessions will suffice.

We have discussed the problem of supraventricular arrhythmias and have offered study designs for each of the three main objectives of medical management in this field. The abolition of an acute attack is an easily approached question. More elaborate, but nonetheless feasible and assured of clear results one way or another, is the question of heart rate control in atrial flutter and fibrillation. In the problem of arrhythmia prevention, the complexity of paroxysmal supra-

ventricular tachycardia is such that the control trials have
to be large and carefully designed in order to produce valid
data. Otherwise, the results may still be equivocal and
subjective. Which may not be so bad, considering the fact that
quinidine, our best chronic antiarrhythmic medication, never
underwent the via dolorosa of today's regulations, and had
it not been with us for over 200 years, might not have been
approved today for want of sufficient studies....

GENERAL GROUP DISCUSSION: ATRIAL ARRHYTHMIAS

Dr. Dreifus: Dr. Kaplinsky has presented several rational programs for
the evaluation of antiarrhythmic agents in the presence of supraventricular
tachycardia.

Dr. Rosen: I have no major objections. I just envision a totally different
approach. I should like to point out that paroxysmal supraventricular
tachycardia is not one arrhythmia but is AV nodal reentry with quantifiable
fast and slow pathways, some utilize Ken bundles which can be either concealed
or manifest, others atrial reentry and sinus node reentry. All of these
varieties have a very precise measureable pathophysiology. The reentrant
limbs in the presence of a Kent bundle are carefully quantifiable in terms
of their ability to conduct or not to conduct. In other words, one can
measure refractoriness and conduction in the anomalous pathway both in an
antegrade as well as retrograde direction. Electrophysiologic studies can
clearly delineate which drugs act in which limb of the surface movement and
quickly provide information for management of these arrhythmias. A communication which will be published very shortly identifies a large series of AV
nodal reentry arrhythmias. Programmed stimulation over several days can
predict which agent will be effective in curing AV nodal reentry rhythms.
As far as the choice of drugs is concerned for paroxysmal supraventricular
tachycardia, one has to consider efficacy mainly that the drug may have the
absolute ability to close a circus movement but may be a most toxic agent
for that patient. For example, quinidine turns out to be a very good drug
for closing AV nodal reentry. Hence, toxicity must be balanced against
efficacy in choosing an agent. Finally, the use of programmed stimulation
to initiate atrial fibrillation in patients who have very infrequent attacks
of paroxysmal atrial fibrillation may be important. Use of antiarrhythmic
agents that may slow the ventricular rate can then be evaluated by placing
the patient in atrial fibrillation after effective administration of the
drug has been accomplished.

Dr. Dreifus: Do you have any comments Dr. Kaplinsky?

Dr. Kaplinsky: These remarks only compliment what I have said since you can find an effective agent in many ways. The basic science is clear but eventually the answer must be obtained during clinical use of these agents. Hence, after elaborate electrophysiologic tests have been performed it is still important to understand how the agent works on a chronic clinical basis. Hence, the studies which I identified are independent of the electrophysiologic studies outlined by Dr. Rosen. Perhaps you will choose a drug according to its electrophysiologic parameters and study the drug in clinical practice using the propoer double blind protocols or other corss over procedures as indicated.

Dr. Dreifus: I have been somewhat troubled by translating the electrophysiologic studies into chronic administration of these antiarrhythmic agents. Sympathetic and cholinergic effects may be quite different once the patient leaves the catheterization laboratory and assumes ordinary life activity. Hence, the action of antiarrhythmic drugs through a precisely controlled situation in the catheterization laboratory may be quite different than its effect while the patient is standing or ambulatory. Obviously these agents must be directed at the most vulnerable part of the reentry circuit, whether it is the atrium or the AV node. Other drugs may specifically affect conduction within anomalous pathways and should be utilized for that purpose.

Dr. Kaplinsky: May I add another short comment. Although it has been a major advance to understand the underlying mechanisms of supraventricular tachycardias you still may eventually find that drugs may be effective regardless of the mechanism. In our experience verapamil may be effective for many varieties of supraventricular tachycardias regardless of the actual mechanism. The important test is what happens when it is given to the patient, particularly using intravenous verapamil.

Dr. Krikler: Can I supplement what Dr. Kaplinsky has said and give some support to Dr. Rosen at the same time. It is important to understand whether the patient's problem may be a result of an unduly frequent number of atrial extrasystoles that might initiate the tachycardia and to what extent is the initiation zone of the tachycardia itself. I feel that it is important to understand these principles in trying to decide whether drug A or B is more suitable for a particular patient. We would for example, consider verapamil worthy of trial perhaps in very full doses and possible even retest to see what has happened to the initiation zone following the use of this agent. Wheras if we see that there are a large number of atrial extrasystoles and especially if failure of prophylactic verapamil were known to be present we would choose amiodarone as a prophylactic agent. One final note, I am sure that you meant digitalis and not quinidine as having been with us for 200 years and having stood the test of time.

Dr. Kline: Dr. Kaplinsky, in frequently-occurring paroxysmal atrial fibrillation would you propose to test the patient in a catehterization laboratory using the extrastimulus technique to initiate atrial fibrillation then administer the agent to determine whether the arrhythmia can be reinitiated and if not, place the patient on chronic follow up study. A second question directed to Dr. Temple, most of our patients with atrial fibrillation have rather advanced heart disease such as amyloid and most testing protocols concurred with the FDA position at the 70 year old age cut off. It is precisely the patients over age 70 who need this medication and we are not then permitted to study them.

Dr. Kaplinsky: I would not try to answer the first question as we do not have any electrophysiologic studies of supraventricular tachycardias. Dr. Rosen may be able to answer that question much better. As you know, we have had verapamil in Europe for at least 7 years. We have given verapamil to many patients over 70 with no problems whatsoever. I feel that it is an excellent agent to control heart rate in the presence of atrial fibrillation even without digitalis regardless of age and regardless of etiology.

Dr. Temple: I suppose the question is whether we have some rule that you can't study people over 70. There is not such a rule of course. The protocols are written, at least initially, to exclude people who might have unexpected problems such as occult renal disease or something like that would produce serious side effects. However, nothing in any protocol is mandated by the FDA as far as older people are concerned. In fact, there is some hullabaloo that studies really aren't conducted frequently enough in elderly patients who are the major recipients of drugs. We are enthusiastic about studies in patients provided the study is done carefully and attention is directed to the clearance of these agents in patients who will be actually taking the drug. If you feel there is an unreasonable constraint in the protocol it would be wise just to ask the FDA. One other comment worth mentioning is that disopyramide was marketed for about 10 years abroad before it entered the United States market. However, not everything was known about that agent when it was introduced to the U.S. marked.

Dr. Kaplinsky: We are studying patients over 70 specifically to determine the pharmacokinetics. Pharmacokinetics in these individuals may be quite different.

HOW SHOULD LONG-TERM SAFETY OF A NEW ANTIARRHYTHMIC DRUG BE DETERMINED?

JOEL S. KARLINER, M.D.

During previous portions of this symposium, much useful information has been presented regarding the electrophysiology of ischemia and of antiarrhythmic drugs. One might characterize what is known about the "electrophysiology" of postmarketing drug surveillance as follows: it is fragmented, abberant and ectopic. A recent report of a United States Senate Committee advocating improved postmarketing drug surveillance echoes similar pleas from the past.[1,2]

When considering the issue of how the long-term safety of a new antiarrhythmic drug should be determined, it is necessary for us to define both "long-term" and "safety". With regard to the former, it is common clinical experience that most patients do not take antiarrhythmic agents for very long periods of time, i.e., for many years. Nevertheless, some agents may be taken for long periods. Common clinical examples are digoxin, quinidine and propranolol. For example, I recently encountered a patient, a 40-year-old physician with systemic arterial hypertension, who had been taking propranolol for nine years. He wished to learn what was known about the long-term safety of this agent. I told him that such information was not currently available in large groups of patients. It may be anticipated that as larger numbers of patients with chronic ischemic heart disease live longer, especially if coronary artery bypass surgery indeed proves to prolong life, antiarrhythmic agents may be taken for much longer periods than had previously been anticipated. Certainly younger individuals with arrhythmias, especially those with preexcitation syndromes, may be expected to t a k e such agents for many years and even decades. For the majority of patients, however, we are probably still dealing with relatively short-term therapy, i.e., one to three or four years. Thus, any considerations of "long-term" safety of such agents must take into account the specific nature of what is meant by "long-term" in the clinical circumstances in which the agent is being employed.

What is meant by "safety?" Here we raise the usual issue of the risk-benefit ratio. For example, one may be more inclined to use an agent with a larger number of side effects if one is treating a potentially malignant arrhythmia compared to the-suppression of a paraoxysmal atrial arrhythmia which produces little or no hemodynamic impairment. A major issue regarding the safety of antiarrhythmic agents is whether such drugs may not themselves induce arrhythmias. It is now recognized that all antiarrhythmic agents, presumably by virtue of their electrophysiologic actions, may themselves induce abnormal cardiac rhythms. One difficulty in assessing this issue is in determining whether time and treatment are confounded. Thus, during the natural history of the disease, some patients will develop arrhythmias or "break through" anti-arrhythmic treatment. Under these circumstances, it may be difficult to attribute an arrhythmia to a drug. For the assessment of arrhythmias, we have a variety of monitoring techniques including long-term ambulatory tape moni-toring as well as exercise testing. Neither of these approaches, however, separate the possible confounding of time and treatment referred to above.

Another question that needs to be answered is: What are the effects of the antiarrhythmic agents on left ventricular performance? Here animal studies, while providing initial useful information, must be corroborated by human investigation. The advent of new or noninvasive techniques, such as echo-cardiography and exercise radionuclide angiography, should help to settle this question fairly rapidly for most new antiarrhythmic agents. By using the radionuclide approach, one can now measure both ejection fraction and left ventricular volume noninvasively so that long-term studies assessing left ven-tricular performance can be undertaken. Although echocardiography appears to be less useful with respect to interventions, we have done some acute studies with afterloading using the ultrasound approach.[3,4]

Long-term safety should, of course, also be assessed by serial evaluation of renal, hepatic, hematologic, serologic and ocular abnormalities. One draw-back to this type of follow-up is that the investigator is often plagued with the necessity to draw blood and to fill out the required forms. Further, some agents could be released selectively (as has been proposed by a number of people in the UK using either "registered" or "recorded" release schemes); such approaches remain to be evaluated. The issue of drug interactions is exceed-ingly important, especially in the usual clinical situation when the practi-tioner has little control over what other medications patients may take. Indeed, one must be certain that the patient is taking the agent. Such

certainty would require periodic measurement of drug plasma or blood levels.
As we all know, some patients may be notoriously unreliable. It is a common
experience to learn that patients may be taking other drugs without informing
the physician in addition to sporadic use of the particular drug under investigation. A recent anecdote illustrates the difficulty of assessing the
patient's responses to drugs. I was consulted by the father of a physician
friend because of recurrent atrial arrhythmias associated with probable chronic
ischemic heart disease. One of the agents prescribed was isosorbide dinitrate.
On a follow-up visit, the patient was asked about his status, and he replied
that he was free of angina. As the treating physician, I made the mistake of
assuming that the patient was taking his medication. I learned later from his
son that the patient was quite pleased that he had "fooled" me, because his
angina had disappeared despite the fact that he never took the prescribed
medication. This patient's victory (by a retired pharmacist!) over the physician illustrates the problem of patient compliance, which we all encounter
every day. Another major problem is that in some instances patients take pro-
prietary medications without informing the physician. These are difficulties
that confound any sort of surveillance scheme that one might hope to undertake.

Table 1. Estimation of sample sizes for detecting adverse reactions*.

EXPECTED PREVALENCE	REQUIRED SAMPLE SIZE (95% CONFIDENCE LIMITS)
10 in a million	400,000
1 in a thousand	4,000
1 in a hundred	400

*Required precision is of the same magnitude as the prevalence.

Table 1 illustrates some relatively simplistic calculations which were
undertaken to t r y to estimate sample sizes needed to detect adverse reactions. One would likely certainly to identify adverse reactions that occur
once in every thousand drug administrations. To do this, one needs only to
have a required sample size of 4,000 to obtain 95 percent confidence limits.
What are some of the possible pitfalls of such a scheme? First we must have a
representative population. Each practitioner and each center may see different
types of patients. Thus, the patient population seen by a referral practi-
tioner or a referral medical center may not be comparable to that seen in a
military hospital or in a large public institution. A population
that was reasonably representative w o ul d probably have to be gathered from

more than one center. How would such information be gathered? Today we rely
on a variety of *ad hoc* schemes such as spontaneous reporting. Physicians
identify adverse reactions, write letters to the editor, inform drug companies
directly, or inform the FDA. Other schemes that have been suggested, and some
of these have been tried, i n clude reporting by hospital pharmacies using
computerized approaches. However, the latter have largely met with moderate
success or to be more honest, with relative failure. Such approaches are ex-
ceedingly expensive and have not worked very well to date. Perhaps we can
learn from other countries, such as the "yellow card" reporting system available in the United Kingdom.

In addition to a representative patient population, other minimal
requirements of a postmarketing surveillance system include baseline laboratory
data (again because of the possible confounding of time and treatment), and
information on all drugs given to the patient. Remington[5] has suggested that
any prospective observational study must include the following elements:[1] The
system must be designed to follow accepted epidemiological principles for data
collection and quality control. [2] The system should include components
making possible direct knowledge of the population at risk. [3] Well-designed
data collection forms must be available. [4] Appropriate quality control
mechanisms must also be an integral part of the study. Whether one can in fact
use the computerized systems available in large medical center pharmacies for
identifying the representative patient population and then for tracking the
requisite number of patients in order to identify adverse reactions will depend
in part on the sample size required. Certainly one should consider attempting
such schemes for the evaluation of a new agent. As indicated above, information on all drugs given to the patient is a key element, and it seems likely
that such information may best be obtained by utilizing computerized data banks
available in hospital pharmacies.

I now wish to raise another issue that I know is quite controversial
within the pharmaceutical industry as well as among physicians. It is conceivable that patients might themselves be helpful in providing an early
warning of adverse reactions. One does not wish to frighten patients, but it
might be made clear in the case of some agents that the particular drug was
being released conditionally because only a relatively small number of patients
(between 1000 and 3000) might have been given the drug, at least in the U.S.A.
Potential benefits of the patient package insert include: [1] improved risk-
benefit assessment; [2] better distribution of information; [3] prevention

of adverse drug reactions; [4] prevention of drug interactions; [5] improved drug administration techniques: [6] improved patient compliance; [7] discussion of sensitive issues; and [8] warnings of inappropriate use. Of course, any such system has potential risks. Included among these are: [1] lack of patient interest; [2] the level of patient education (the issue of bilingual or multilingual forms must be considered): [3] potential increased cost of medication; [4] the requirement for increased physician time to deal with the patient package insert; and [5] the spurious induction of side effects where none in fact exist. An additional approach that might be employed is that pharmaceutical advertising should encourage both the physician and the patient to report adverse reactions. Although this suggestion is also a controversial one, it seems to me that it might lead to a better early-warning system than we presently have.

Finally, to quote Melmon and Morelli, "Continuing vigil must be maintained for unusual or changing effects produced by a drug even though the drug has been safely given for long periods."[6]

REFERENCES

1. Culliton BJ and Waterfall WK. Post-marketing surveillance. Br Med J 280: 1175-6, 1980.
2. Wilson AB. Post-marketing surveillance of adverse reactions to new medicines. Br Med J 2: 1001-3, 1977.
3. Crawford MH, Karliner JS and O'Rourke RA. Favorable effects of oral maintenance digoxin therapy on left ventricular performance in normal subjects: echocardiographic study. Am J Cardiol 38: 843-7, 1976.
4. Ryan WF and Karliner JS. Effects of tocainide on left ventricular performance at rest and during alterations in heart rate and systemic arterial pressure: an echocardiographic study. Br Heart J 41: 175-81, 1979.
5. Remington RD. Post-marketing drug surveillance: a comparison of methods. Am J Pharm 150: 72-80, 1978.
6. Melmon KL and Morelli HF. Drug reactions. In: Melmon KL and Morelli HF, ed. Clinical Pharmacology. Basic Principles in Therapeutics. 2nd ed. New York: Macmillan, 1978: 977.

GENERAL GROUP DISCUSSION: LONG-TERM SAFETY

Dr. Temple: One question. The numbers you gave for the number of patients
needed to be exposed to detect an adverse reaction. Those numbers are sur-
prisingly low. Do I understand that the number needed is to have at least
a 95% chance that the reaction will occur?

Dr. Karliner: If you are looking for any effect.   I can give you a specific
reference for this.

Dr. Temple: It is important though in thinking of how practical those numbers
are to raise the question of how likely that the event will be recognized
as drug related. We have tried to run some calculations like this through and
also for things that have a background rate. Of course you are looking at
several problems. It is hard to know whether the event you see is drug related
or not. Take for instance myocardial infarction in a particular patient.
If the drug caused an adverse reaction of 1 in 10,000 in the treated population, obviously the adverse effect would never be detedted short of a
clinical trial of the size that would stagger anybody.

Dr. Temple: I was just using it as an illustration of difficulty, not of
real importance. You wonder how many reports we get directly. The answer
is not too many. This is probably because our system works through the drug
companies. If reports came directly to the regulatory agency we may see
a different incidence. The numbers that we currently give are somewhere
around 10,000 or 12,000 total per year of which only 1,000 to 2,000 come
directly to us. Just another comment. There was a patient package insert
provided voluntarily by Upjohn for Monoxidil. It is a good illustration
for anyone who wants to see what they might look like. It was developed
because that seemed to be a drug where the patient could help in detecting
some adverse events early. The other thing that everyone should know is
that there is a proposal in the September 1980 Federal Register with 10
sample patient pacage inserts. They were developed fairly quickly. I
am not sure that they are the best that can be developed. There is a

fairly short comment period allowed on them. If anyone wants to tell us
what they think of the patient package insert program and specifically the
ones that were proposed in the Federal Register, please comment.

Participant: Once the drug has been determined efficacious, what percentage
of side effects are we going to accept. There is no drug that I know of
that doesn't have side effects.

Dr. Karliner: That is why I showed the different orders of magnitude.
It depends on what you are looking for. If you are looking for the percent
adverse reactions or the severity of the reaction. The severity of the
reaction that you would tolerate would probably be in direct proportion to
the severity of the disease you are treating. I was wondering if any of
our colleagues from abroad have anything to add in relation to drug surveillance in their own countries?

HOW SHOULD ONE MANAGE EMERGENCY DRUG REQUESTS AND THEIR DATA?

STEWART J. EHRREICH, Ph.D.,
DEPUTY DIRECTOR, DIVISION OF CARDIO-RENAL DRUG PRODUCTS
BUREAU OF DRUGS, FOOD AND DRUG ADMINISTRATION

ROBERT LINKOUS, B.S.,
CONSUMER SAFETY OFFICER, DIVISION OF CARDIO-RENAL DRUG PRODUCTS
BUREAU OF DRUGS, FOOD AND DRUG ADMINISTRATION

1.   INTRODUCTION

The Food and Drug Administration is aware that there may be good reason to use an investigational drug in patient care, i.e., not in a formal investigation, before complete data on effectivenss and safety are available. The usual reason is the combination of a patient with a life-threatening disease who has exhausted all standard therapy and the availability of a promising new agent with some evidence of usefulness in the condition. A request for use of a drug in such cases is usually called a request for "emergency" or "compassionate" use. Patients with life-threatening cardiac arrhythmias provide a particularly common source of these requests, and the gravity of the situation often requires quick action. The problem is thus not only to obtain permission to treat the patient with the experimental compound, but to find out how the drug can be obtained in as short a time as possible.

Emergency uses of drugs are a source of some discomfort to both FDA and the pharmaceutical industry: to FDA because these uses cannot be closely monitored and because information about the drug is incomplete; to industry because very sick patients may die or have adverse events and raise troubling questions about the drug. Nonetheless, FDA and the pharmaceutical industry have always felt that a seriously ill patient cannot be denied that medication which may offer a reasonable possibility of benefit. It is essential however, that physicians using drugs under these circumstances carry out their obligations to their patients, to the drug manufacturer, and to FDA by monitoring patients closely and supplying needed information.

There are established procedures in our Division and in the rest of the Bureau of Drugs, for considering emergency request promptly. If an emergency occurs during non-business hours there are ways to contact the appropriate individuals, but this is a more difficult and every effort should be made to reach us between 8:00 a.m. and 5:30 p.m.

Emergency use of a drug can be carried out either under an emergency protocol developed by the drug manufacturer, if such a protocol exists, or under an application by the treating physician. Most antiarrhythmic drugs, because of their nature, do have existing emergency protocols including entry criteria, monitoring requirements, etc. Whenever possible patients will be treated under such protocols, rather than under a separate individual investigator application, as it is far easier for us and it keeps all the data together. In addition, the investigator usually need contact only the manufacturer to use the drug under these protocols.

A summary of the protocols available for commonly used investigational antiarrhythmic agents is provided below. In addition, there are the names of the appropriate individuals to contact in each case. These protocols may be amended or terminated and the individuals named may also change, but the information should be of help as a starting point.

2.   MECHANISMS FOR OBTAINING INVESTIGATIONAL (NON-APPROVED)
      ANTIARRHYTHMIC AGENTS

2.1   Does an emergency protocol exist?

Figure I illustrates the procedure for obtaining permission to use an investigational agent in an emergency situation.

Once a physician concludes that his patient needs an investigational agent, he should contact either the drug manufacturer or

consumer safety officer within the Division of Cardio-Renal Drug
Products. If an emergency protocol exists, FDA will ask the investigator
to call the pharmaceutical company,whereupon the company can make
arrangements for the drug to be shipped at once if the patient meets the
emergency protocol entrance criteria. Sometimes a lengthier written
submission will be requested. The investigator must agree to follow the
company's protocol as closely as possible and to report fully all details
of the case and all resulting data should be sent to the company. They
will handle the necessary paper work for FDA purposes from that point
on.

Any physician using drug under any emergency protocol should be
certain he has obtained as much information as possible about the drug;
at a minimum he should ask the drug manufacturer to provide the
Investigators' Brochure, a summary of available animal and clinical
data. It may also be helpful to update this by discussions with the drug
monitor.

In the event that no emergency protocol exists, the manufacturer
may be willing to request a single emergency use under its own IND or may
ask the physician to file one himself. In that case, FDA will need to
review the proposal.

2.2   Mechanism to obtain a "compassionate IND"

In the absence of an existing emergency protocol, the FDA medical
officer, supervisory medical officer, or Division Director may determine
that the proposed use should be permitted. The drug manufacturer will
then be told he may provide the drug and describe the case in writing to
us or, if the physician obtains his own IND, an IND number will be
obtained from FDA to identify the drug investigator and purpose of the
study, which is called a "compassionate IND". Once the number is given,
the drug will beshipped to the investigator by the company. Such an IND
may list specific patients or specific charcteristics of the patients who
will be treated. Only those patients indicated in the IND are to be
treated and unused drug is to be returned to the company. The

investigator is <u>not</u> authorized to administer the agent to other kinds of patients or to transfer the drug to another investigator. The investigator is held accountable for the entire supply of the drug which he received.

2.3 Supplying information on the completed investigation or "compassionate use"

If patients have been treated in an emergency situation the investigator will not have been able to provide the usual required information ahead of time so that, as soon as possible, he should provide the completed FDA form 1571 (for his own IND) or 1572 or 1573 if he joins the manufacturer's IND; these forms will include the study protocol used and, if available, results obtained. If more time is available, forms 1571, 1572, and/or 1573 are filed ahead of time.

3. CURRENT EMERGENCY PROTOCOL STATUS OF NEW ANTIARRHYTHMIC AGENTS

Table I gives the current status of the present antiarrhythmic agents with respect to existence of emergency protocols.

Amiodarone is the only agent listed which does not have an emergency protocol. The drug is not under study by its manufacturer but has been made available under individual investigator "compassionate" IND status for many years.

4. ANALYSIS OF DATA OBTAINED FROM EMERGENCY PROTOCOLS

Much of the data derived from emergency protocols comes from studies with few patients per investigator and has provided little useful information on effectiveness, some on safety. Emergency protocols typically lack the sophistication of approach and analysis needed to be useful. Perhaps this need not always be the case.

Dr. Temple's earlier remarks suggest that even in emergency situations it may be possible to design an adequate study so that the data generated would contribute useful information in the ultimate evaluation of the drug's safety and effectivness for marketing.

GENERAL GROUP DISCUSSION: EMERGENCY DRUG REQUESTS

Dr. Temple: The new drug law was written to be broad in its powers. It
gives the Commissioner or the Secretary the flexibility to regulate investigational use of drugs. Some of the uses of drugs cannot be merely considered
investigational in the usual sense as they are actually patient care.
Dr. Sami: What if the FDA approved the use of a drug in a particular patient
and the pharmaceutical company said no. Is there any standard comment on
this.
Dr. Ehrreich: Well if the drug company said no, you're not going to get the
drug.
Dr. Temple: We are often asked can we lean on them or something. We are
not really willing to do that. The drug belongs to the company. They are
very willing to help in most cases. They are somewhat nervous about proliferation of individual uses under settings that they cannot control very
well and cannot assess the results. Furthermore, we have had some emergency
reugents for drugs that we have not even heard of. We would try to dis-
courage too early use of agents that have not been thoroughly evaluated.
There are several other emergency protocols available. One is available
for Lorconide, however there is no formal protocol.
Dr. Zipes: I would like to support the position of some of the drug companies
to have the option of saying no. If there are 40 physicians treating 40
patients under an emergency protocol we are very unlikely to get data compared
to one physician treating all 40 of those patients. Unfortunately, not
all of the patients can be transported to a center, especially a patient with
recurrent ventricular tachycardia and fibrillation. I am surprised that the
pharmaceutical companies have not been more rigid in releasing investigational
drugs. Transferring patients to a center for treatment sounds rather non-
humanitarian but in fact, it is probably not a bad approach.
Dr. Jaffe: I think there are two other approaches which Dr. Ehrreich did
not mention. One system mentioned by Dr. Zipes of shipping the patient

to a center rather than the drug, the second is what we like often to do at Merck is to suggest to the physician that even if the FDA has given permission for an IND, that one of our expert investigators be consulted on the use of the drug. If our expert investigator concurs that the patient is a proper candidate and that the patient cannot be transferred, the expert investigator is willing to accept the other physician as a secondary investigator on his own protocol. This may reduce some paper work for the FDA. It certainly gives the pharmaceutical company a good deal of confidence that someone expert in the field of this agent is following the situation. However, if the drug is well along it is progress to release but there are various reasons for some delay and reasonable information is available for its use, the drug can be made available to the treating physician. However, in the early investigational stages of a new drug, I would encourage the FDA to tightly control the proliferation of these agents. These agents should be restricted to experienced investigators.

Dr. Rosen: We have had the experience that a physician was treating a patient with an experimental agent for an inappropriate indication. I would encourage the pharmaceutical company to be reasonably sure the the physician was using the agent for a precise indication or have it overviewed by an experienced investigator for that agent. On the other hand, we have had difficulty in acquiring a humanitarian consent for a drug because we have been considered a research laboratory. Furthermore, programmed stimulation to test these agents has been considered by the FDA as research only.

TABLE 1

DRUG	DOES EMERGENCY PROTOCOL EXIST	COMPANY AND CONTACT	MAXIMUM DOSE	ROUTE	INDICATIONS
Verapamil	Yes	Knoll Pharm. Steve Svokos, Ph.D. (201) 877-8300	240-480 mg/day 0.75 mg/kg - 1.5 mg/kg	Oral IV	Life-threatening arrhythmia, Angina at rest, Angina at effort, IHSS
Amiodarone	No	Sanofi (Labaz) Ms. McCafferty New York, New York	Usual dose 600 mg/day Maximum dose 2400 mg/day	Oral	Life-threatening arrhythmia uncontrolled by available therapeutic agents
Ethmozin	Yes	Endo Labs Ed Adams Garden City, New York (516) 832-2124	12.5 mg/kg/day	Oral	Same as above
Aprindine	Yes	Lilly Research Charles Matsumoto, Ph.D. (317) 261-2727	1st day loading dose 400 mg 2nd day 30 mg 3rd day 200 mg 4th day ? titrate patient	Oral	Same as above
Mexitil (Mexilitine)	Yes	Boehringer Ingelheim Ltd. Dr. R. Muntes (203) 438-0311 (X289)	100 mg t.i.d. starting, up to average maximum of 400 mg t.i.d.	Oral	Life-threatening arrhythmia refractory to other agents
Tocainide	Yes	Astra Pharm., Inc. David Blois, Ph.D. (617) 620-6200	Starting dose 600 mg b.i.d. then 600 mg t.i.d., if necessary then contact company for consultation if necessary	Oral	Life-threatening arrhythmia refractory to other agents
Encainide	Yes	Mead Johnson Larry Versteegh, Ph.D. (812) 426-6049	Usual dose 0.9-1.05 mg/kg (shows elongation of PR interval) up to 2.0 mg/kg	Oral IV	Life-threatening arrhythmia refractory to other agents

FIGURE 1

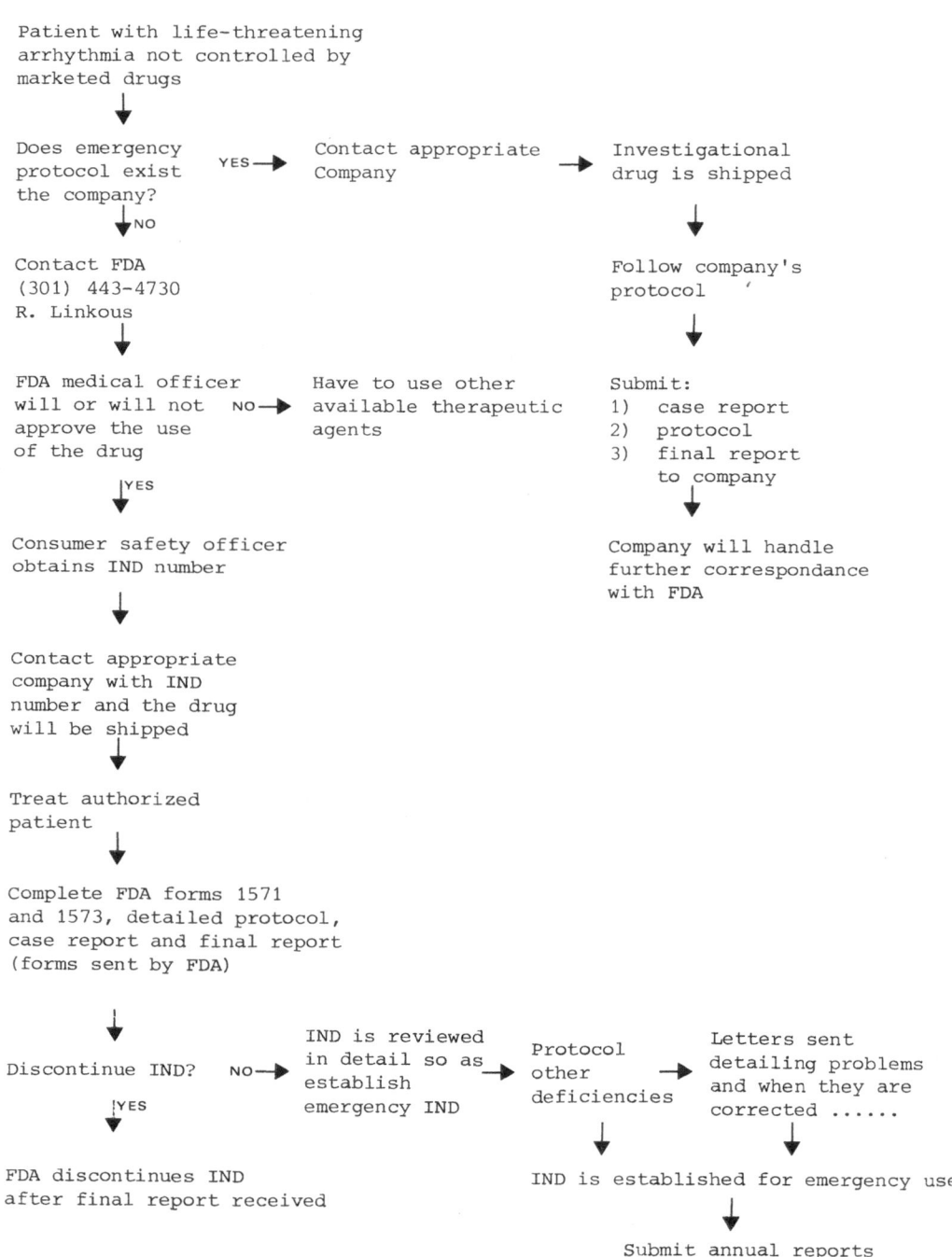

HOW DOES ONE EVALUATE AND USE OUTSIDE U.S.A. DATA IN THE NEW DRUG APPLICATION?
AUGUST M. WATANABE, M.D.

The problem of how to evaluate and utilize foreign data in the development and clinical application of drugs in the U.S.A. is a very complex one which requires consideration of political, social and economic as well as scientific issues. Because this will be a brief overview, I will not be able to cover in detail the recent history of drug development in U.S.A., upon which the need for consideration of this topic is based (1). Rather, I will focus on the evidence that reliance on foreign data might speed the availability of certain drugs in the U.S.A. and, second, to offer some consideration of specific things that would need to be done to utilize foreign data in our drug development process. In this short paper I will not be able to offer any definitive recommendations, but hopefully will be able to identify some of the important issues and perhaps raise some questions which might lead to future constructive approaches.

The fact that this subject is on the program of this symposium suggests that certain drugs develop faster and are available sooner for clinical use in certain foreign countries than in the U.S.A. - that is, that there is a so-called drug lag in the U.S.A. The evidence for a drug lag can be found in several studies, conducted by industry (1), by academia (2,3), or by the federal government itself (4). A recent example of the latter is the general accounting office's (GAO) report of a two year study of the problem, entitled "FDA Drug Approval - A Lengthy Process that Delays the Availability of Important New Drugs" (4). In this study, the GAO examined the drug approval process both in the U.S.A. and in selected foreign countries. Based on the results of this GAO study, let us examine how long it takes for a new drug application to be approved by the FDA. The GAO study examined the year 1975 as a test year (4). 132 new drugs were submitted for approval that year. As of May 1979, the time of the GAO study (four years later), 69 or 52% of the new drugs had been

approved (4). Of those approved, the average duration required for approval
was 20 months, and of this duration FDA accounted for an average of 17
months and the applicant drug company an average of 3 months (4). Thus,
it does indeed appear to take quite a long time for new drug applications
to be approved in the U.S.A., and a major component of this long delay
seems to be contributed by the FDA. The possible reasons for this delay
are discussed in the GAO study (4).

Let us now examine whether the new drug approval process is faster in
European countries. In Table 1 I have listed three drugs of interest to
cardiologists which were among a list of 14 agents specifically studied
by the GAO (4).

Table 1

TIME (MONTHS) REQUIRED TO APPROVE SELECTED CARDIAC DRUGS

PROPRANOLOL

FOR ARRHYTHMIAS	SWITZ. (4)	U.K. (5)	NOR. (9)	SWED. (16)	U.S. (17)	CAN. (23)
FOR ANGINA	SWITZ. (4)	U.K. (5)	NOR. (9)	CAN. (11)	SWED. (16)	U.S. (17)
FOR HYPERTENSION	SWITZ. (4)	NOR. (14)	SWED. (16)	U.S. (18)	CAN. (19)	
DISOPYRAMIDE	SWITZ. (17)	CAN. (19)	NOR. (36)	U.S. (54)	SWED. (80)	
PRAZOSIN	U.K. (6)	SWITZ (10)	NOR. (27)	CAN. (30)	U.S. (40)	

ADAPTED FROM GAO REPORT

The countries are listed in chronological order according to the duration
in months required for approval. Notice that the U.S.A. was last or
second last for each of the drugs and/or indications listed. The quickest
approval for any of these drugs in the U.S.A. was for propranolol for
arrhythmias and angina - this took 17 months. The longest time required
for approval of one of these drugs in the U.S.A. was for disopyramide -
this took 54 months (4 1/2 years). Another way of looking at the question
of drug lag is to examine when and where given drugs first became available.
In Table 2 I have listed the dates when drugs were first approved and the
dates approved in the U.S.A. (4). Each of these drugs first became available in the United Kingdom. It took from approximately 2 1/2 to nearly
12 additional years for the drugs to be approved, at least for certain
uses, in the U.S.A.

Table 2

AVAILABILITY OF NEW CARDIAC DRUGS

DRUG	DATE & LOCATION FIRST AVAILABLE		DATE AVAILABLE IN U.S.A.	LAG
PROPRANOLOL				
FOR ARRHYTHMIAS	JUNE 1965	U.K.	NOV. 1967	2 YR, 5 MO
FOR ANGINA	JUNE 1965	U.K.	NOV. 1967	2 YR, 5 MO
FOR HYPERTENSION	OCT. 1965	SWITZ.	JUNE 1976	11 YR, 8 MO
DISOPYRAMIDE	JULY 1972	U.K.	AUG. 1977	5 YR, 1 MO
PRAZOSIN	OCT. 1973	U.K.	JUNE 1976	2 YR, 8 MO

ADAPTED FROM GAO REPORT

Thus, the data suggest that there is indeed a so-called drug lag in the U.S.A. It is worthwhile to examine some of the possible reasons why drugs are approved so much more rapidly in European countries than in the U.S.A., for in these reasons might be found methods by which we could speed the process here and also justification for relying on foreign data in our new drug approval process. As I mentioned earlier, these are complex issues that involve scientific, social, and political considerations (4,5). Any list of reasons is likely to be incomplete and simplistic. Nevertheless, for the purposes of this discussion, I have listed in Table 3 several factors identified by the GAO study (4) and by the FDA (5) that contribute to the rapidity of NDA approvals in foreign countries and the slow pace of approval in the U.S.A.

Table 3

WHY THE DISPARITY IN TIME REQUIRED FOR NDA: U.S.A. vs. FOREIGN COUNTRIES

SPEEDS THE PROCESS IN FOREIGN COUNTRIES	SLOWS THE PROCESS IN U.S.A.
• POST-MARKETING SURVEILLANCE	• INTENSIVE CONGRESSIONAL & CONSUMER SCRUTINY
• EXTENSIVE USE OF EXPERT COMMITTEES	• ADVERSARY RELATIONSHIP BE-TWEEN FDA AND INDUSTRY
• ACCEPTANCE OF FOREIGN CLINICAL STUDIES	• VERY CONSERVATIVE APPROACH TO DRUG REGULATION
• CONTINUED GOVERNMENT CONTROL OVER MARKETED DRUGS	
• RESTRICTED DISTRIBUTION	
• RECERTIFICATION REQUIREMENT	

The first and last factors that contribute to the rapidity of approval in European countries have largely to do with the nature of the health care delivery systems in the countries studied. Most of the countries studied have some form of national health care systems with governmental controls which facilitate post-marketing surveillance, restricted distribution, and recertification requirements for certain drugs (4). For these reasons, the governmental regulatory agencies are willing and able to release new drugs perhaps sooner and with less data than if they had to work under a system such as ours, in which post-marketing surveillance is limited and spotty at best, and in which present laws do not allow restricted distribution or require recertification. Two other characteristics of the foreign countries are that they rely heavily on expert committees to determine safety and efficacy and they utilize data from foreign clinical trials more extensively than we do (4). When considering why the process takes more time in the U.S.A. than in European countries, one can first go down the list of characteristics of foreign countries and find that we do not have these traits. Post-marketing surveillance does not work here, largely because physicians do not report adverse drug experiences (4). Expert committees are used only sparingly; they meet infrequently and they review only selected drugs upon request of the FDA. Data from foreign clinical trials are used to only a limited extent (5). FDA control over marketed drugs is limited. In addition, the traits we do have tend even more to slow the drug approval process (Table 3). The items listed as slowing the process in the U.S.A. can be illuminated by remembering the main charge of Congress to the FDA as embodied in the present drug laws: The present laws emphasize the responsibility of regulators to ensure the safety of drug research and the safety and effectiveness of new drug products. There is no charge to the regulators to foster innovation or to facilitate patient access to new drugs (1).

The points listed in Table 3 are also instructive in our consideration of the question in the topic assigned to me, "How does one evaluate and use outside U.S.A. data in the NDA?" First, it should be noted that one of the reasons that the process of approving new drugs requires less time in foreign countries is that they utilize foreign data (4). Perhaps we should learn from this experience of our foreign colleagues and try to adopt the best of their methods for utilizing foreign data to their advantage. Some countries, such as the Netherlands, Norway and Switzerland, utilize foreign data from certain sources even without domestic verification (4). Others require some degree of domestic verification. Thus, some of our foreign colleagues have apparently developed methods by which they can ensure the quality of other countries' data and utilize such data in their own NDA's. A second important point is that foreign clinical data include substantial information from post-marketing surveillance (4). These are perhaps the most valuable of the clinical data, as these are the data collected in the "real world" of patients and should indicate the true safety and efficacy of drugs. Moreover, these are the type of data that we, in our present system, have the least of and have in the least reliable and least complete form. Thus, if we could ensure the quality and validity of these post-marketing surveillance data, they should be of substantial value to our NDA's.

Additional specific considerations on use of foreign clinical data are listed in Table 4.

Table 4

SPECIFIC CONSIDERATIONS REGARDING U.S.A. ACCEPTANCE OF
FOREIGN CLINICAL DATA

- FDA SHOULD CLARIFY OFFICIAL POLICY

- INTERNATIONAL ORGANIZATIONS (SUCH AS WHO) SHOULD BE UTILIZED AS FORUM FOR DEVELOPMENT OF:

    - COMMON NDA'S

    - COMPATIBLE GUIDELINES FOR TOXICOLOGY TESTING

    - COMPATIBLE GUIDELINES FOR CONDUCT OF CLINICAL TRIALS

    - COOPERATIVE APPROACHES FOR DETECTING AND REPORTING ADVERSE EXPERIENCES

- ADEQUATE FOREIGN DATA SHOULD BE UTILIZED TO DECREASE THE NUMBER OF OR THE SIZE OF STUDIES DONE IN U.S.A.

- PRIORITY SYSTEM - HEAVIER RELIANCE ON ADEQUATE FOREIGN DATA ON DRUGS USEFUL FOR POTENTIALLY LETHAL PROBLEMS (BREAKTHROUGH DRUGS)

First, according to the GAO study most pharmaceutical houses are confused about the true FDA position on use of foreign clinical data (4,5). Whereas certain policies of allowing use of foreign data have been stated, in actual fact and practice it seems that extensive duplicative domestic studies are required (4,5). The FDA should clearly state its policies and guidelines regarding the use of foreign data so that the drug industry can utilize such data to its best advantage. If possible, via the help of international organizations, guidelines that transcend national boundaries should be established so foreign studies are compatible with ours and our studies compatible with foreign studies. Thus, not only would their data be more useful to us, but our data would also be more useful to them. In the cases where foreign studies are deemed adequate, (according to criteria set by FDA), those data should be utilized in our NDA's to allow speedier approval of the drug in this country. The degree of reliance on foreign data should perhaps be influenced by how important the new drug is - that is, if it is a potential lifesaving agent, our utilization of the foreign data in the NDA should be more substantial so that the drug can be approved here faster (5).

These are general thoughts meant to provoke further consideration and dialogue about the question, and not meant to be final or definitive recommendations. The main message is that it does indeed take substantially longer to develop new drugs here than most other developed countries (4). It is not clear that this longer time for approval has been beneficial to U.S.A. citizens, for example by protecting Americans from toxic agents. If we could speed the process safely, Americans should benefit from quicker access to important new drugs. Perhaps one means to speed the process here would be to rely more on foreign clinical data.

ACKNOWLEDGEMENTS

I thank Mr. Michael Romansky for assistance in collecting and interpreting resource materials, particularly those originating from the federal government. I gratefully acknowledge the secretarial assistance of Ms. Terri Butcher.

REFERENCES

1. Laubach, G.D.: Federal regulation and pharmaceutical innovation. Proceedings of the Academy of Political Science 33:60-80, 1980.
2. Wardell, W.M., Hassar, M., Anavekar, S.M., Lasagna, L.: The rate of development of new drugs in the United States, 1963-1975. Clin. Pharmacol. Therap. 24:133-145, 1978.
3. Wardell, W.M., DiRaddo, J., Trimble, A.G.: Development of new drugs originated and acquired by United States-owned pharmaceutical firms, 1963-1976. Clin. Pharmacol. Therap. 28:270-277, 1980.
4. FDA drug approval - A lengthy process that delays the availability of important new drugs. Report by the Comptroller General to the Subcommittee on Science, Research, and Technology, House Committee on Science and Technology. U.S. Government Printing Office, Washington, D.C., 1980.

5. Oversight - The food and drug administration's process for approving new drugs. Hearings before the Subcommittee on Science, Research, and Technology, House Committee on Science and Technology. U.S. Government Printing Office, Washington, D.C., 1979.

GENERAL GROUP DISCUSSION: OUTSIDE U.S. DATA

Dr. Dreifus: Is there further discussion?

Dr. Yoshio Watanabe: I would like to strongly support the conclusions of
Dr. Gus Watanabe. In Japan we have an extremely considervative ministry of
health policy for the approval of new drugs. Actually we do not have aprindine, amiodarone, mexilitene, tocainide, or encanide. Actually we have
nothing other than verapamil so we are in a similar position to those investigators in the United States. In Japan we have had several unfortunate incidences of drug induced disease. I suspect the ministry of health in Japan
may take the standards of the FDA in the United States. I hope it is not
true, but if so, I hope that the FDA in the United States sets a better
standard for our government to expedite approval of many important and
useful drugs in the treatment of cardiac arrhythmias.

Dr. Dreifus: Would anyone like to comment on the so-called drug lag?

Dr. Temple: I am not sure I know where to begin. I think it is dangerous
to let accountants discuss such an important subject. The General Accounting
Office is unable to deal with many proglems because they are not medically
sophisticated. They do not understand the quality of the applications which
are before the FDA. Hence, their conclusions cannot reflect all of the
problems in drug approval. Their conclusions concerning the time for drug
approval once an application has been filed may not be truly representative.
Perhaps Dr. Watanabe only identified certain cardiovascular drugs of interest
to this audience. Of the 5 countries which the General Accounting Office
examines, the only one that was substantially different from the United States
was Great Britain where the approval time for a new drug from the time of
application or the equivalent was approximately 5 months. All of the other
countries that they examined were in the neighborhood of 16 to 24 months.
This is relatively little different from our experience. Now for the
particular drugs which you identified. It is obvious that at least half of
the audience thinks that we acted too quickly on disopyramide, not too

slowyly. Furthermore, I can tell you that the initial submission of this agent was totally inadequate. However, eventually adequate studies were performed.

Whether one should throw into the drug lag mixture the question of additional indications I think is really debatable because the physician who believes the literature reports can just use the agent for a new indication as he is not barred in any way from doing just that. The question of use of foreign data is becoming somewhat clear. There are a number of drugs that have been approved principally on the basis of foreign studies. Metoprolol was approved after only 2 small controlled U.S. trials. The agent was approved largely on the basis of data collected in Scandinavia, Great Britain, and Australia. Cimethidine was approved principally on the basis of data collected in western Europe although in all of these instances there were repeated studied in United States. The policy of asking from some domestic studies as practiced in the United States is not very different from what most foreign countries require. It is also my impression that Japan not only requires additional studies to be conducted in Japan, but will not accept toxicology studies from the rest of the world. Perhaps that is not true and the situation may be changing. We have accepted long term toxicology as well as short term toxicology conducted abroad for a long time. I don't think we have any ambiguity about this. Furthermore, it is not correct that post marketing surveillances better in foreign countries, it is probably worse. Tritrinifin was marketed for 4 years in France and I need not remind you what they missed. I feel the available information on disopyramide in the 2 years of marketing in this country is far better than that available in the rest of the world for 10 years. I agree with you that it would be extremely helpful in specific cases for early approval of drugs if they were limited in distribution in some way. That would apply to a new antiarrhythmic agent where you did not feel quite comfortable in letting the agent out for general use. Restriction to several centers might make the drug available earlier. This has been tested in the supreme court but we do not have the authority to do that.

Dr. Gus Watanabe: Dr. Temple, I thought you would have a few things to say. I'd like to reiterate that I am not attacking the FDA either personally or in my role as Chairman of the American Heart Association and American College Cardiology committee on cardiovascular drugs. I think that one could spend 2 days discussing some of the arguments of whether or not drugs

should be approved more rapidly in this country and the reasons for this
apparent delay. I did rely heavily on that GAO report from my data and I
did extract the data from that report which incidentally is a body of the
federal government. As far as post-marketing surveillance, there does seem
to be a substantial difference in the quality of that procedure at least
comparing the United States with certain of the European countries such
as Great Britain where they have a National Health Care Service. In Great
Britain, they have physicians who are specifically assigned to follow up
on adverse reports, study them to see if indeed there is cause and effect
between the adverse effect and the administration of the drug and where they
apparently have very good compliance because the information is kept con-
fidential. In Great Britain, physicians don't worry about legal suits.
Furthermore, there is a system for feeding the information back to the
physicians. I think the FDA is doing a fairly good job given then current
charge and I think they are moving in the right direction.

Dr. Cleaver: As a representative or employee of a pharmaceutical company
whose primary work is done overseas in Western Europe, we have to deal with
the regulatory agencies of countries all over the world including the U.S.
We have found that the FDA is probably the most approachable of any of the
regulatory agencies around the world. Although the other agencies may
approve or disapprove on less data, it is generally very difficult to find
out why. The FDA is one of the most straight forward agencies and has the
most reasonable approach. They will give you answers if you ask. From that
point of view, I think the FDA is a model for most other countries. One
other point that I would like to make about submission of foreign data.
We have found that the FDA pretty generally will accept foreign data if
it is presented in decent shape. We have a severe problem getting physicians
in foreign countries to fill out case record forms which is the cornerstone
of our regulatory system. It has been a very long and harrowing experience
in many countries and we haven't made very much progress in the last 8 years.

Dr. Gus Watanabe: I would like to make another brief comment. Dr. Marvin
Jaffe who is here from Merck indicated that their company, and I am sure
that this is true of several of the other multinational countries, has
developed perspective multinational studies so that the protocols are conducted prospectively according to criteria that would be satisfactory to the
FDA. Hence, studies done in Europe and perhaps in Japan could be very
useful in the NDA. If we could make this unifersal among more companies

then it would be even more effective.

PARTICIPANTS

Gunnar Aberg, Ph.D.
Ciba-Geigy Pharmaceuticals

William B. Abrams, M.D.
Executive Director, Clinical Pharmacology
Merck Sharp & Dohme

Barry L. Alpert, M.D.
Assistant Professor of Medicine
University of Pittsburgh

Cynthia B. Altman, M.D.
Associate Director, Clinical Investigation
Smith Kline Corporation

Jeffrey L. Anderson, M.D.
Assistant Professor of Medicine
University of Michigan

Elliott Antman, M.D.
Co-Director, S.A. Levine Cardiac Center
Peter Bent Brigham Hospital

Keiko Aogaichi, M.D.
Research Physician
Hoffman-LaRoche, Inc.

Ronald Aronson, M.D.
Assistant Professor of Medicine
Albert Einstein College of Medicine

Tania Assaykeen, Ph.D.
Associate Director, Clinical Research
Astra Pharmaceutical Products, Inc.

Marie-France Aymard, M.D.
Hoffman-LaRoche, Inc.

K. Balakumaran, M.D.
Laboratory for Experimental Cardiology
Erasmus University Rotterdam

Franz Bender, Prof. Dr. Med.
Head of the Department of Cardiology
University Hospital of Munster

James L. Bergey, Ph.D.
Supervisor, Antiarrhythmic Section
Wyeth Labs Inc.

Klaus-Peter Bethge, M.D.
Division of Cardiology
Hannover Medical School
West Germany

J. Thomas Bigger, Mr., M.D.
Professor of Medicine and Pharmacology
Columbia University

Selvyn Bleifer, M.D.
Associate Clinical Professor of Medicine
University of California at Los Angeles

David W. Blois, Ph.D.
Director, Drug Regulatory Affairs
Astra Pharmaceutical Products, Inc.

Guenter Breithardt, M.D.
University of Duesseldorf

Kenneth Cleaver
Manager of Clinical Research
Janssen Pharmaceutica

Dr. Ronald W.F. Campbell
Consultant Cardiologist
Freeman Hospital
Newcastle-Upon-Tyne, England

Britt Canada
Department of Medical Computer Sciences
University of Texas H.S. Ctr.

Paul L. Canner, Ph.D.
Division of Clinical Investigation
University of Maryland

Manuel Cardenas, M.D.
Chief, Coronary Care Unit
Instituto N. de Cardiologia Mexico

Joan Carter, Vice President
United Medical Corporation

Francis Chardo, M.D.
Staff Cardiologist
Rancocas Valley Hospital

Vernon M. Chinchilli, Ph.D.
Mathematical Statistician
Food and Drug Administration

Bernard J. Clark, M.D.
Director, Clinical Research
Lederle Laboratories

Dr. Leonard Cook
Director of Pharmacology
Hoffman-LaRoche Inc.

David L. Copen, M.D.
Chief of Cardiology
Danbury Hospital

Nancy Corkum
Knoll Pharmaceutical Co.

Stanley Cortell, M.D.
Professor of Clinical Medicine
Columbia University

Terrance C. Coyne, M.D.
Director, Medical Research
Riker Laboratories, Inc.

J. Richard Crout, M.D.
Director, Bureau of Drugs
Food and Drug Administration

Daniel David, M.D.
Cardiology Research
Lankenau Hospital

Joan L. Davies, Sc.M.
Clinical Epidemiology Unit
Hospital of the University of Pennsylvania

Robert DiBianco, M.D.
Assistant Chief, Cardiology Section
VA Medical Center, Washington, D.C.

James V. Dingell, Ph.D.
Cardiac Diseases Branch
National Institutes of Health

James E. Doherty, M.D.
Professor of Medicine and Pharmacology
University of Arkansas College of Medicine

Leonard S. Dreifus, M.D.
Professor of Medicine & Physiology
Jefferson Medical College
Chief, Cardiovascular Division
Lankenau Hospital

Kenneth L. Duchin, Ph.D.
Assistant Clinical Pharmacology Director
E.R. Squibb & Sons, Inc.

Stewart J. Ehrreich, Ph.D.
Deputy Director
Division of Cardio-Renal Drugs
Food and Drug Administration

Gerald F. Eisen
Senior Clinical Research Associate
Janssen Pharmaceutica

Toby R. Engel, M.D.
Professor of Medicine
The Medical College of Pennsylvania

Alfred Fasola, M.D.
Lilly Labs for Clinical Research
Wishard Memorial Hospital

Charles L. Feldman, Sc.D.
Research Professor of Cardiovascular Medicine
University of Mass Med. School

Nancy Feliciano
Ciba-Geigy

Ross Fletcher, M.D.
Director, Cardiology Division
VA Hospital
Washington, D.C.

James R. Foster, M.D.
University of North Carolina
Medical School

Peter L. Frommer, M.D.
Deputy Director
National Heart, Lung & Blood Institute

Curt D. Furberg, M.D.
Chief, Clinical Trials Branch
National Heart, Lung & Blood Institute

Arthur Garson, Jr., M.D.
Assistant Professor of Pediatrics and Medicine
Baylor College of Medicine and
Texas Children's Hospital

Lisa B. Gehrie, M.D.
Assistant Director, Clinical Research
Ciba-Geigy Pharmaceuticals

Leonard M. Gonasun, Ph.D.
Associate Director, Clinical Research
Sandoz Inc.

Juan R. Guerrero, M.D.
Medical Director
Knoll Pharmaceutical Co.

Hamid A. Hai, M.D.
Director, Cardiac Arrhythmias Center
Associate, Northwestern University

Ag C. Hanzas
Knoll Pharmaceutical Company

Richard H. Helfant, M.D.
Chief, Division of Cardiology
Presbyterian-University of Pa. Medical Center

Harry M. Helfrich, Jr., M.D.
Associate Director, Clinical Investigation
Smith Kline and French

Irving M. Herling, M.D.
Co-Director, Critical Care Unit
Likoff Cardiovascular Institute

Morrison Hodges, M.D.
Director, Cardiology
Hennepin County Medical Center

Brian F. Hoffman, M.D.
David Hosack Professor of Pharmacology
Chairman, Pharmacology Department
Columbia University

Nicholas Holford, M.D.
Associate Physician, Medicine & Clinical
Pharmacology
University of California at San Francisco

William L. Holmes, Ph.D.
Chairman, Department of Research
Lankenau Hospital

Leonard N. Horowitz, M.D.
Assistant Professor of Medicine
Hospital of the University of Pennsylvania

Hiroyuki Iinuma, M.D.
Cardiology Research
Lankenau Hospital

Ken Jady, M.D.
Medical Advisor
Boehringer Ingelheim Ltd.

Marvin E. Jaffe, M.D.
Vice President, Clinical Research
Merck Sharp & Dohme

Borje Johansson, M.D. Professor
AB Hassle
Sweden

Mark E. Josephson, M.D.
Associate Professor of Medicine
University of Pennsylvania School of Medicine

Elieser Kaplinsky, M.D.
Associate Professor of Cardiology
Meir General Hospital, Israel

Joel S. Karliner, M.D.
Associate Professor of Medicine
University of California, San Diego
Director, Clinical Cardiology
University Hospital, UCSD

Peter P. Karpawich, M.D.
Fellow in Pediatric Cardiology
Baylor College of Medicine and
Texas Children's Hospital

Robert E. Kates, Ph.D.
Assistant Professor of Medicine
Stanford University Medical Center

Harold L. Kennedy, M.D., MPH
Director of Ambulatory Monitoring and
Arrhythmia Clinic
Memorial Hospital of Long Beach

J.R. Kilborn, M.D., Ph.D.
Head of Cardiovascular Group
Laboratoires D'Etudes et de Recherches Synthelabo

Edward Kirsten, Ph.D.
Director, Clinical Pharmacology
Knoll Pharmaceutical Co.

Michael Klein, M.D.
Associate Professor of Medicine
Boston University Hospital

Dr. Larry Klevans
Assistant Research Group Chief
Pharmacology I
Hoffman-LaRoche Inc.

John B. Kostis, M.D.
Professor of Medicine
College of Medicine and Dentistry
of New Jersey-Rutgers Medical School

Helena Chmura Kraemer, Ph.D.
Associate Professor of Biostatistics in Psychiatry
Stanford University

Dennis Krikler, M.D.
Consultant Cardiologist
Royal Postgraduate Medical School
London, England

William Krol, Ph.D.
Maryland Medical Research Institute

Atul R. Laddu, M.D.
Associate Director of Clinical Investigation
Ives Laboratories

James C. Laidlaw, M.D.
Clinical Professor
University of Virginia

Ezra Lamdin, M.D.
Director, Marketed Drugs
ICI Americas Inc.

Norman W. Lavy, M.D.
E.R. Squibb & Sons, Inc.

Ralph Lazzara, M.D.
Chief of Cardiology
Oklahoma University Health Science Center

Raymond Lipicky, M.D.
Cardio-Renal Division
Food and Drug Administration

Robert A. Long, Ph.D.
Clinical Research Scientist
Burroughs Wellcome Co.

Robert J. Loring, Vice President
Cardio Data Systems

Reginald Low
University of California, Davis

Benedict R. Lucchesi, Ph.D., M.D.
Director, Upjohn Center for
Clinical Pharmacology
University of Michigan

Jerry C. Luck, M.D.
Assistant Professor of Medicine
Medical College of Pennsylvania

Sara A. Mahler, M.D.
Associate Medical Director
Endo Laboratories, Inc.

Prof. A. Masbernard
Prof. Agrege Valde Grace
Sanofi, FRANCE

Todor Mazgalev, Ph.D.
Cardiology Research
Lankenau Hospital

Elizabeth A. McCafferty
Director, REgulatory Affairs
Sanofi, Inc.

Bernard McDonagh, Ph.D.
Manager, Research Data Operations
Riker Laboratories

E.F. McNichols, M.D.
Associate Director, Clinical Research
Riker Laboratories

Milenko Medakovic, M.D.
Schering Corporation

Eric L. Michelson, M.D.
Director, Clinical Research Unit
Lankenau Hospital

Howard Miller, M.D.
Director, Clinical Research
Mead Johnson & Co.

E. Neil Moore, D.V.M., Ph.D.
Professor of Physiology in Medicine
School of Veterinary Medicine
University of Pennsylvania

Terrance J. Moran, M.D.
Director of Coronary Care Unit &
Cardiac Rehabilitation
Harbor-UCLA Medical Center

Joel Morganroth, M.D.
Chief, Cardiac Research and Education
Lankenau Hospital
Associate Professor of Medicine
Jefferson Medical College

Masahito Naito, M.D.
Cardiology Research
Lankenau Hospital

Susan K. Nunchuck, M.S.N.
Clinical Research Associate
Mead Johnson & Co.

Carolyn O'Connor
Clinical Data Inc.

Carol M. Ordille, Ph.D.
Manager, Biostatistics, Pharmaceuticals
E.I. duPont deNemours & Co., Inc.

Eugene Passamani, M.D.
Medical Project Officer
National Heart, Lung & Blood Institute

Gerd Petrik
Helopharm
West Germany

James Pickands, III, Ph.D.
Associate Professor of Statistics
& Operations
University of Pennsylvania

Rene A. Pingeon, M.D.
Director, Clinical Research International
Merck & Co., Inc.

Bertram Pitt, M.D.
Director, Cardiovascular Division
University of Michigan

Philip J. Podrid, M.D.
Research Associate, Harvard Medical School
Associate in Medicine, Peter Bent Brigham Hospital

Edward L.C. Pritchett, M.D.
Assistant Professor of Medicine
Duke University Medical Center

Elliot Rapaport, M.D.
Chief, Cardiology Service
University of California at San Francisco

Philip R. Reid, M.D.
Associate Professor of Medicine
Johns Hopkins Hospital

Joseph Reiser, Ph.D.
Assistant Professor of Medicine and Physiology
Hahnemann Medical College & Hospital

Robert D. Reynolds, Ph.D.
Senior Research Investigator
American Critical Care

Barry A. Rofman, M.D.
Director, Clinical Research
Merck Sharp & Dohme

Michael Romansky
Washington, D.C.

Kenneth M. Rosen, M.D.
Director, Investigational Drugs
ICI Americas Inc.

Shirley Roth, R.N.
Clinical Research Associate
Mead Johnson & Co.

Jeremy N. Ruskin, M.D.
Director, Clinical Electrophysiology Laboratory
Massachusetts General Hospital

Magdi Sami, M.D.
Assistant Professor of Medicine in Cardiology
McGill University

Martin Schlepper, M.D
Professor of Cardiology
Kerckhoff-Klinik
West Germany

Ludger Seipel, M.D.
Professor of Medicine
University of Duesseldorf

Herbert J. Semler, M.D.
Transtelephonic Monitoring of
Cardiovascular Drugs

Harold Shlevin, M.D.
Department of Biological Research
G.D. Searle & Co.

Steven Singh
Washington, D.C.

Bruce J. Sobol, M.D.
Director, Medical Research
Boehringer Ingelheim Ltd.

Peter Somani, M.D.
Professor of Pharmacology and Medicine
University of MIami School of Medicine

Joseph F. Spear, Ph.D.
Professor of Physiology
University of Pennsylvania

H.C. Stanton, Ph.D.
Director, Biologic Research
Mead Johnson Pharmaceutical Division

Israel M. Stein, M.D.
President/Medical Director
Clinical Data, Inc.

Girt Steinbeck, M.D.
Germany

Dr. Kurt Stoepel
Bayer, AG
Germany

R.W. Stoll, M.D.
Associate Director, Clinical Research
Abbott Laboratories

Jeffrey A. Stritar, M.D.
Assistant Clinical Research Director
E.R. Squibb & Sons., Inc.

John Stump, M.D.
Research and Development, Pharmaceuticals
E.I. duPont deNemours & Co.

Robert Temple, M.D.
Director, Cardio-Renal Division
Food and Drug Administration

J. Gerald Toole, M.D.
Associate Director of Clinical Therapeutics
Warner-Lambert/Parke-Davis

Junichi Toyama
Nagoya University
Japan

Paul Troup, M.D.
Division of Cardiology
Milwaukee County Medical Complex

Ilhan Tuzel, M.D.
Director, Cardiovascular Research
Hoffman-LaRoche, Inc.

Pedro R. Urquilla, M.D.
Associate Director of Medical Research
Miles Laboratories

Jean-Pierre Van Durme, M.D., Ph.D.
Lecturer in Cardiology
University Hospital, Gent Belgium

Svetislav K. Vanov, M.D., Ph.D.
Director of Medical Research III
Miles Laboratories, Inc.

Louis Vasquez, M.D.
American Critical Care

P.D. Verdouw, Ph.D.
Laboratory for Experimental Cardiology
Thoraxcenter, Erasmus University

Larry R. Versteegh, Ph.D.
Mead Johnson & Co.

Andre D. Waleffe, M.D., Ph.D.
Laboratory of Clinical Electrophysiology
 and Pharmacology
University of Liege

G.A. Walker, Ph.D.
Biostatistician
Abbott Laboratories

August Watanabe, M.D.
Professor of Medicine and Pharmacology
Indiana University School of Medicine

Yoshio Watanabe, M.D.
Fujita-Gakuen University
Japan

Debbie Weida
Sr. Regulatory Affairs Coordinator
Riker Laboratories

Hein J.J. Wellens, M.D.
Professor of Cardiology
University of Limburg

Nanette K. Wenger, M.D.
Professor of Medicine
Emory University School of Medicine

Thomas L. Wenger, M.D.
Senior Clinical Research Scientist
Burroughs Wellcome Co.

Park W. Willis, III, M.D.
Chief of Cardiology
Michigan State University School of Medicine

Richard R. Wilson, M.D.
Associate Director
Cardiovascular-Renal Clinical Research
G.D. Searle

Roger A. Winkle, M.D.
Associate Professor of Medicine
Stanford University

R.A. Wolbach, M.D.
Assistant Director, Clinical Research
Abbott Laboratories

Raymond L. Woosley, M.D., Ph.D.
Associate Professor of Medicine and Clinical Pharmacology
Vanderbilt University Medical Center

Christopher R.C. Wyndham, M.D.
Director of Electrocardiography and Electrophysiology
Baylor College of Medicine

Michael D. Young, M.D., Ph.D.
Senior Vice President for Scientific Affairs
Astra Pharmaceutical Products, Inc.

Douglas P. Zipes, M.D.
Professor of Medicine
Director of Cardiovascular Research

Ruben A. Zito, M.D.
Assistant Professor of Medicine
Yale University School of Medicine